T0323412

Positive Neuroscience

Positive Neuroscience

EDITED BY

JOSHUA D. GREENE

INDIA MORRISON

MARTIN E. P. SELIGMAN

OXFORD
UNIVERSITY PRESS

Oxford University Press is a department of the University of Oxford. It furthers
the University's objective of excellence in research, scholarship, and education
by publishing worldwide. Oxford is a registered trade mark of Oxford University
Press in the UK and certain other countries.

Published in the United States of America by Oxford University Press
198 Madison Avenue, New York, NY 10016, United States of America.

Library of Congress Cataloging-in-Publication Data
Names: Greene, Joshua David, 1974– editor. | Morrison, India, editor. |
    Seligman, Martin E. P., editor.
Title: Positive neuroscience / edited by Joshua D. Greene, India Morrison,
    and Martin E. P. Seligman.
Description: New York : Oxford University Press, 2016. | Includes index.
Identifiers: LCCN 2015041438 (print) | LCCN 2015044606 (ebook) |
    ISBN 9780199977925 (hardcover : alk. paper) | ISBN 9780199977932 (UPDF) |
    ISBN 9780199977949 (EPUB)
Subjects: LCSH: Affective neuroscience. | Neuropsychology. | Positive
    psychology. | Social psychology.
Classification: LCC QP401 .P68 2016 (print) | LCC QP401 (ebook) |
    DDC 612.8—dc23
LC record available at http://lccn.loc.gov/2015041438

CONTENTS

ACKNOWLEDGMENTS

The research described in these pages was supported by the Positive Neuroscience Project, spearheaded by Martin E. P. Seligman through the University of Pennsylvania's Positive Psychology Center and supported by a generous grant from the John Templeton Foundation.

CONTRIBUTORS

Daniel L. Ames, University of California Los Angeles
Adam K. Anderson, Cornell University
Jessica R. Andrews-Hanna, University of Colorado Boulder
Yoni K. Ashar, University of Colorado Boulder
Tony W. Buchanan, St. Louis University
William A. Cunningham, University of Toronto
Sona Dimidjian, University of Colorado Boulder
Lindsey A. Drayton, Yale University
Joshua D. Greene, Harvard University
Britta K. Hölzel, Harvard Medical School
Sara W. Lazar, Harvard Medical School
Psyche Loui, Wesleyan University
Vincent Man, University of Toronto
Abigail A. Marsh, Georgetown University
Jennifer Mascaro, Emory University
Iris B. Mauss, University of California Berkeley
Kateri McRae, University of Denver
Hans L. Melo, University of Toronto
Mohammed R. Milad, Harvard Medical School
Jason P. Mitchell, Harvard University
India Morrison, Linköping University
Stephanie D. Preston, University of Michigan
James K. Rilling, Emory University
Laurie R. Santos, Yale University
Martin E. P. Seligman, University of Pennsylvania

Beau Sievers, Dartmouth College
Alexander Todorov, Princeton University
Tor D. Wager, University of Colorado Boulder
Thalia Wheatley, Dartmouth College
Jamil Zaki, Stanford University

Introduction

JOSHUA D. GREENE AND INDIA MORRISON ■

As primates go, humans are pretty good. We do horrible things, of course, but increasingly less so (Pinker, 2011), thanks to our unmatched ability to form cooperative relationships, to value one another's well-being, and to build social structures that expand the scope of human flourishing. Happily, these laudable behaviors are not rare occurrences, but rather the predictable products of healthy human brains. We seem built not just to survive, but to thrive—each of us born with a capacity for experiencing happiness and seeking meaning. How the brain produces these capacities and behaviors remains mysterious. This is largely because human flourishing is distinctively human, and most of what we know about brains comes from decades of research on nonhuman animals. Only in the last 20 years, with the advent of noninvasive functional neuroimaging, have healthy human brains become widespread objects of scientific study. And neuroscientific research aimed at understanding the biological bases of human flourishing is newer still. This volume brings together some of the most exciting new ideas and findings from this rapidly growing field.

Since this project began, the research from the scientists represented in this volume on the neuroscience of human flourishing has itself flourished, yielding surprising findings, deep insights, and new questions for each contributor and the next generation of positive neuroscience researchers. Most of this research has now been published in scientific journals (including some of the world's top neuroscience and general science journals). Here we bring this work together in one place, and in a format suitable for both students and seasoned scientists. The research described herein falls into three broad categories.

Part I (Social Bonds) describes the mechanisms that enable humans to connect with one another. In Chapter 1, India Morrison discusses research on the neuroscience of touch as a means for emotional communication, beginning with work on a newly discovered mammalian nerve type that may be specially attuned for touch in social interactions. In Chapter 2, James Rilling and Jennifer Mascaro describe research showing that the brains of men who are active parents differ from those of other men, consistent with patterns identified by research on nurturing behavior in nonhuman animals. In Chapter 3, Thalia Wheatley and Beau Sievers explain how human brains resonate with one another, enabling people to feel each other's pain, communicate through music, and form social bonds.

Part II (Altruism) focuses on the neural mechanisms underlying our ability and willingness to confer costly benefits on others. In Chapter 4, Jamil Zaki and Jason Mitchell discuss research showing that human brains represent the value of altruistic behavior just as they represent the value of self-serving behavior, using general-purpose neural machinery that we share with other mammals. In Chapter 5, Lindsey Drayton and Laurie Santos consider the range of altruistic behaviors observed across animal species and conclude that human altruism has some features that are shared with other species but other features that appear to be uniquely human. In Chapter 6, Tony Buchanan and Stephanie Preston present a biologically based theory explaining why empathic feelings sometimes do and sometimes do not translate into altruistic action. In Chapter 7, Vincent Man, Daniel Ames, Alexander Todorov, and William Cunningham focus on the amygdala, a neural structure widely known for its role in fear and other forms of self-preserving behavior. They present evidence that, in humans, the amygdala's operations can be directed toward the goals of others, given the right motivation. In Chapter 8, Yoni Ashar, Jessica Andrews-Hanna, Sona Dimidjian, and Tor Wager present a model of compassion and compassionate behavior according to which distinct neural systems are responsible for the generation of compassion-related feelings, for inferring the contents of other minds, and for the representation of others' suffering as related to oneself. In Chapter 9, Abigail Marsh discusses her research examining the distinctive neural and behavioral qualities of a group of extraordinary altruists, people who voluntarily donated kidneys to strangers.

Part III (Resilience and Creativity) examines the mechanisms by which human brains overcome adversity, create, and discover. In Chapter 10, Kateri McRae and Iris Mauss discuss the brain's ability to reappraise traumatic life events and generate positive emotions that promote recovery and growth. In Chapter 11, Britta Hölzel, Sara Lazar, and Mohammed Milad argue that mindfulness meditation may promote resilience by bolstering the brain's ability to extinguish counterproductive fear responses. In Chapter 12, Psyche Loui explains how patterns of structural and functional connectivity across disparate brain regions give some people exceptional musical abilities and give music its emotional power. Finally, in Chapter 13, Hans Melo and Adam Anderson explain how positive emotions motivate exploratory behavior that builds cognitive resources and enables flexibility, creativity, and resilience.

At the outset of the Positive Neuroscience Project, it was not clear how, if at all, the specific research projects chosen for support would cohere. As the foregoing summary suggests, there is, in fact, a great deal of biological convergence and thematic overlap among the ideas and results presented, much of which we could not have anticipated. For example, Wheatley and Siever's work on social resonance (Part I) dovetails both thematically and anatomically with Psyche Loui's research on the neural bases of musical creativity and emotional experience (Part III). Likewise, within Part II, Man, Ames, Todorov, and Cunningham's focus on the amygdala as an unlikely locus of altruistic processing is reprised in Abigail Marsh's finding that altruistic kidney donors have (on average) exceptionally large and responsive amygdalas. We leave it to readers to discover their own connections as they work through this exceptionally rich and illuminating body of work.

REFERENCE

Pinker, S. (2011). *The better angels of our nature: Why violence has declined.* New York: Viking.

PART I

Social Bonds

Affective and Social Touch

INDIA MORRISON ■

The novelist Margaret Atwood has written: "Touch comes before sight, before speech. It is the first language and the last, and it always tells the truth" (Atwood, 2000, p. 256). Many of us share Atwood's intuitive idea of the primacy of touch. But we might also share an intuition that Atwood was not thinking of "discriminative" touch when she wrote those words—the practical tactile abilities that enable you to identify a quarter among the other coins in your pocket or to determine precisely where a fly has landed on your skin. Neuroscience has made much progress in mapping out these discriminative functions. Yet until recently, neuroscience was unequipped to address the kind of *affective* touch evoked by Margaret Atwood: thrilling, tingling, tickling, titillating, and sometimes even burned into memory for a lifetime.

Despite this, students of neuroscience have not learned about affective touch, simply because affective touch has been absent from neuroscience textbooks. Is this because the discriminative, coin-fingering, spider-detecting variety of touch is sufficient to account for affective touch as well? Or could it be that something has been overlooked?

This chapter takes the view that something *has* been overlooked. It discusses recent advances in our neuroscientific understanding of affective touch and its underlying neural mechanisms. Its central pillar is the hypothesis that affective touch operates predominantly in the domain of social interactions and has an impact on behavior. The affective touch research discussed here inspires the idea that human touch is a special tactile experience that is not only inherently hedonic and rewarding but also does useful work. Possible functional roles of pleasant, social touch might be to buffer stress and to foster and maintain relationships.

AFFECTIVE TOUCH STARTS IN THE SKIN

The available experimental evidence from psychology and animal behavior corroborates the idea that affective touch is of central importance in a variety of social interactions, including those in the early development of humans and other mammals (Ainsworth, Blehar, Waters, & Wall, 1978; Bowlby, 1973; Brossard & Decarie, 1968; Harlow, 1958; Hertenstein, 2001; Hertenstein & Campos, 2001; Liu et al., 2007; Menard, Champagne, & Meaney, 2004; Pelhez-Nogueras et al., 1996; Rubin, 1963; Stack & Muir, 1992). In everyday adult life, even brief, casual touches from strangers can affect how we evaluate people or situations and influence our behavior toward them (Burgoon, Walther, & Baesler, 1992; Crusco & Wetzel, 1984; Fisher, Rytting, & Heslin, 1976; Hertenstein et al., 2006; Hornik, 1992; Joule & Guégen, 2007; Kleinke, 1977). Could affective touch represent a channel of tactile information, distinct from the "usual" kind of discriminative touch sense that helps you manipulate objects or feel when a fly has landed on your knee? If that is the case, it is plausible that affective touch is underpinned by distinct neural pathways, perhaps even involving special nerves.

Gentle stroking may indeed be encoded by a distinct neural pathway that begins in the nerves of the skin. In 1939, Ingve Zotterman discovered that a subtype of C afferent nerves in the skin of a cat discharged when the tactile receptive field was gently touched or stroked (Zotterman, 1939). He recorded directly from the nerve of a live cat using an electrode needle hooked up to an amplifier. The touch-sensitive C afferent nerves he identified continued to spike even after the stimulus stopped: "The smallest spikes . . . in the after-discharge following a firm stroke, may also appear in response to a very gentle touch, especially when the stimulus is repeated with short intervals," he wrote. "In such cases they form a weak after-discharge, which is very well heard from the loudspeaker as the low frequencies building up the spike of these potentials give rise to sounds reminiscent of distant kettle-drums" (p. 9). In the following decades, similar observations were reported in other nonhuman animals (e.g., Bessou, Burgess, Perl, & Taylor, 1971; Iggo, 1960; Iggo & Kornhuber, 1977). In 1990, equivalent nerves were discovered in humans (Nordin, 1990) and were eventually referred to as tactile C (CT) afferents.

As a class, C afferents are thin and unmyelinated, and have a slow conduction velocity of about 1 meter per second (in contrast to the thick, myelinated discriminative Aβ afferents, which zap touch impulses along the axon at a much speedier 35–75 meters per second). Several further properties set CTs, or "low-threshold mechanoreceptive C" (C-LTM) afferents, apart. First of all, CTs are found only in hairy skin. Mammals have two general types of epidermal skin, each with a slightly different composition of nerve receptors. Hairy skin, which covers most of the body even where the hair is not obvious, contains both Aβ *and* CT nerves. Glabrous skin is the smooth skin of the palms, soles, and lips, and contains Aβ but *not* CT nerves. Another salient property of CTs is that they are so sensitive to skin deformation that touching the skin with a force as low as 0.22 grams—about the weight of a small monarch butterfly—causes the signals to fire along the nerve axon with high frequency (around 100 impulses per second; Vallbo, Olausson, Wessberg, & Norrsell, 1993, Wessberg, Olausson, Fernstrom, & Vallbo, 2003). As Zotterman had noticed, they also exhibit after-discharge, firing after the stimulus has been removed.

Data about these properties of CT afferents come from microneurography studies. Microneurography is the technique of recording directly from peripheral nerve fibers, and it was pioneered in the first half of the 20th century by neurophysiologists like Yngve Zotterman. In this technique, the different afferent types in a nerve bundle (say, in the arm) can be identified based on characteristic firing properties—such as CTs' "distant rumble of kettle-drums"—and other signature properties like the latency, magnitude, and habituation of responses to stimulation of the receptive field.

So far, the properties of CTs appear to render them suboptimal for conveying the fast, reliable signals essential for discriminative tactile function. But could these unique features point to another functional role in encoding touch? Part of the answer comes from two rare patients who lost Aβ afferent function in adulthood as the result of illnesses that selectively attacked myelinated nerves. These patients still have unmyelinated afferents, including CTs. They can detect soft brush stroking on the forearm skin (Cole et al., 2006; Olausson et al., 2002, 2008), but not on the glabrous skin of the palm where CTs are absent. This indicates that they can feel tactile sensation based on CT activation, reporting it as being rather vague (consistent with the lower acuity of CT receptive fields compared to Aβs). But intriguingly, they also rated the stroking as *pleasant* (Olausson et al., 2002).

Further evidence for a CT–pleasantness relationship comes from microneurography studies in healthy volunteers. Because human volunteers can tell the experimenter how the tactile stimulation feels, experimenters can investigate how CT firing may relate to any aspects of subjective sensation. Line Löken and colleagues (2009) recorded CT afferent responses at six different speeds from glacially slow (0.1 cm per second) to very brisk (30 cm per second). Thick, myelinated Aβ afferents also respond to touch moving over the skin surface, but whereas their discharge scales linearly with speed of stroking (increasing as speed increases), mean CT discharge frequency shows a ∩-shaped tuning curve for stimulus velocity. So CTs *decrease* firing at very slow speeds (around 0.3 cm per second, about as fast as an unhurried snail) and very fast speeds (around 30 cm per second, about as fast as an irritated cat's tail-swish), but they *increase* firing at intermediate speeds (around 3 cm per second, about as fast as a caress). In other words, they are most excited by stroking in the middle speed range. This tuning curve for stroking speed implies a potential "middle-pass" information filter: It lets through intermediate speeds, but not very fast or slow ones.

What might be so special about intermediate speeds? Intermediate, caress-like speeds may be the most affectively potent. CT firing frequency correlated highly with the participants' ratings of how pleasant the touch felt, increasing their activity for speeds that were experienced as most pleasant (Löken, Wessberg, Morrison, McGlone, & Olausson, 2009). More recent findings suggest that CTs are also sensitive to temperature information—but intriguingly, their responses to different temperatures seem to depend on stroking speed (Ackerley et al., 2014). Their firing increases most to 3 cm/s stroking by a skin-temperature (32°C) probe, compared to stroking at other speeds and by warmer or colder probes. This suggests that CTs prefer caress-speed stroking at "creature temperature," which is also rated as most pleasant.

Taken together, the properties of CT afferents point to a relationship between caress-like stroking and positive evaluation. This has led to a working hypothesis about their functional role. The "social touch hypothesis" (Morrison, Löken, & Olausson, 2010; Olausson, Wessberg, Morrison, McGlone, & Vallbo, 2010) postulates that slow, gentle touch is highly likely to occur during close affiliative interactions with members of one's species—between a parent and offspring, between siblings, between friends and allies, and not least between mates. Such affective touch may constitute a distinct domain of touch, drawing on a functionally and qualitatively different kind of information than that coded by Aβ afferents, and requiring specialized functional organization in both the periphery and the central nervous system. CT afferents and their middle-pass filtering may thus "tag" tactile stimulation that is likely to signal close, affiliative body contact with others, packaging it for further affective evaluation in the brain.

BRAIN PROCESSING OF AFFECTIVE TOUCH

From the nerve receptors in the skin, unmyelinated C afferents synapse in neural populations in the dorsal horn of the spinal cord (e.g., Andrew, 2010; Craig, 1995). There is little direct evidence about where CTs might go from there, especially in humans, but it is likely that the CT pathway ascends to the thalamus via the spinothalamic tract. In contrast, Aβ tactile afferents associated with discriminative function follow a pathway up to the brain via the dorsal column of the spinal cord. These two pathways terminate in relatively distinct sets of thalamic nuclei, which project in turn to relatively distinct sets of cortical regions (Figure 1.1).

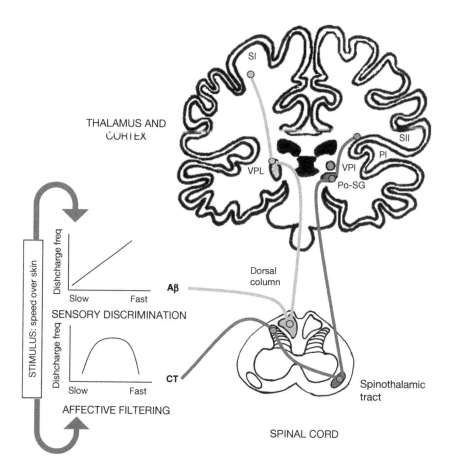

Figure 1.1 Schematic diagram of affective and discriminative pathways for dynamic touch on hairy skin dependent on stroking speed. Large, myelinated Aβ afferents discharge with greater frequency as speed increases, indicating a role in accurate discrimination of stimulus speed. In contrast, thin-diameter, unmyelinated tactile C (CT) afferents may serve as a "filter" for medium speeds, decreasing discharge frequency with slow and fast speeds but increasing for intermediate velocities. Aβ afferents synapse mainly in the dorsal column of the spinal cord (lighter gray pathway), whereas CT afferents probably project via the spinothalamic trace (darker gray pathway). These relatively distinct pathways have different dominant projections in different nuclei of the thalamus. Major thalamic nuclei shown here are ventral postlateral nucleus (VPL), ventroposterior inferior nucleus (VPI), and posterior-suprageniculate complex (Po-SG), which includes ventral medial posterior nucleus (VmPO). The major cortical target of the "discriminative" (lighter gray) pathway is primary somatosensory cortex (SI). The "affective" (darker gray) pathway projects predominantly to posterior insular cortex (PI) and secondary somatosensory cortices (SII). Each of these areas is interconnected with wider cortical networks.

NOTE: the dorsal column pathway decussates (crosses) to the opposite hemisphere at the brainstem level, but it is shown projecting to the ipsilateral hemisphere here for purposes of illustration.

Neuroimaging cannot shed light on the exact course the CT pathway takes before the level of its thalamic projections, but it can easily measure blood-oxygen-level-dependent responses in the cortex of the brain. A number of functional magnetic resonance imaging studies have suggested that a main cortical target of the CT pathway is an area of the brain called the posterior insula (Björnsdotter et al., 2009; Krämer et al., 2007; Lovero, Simmons, Aron, & Paulus, 2009; Morrison, Björnsdotter, & Olausson, 2011, Morrison, Löken, et al., 2011; Olausson et al., 2002). This is consistent with a proposed pathway for all C afferents in rodents and nonhuman primates (Craig, 2002). The posterior insula is activated by a broad range of visceral and somatosensory stimulation in humans (Kurth, Zilles, Fox, Laird, & Eickhoff, 2010), and it is highly connected with sensorimotor cortices (Cauda et al., 2011; Deen et al., 2011). Many individuals with autism spectrum disorders find stroking aversive (Cascio et al., 2012) and show decreased insular activation for pleasant textures compared to controls (Cascio et al., 2008, 2012).

Insular cortex is folded inward, like the inside of a sock puppet's mouth, and the parietal operculum forms the sock puppet's upper lip. Opercular somatosensory areas and posterior insula are highly interconnected and functionally related, and granular fields of the insular cortex are probably continuous with secondary somatosensory (SII) regions of the operculum. When participants were stroked by a human hand as opposed to a velvet-tipped stick, both insula and SII showed larger activations (Kress, Minati, Ferraro, & Critchley, 2011).

What if a person lacked typical CT innervation in their skin but had typical Aβ innervation. Might the person's perception of gentle stroking be different and, if so, might we expect cortical engagement to differ as well? A small population of individuals in northern Sweden may shed light on this question. They carry an extremely rare mutation that results in a severe reduction in the density of thin, unmyelinated afferent nerves in the skin, including CTs (Einarsdottir et al., 2004; Minde et al., 2004, 2009). Carriers perceive CT-optimal stroking speeds as less pleasant than do matched controls, as well as differing in their rating patterns across stroking speeds (Figure 1.2).

Unlike controls, their posterior insula is not modulated by stroking speed (Morrison, Löken, et al., 2011). Carriers also showed significantly reduced white matter volume in a tract from thalamus to posterior insula (Figure 1.2). These findings are consistent with a reduced input from the CT pathway to the posterior insula.

However, these mutation carriers cannot be regarded as affective touch "knockouts," that is, an otherwise neurologically typical phenotype minus a proportion of CT afferents. Although they rate stroking as less pleasant than controls on average, many individuals' ratings lie on the positive side of the rating scale's neutral midpoint (Figure 1.2). This suggests that a compensatory

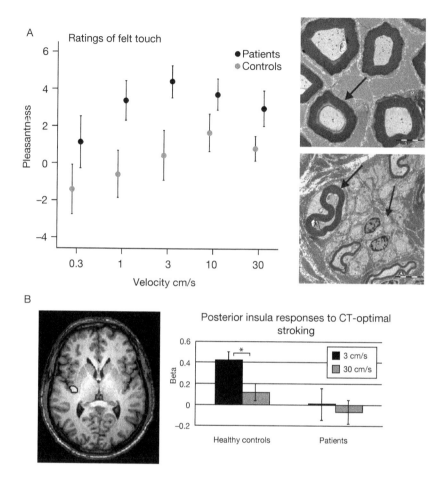

Figure 1.2 (A) Upper-left panel shows mean visual-analogue scale (VAS) scores of pleasantness in relation to brush stroking velocity (0.3, 1, 3, 10, and 30 cm/s) for carriers of a nerve growth factor beta (NGFB) mutation (*n* = 10; closed circles) and matched controls (*n* = 10, open circles). The controls show the typical inverted-U-shaped rating pattern associated with tactile C afferents (CTs). Upper-right panel shows electron microscopy cross-section of nerve fibers from a carrier's sural nerve (top) showing severe reduction of C fibers, compared with a control biopsy (bottom). Top arrow indicates an Aβ fiber; on bottom image left arrow indicates an Aβ fiber, and the right arrow indicates a single unmyelinated C fiber. (B) Left panel shows location of posterior mask based on the contrast between 3 cm/s (CT-optimal) and 30 cm/s stroking (CT nonoptimal) in controls. At the whole-brain level, 3 cm/s stroking did not activate this region in carriers. Right panel shows blood-oxygen-level-dependent (BOLD) modulation in this region by stroking speed for controls and carriers.

(Reproduced with permission from Morrison, Löken, et al., 2011.)

mechanism may be at work in processing caress-like touch in affective, evaluative terms—perhaps a little differently or less efficiently than the CT-insula pathway.

Although the insula might provide an important contribution to stimulus processing, and may even be critical for the efficient integration of somatosensory and affective information, its activity probably does not singlehandedly exhaust the hedonic and social content of affective touch. Rather, it is probably part of a brain-wide network of different areas specializing in different aspects of social touch processing. For example, the superior temporal gyrus is engaged by affective touch (Bennett et al., 2014; Gordon et al., 2011). Neurotypical individuals who nonetheless score high on some measures associated with autism spectrum disorder show reduced activation in the superior temporal sulcus during skin stroking (Voos et al., 2013). Studies involving tactile massage have implicated another important limbic region, the perigenual anterior cingulate cortex, associated with emotional processing (Lindgren et al., 2012; Sliz et al., 2012).

It is also possible that somatosensory areas associated with the discriminative aspect of touch also contribute to the processing of affective or social touch stimuli. Although the "middle-pass filter" of the CT pathway may privilege certain information based on speed (and perhaps temperature), any tactile stimulation anywhere on the body will also activate the large myelinated Aβ afferents that project to somatosensory cortices. Primary somatosensory cortex (SI) can distinguish between videos of male and female strokers during tactile stimulation of the leg (Gazzola et al., 2012). A recent meta-analysis of published neuroimaging studies indicates that SII on the parietal operculum has a high probability of being activated by *both* discriminative *and* pleasant touch (Morrison, in press). This indicates that whereas posterior insula shows functional specificity for pleasant or CT-related touch stimulation, both dimensions of touch may converge in the operculum (see also Ebisch et al., 2011).

FUNCTIONAL ROLES OF SOCIAL TOUCH

Why are we disposed to seek touch contact with others in the first place? Affective touch may not exist to give us lovely warm feelings just for the heck of it, but it may play a distinct functional role in social interactions. What this role may be is currently speculative, because there is very little direct evidence to draw on. Research has just begun to approach this question. But it is reasonable to propose that affective, social touch may simply be *calming*. It may signal that it is all right to relax, that things are more or less safe, and that one need not be on the alert for danger. More specifically, it could alleviate mild, short-term stress by applying the brake to sympathetic nervous system arousal. In this perspective, social touch interactions would give rise to functional neural changes, such as hemodynamic changes in the brain, as well as behavioral changes, such as relaxed vigilance and enhanced prosocial behavior.

Adaptive autonomic responses to mild and short term stressors (like talking to a stranger, holding your breath, or reading your bills) facilitate the body's ability to regulate multiple complex systems such as blood pressure, heart rate, and oxygen consumption. This is useful, but it imposes cumulative physical and chemical wear and tear on bodily tissues—for example, the stretching of blood vessel walls as they expand rapidly. Autonomic arousal is mediated by the sympathetic branch of the autonomic nervous system, the effects of which can be dampened by the parasympathetic branch—sometimes on a scale of milliseconds. A primary neural correlate of parasympathetic influence on sympathetic cardiac modulation, for example, is the nucleus ambiguus in the brainstem's ventral vagal complex (Porges, 2007). Other corticolimbic candidate sites for parasympathetic modulation are the central nucleus of amygdala, periaqueductal gray (Porges, 2007), anterior insula (Craig, 2002), and medial prefrontal cortex, especially portions of the anterior cingulate (Owens, Sartor, & Verberne, 1999). Positive social interactions may play a large role in buffering such processes, possibly via cortical influences on brainstem autonomic nervous system structures.

So far, the idea that affective touch may counter the effects of mild stress is just a conjecture, but recent evidence from mice suggests that this conjecture is pointing in the right direction. Vrontou et al. (2013) isolated mouse CT, or CTLM, neurons through a combination of genetic manipulation and calcium imaging of the spinal cord. This in itself was an advance, but this study was also able to make a link between CTLM neural activity and the mouse's behavior. They did this by giving the mice an injection that selectively depolarized the CLTMs (which expressed a molecule called MrgprB4+), causing them to fire, but having no effect on other neuron types. First, though, they presented the mice with two chambers and observed which chamber each mouse preferred to spend time in. Then they injected the mice with the CTLM-activating compound when they spent time in the *nonpreferred* chamber. In its preferred chamber, each mouse received neutral saline injections. This "place-conditioning" procedure overturned the mouse's previous poor opinion of the nonpreferred chamber, and the mice began spending more time in the place they had not been so keen on before. If CLTMs are indeed involved in grooming or other forms of social touch, this would imply that their activation has calming power in less-than-wonderful contexts. Real-life analogues to the nonpreferred chamber could be minor stressors, like fights or frights.

Related to its possible role as a stress buffer, affective touch may serve as a foundation for affiliative behavior. The most salient example of this in mammals is allogrooming—grooming others. Allogrooming may reflect a generalized form of pair-bonding usually seen in mate or mother–offspring pairs (Dunbar, 2010), in which touch plays a demonstrably vital role in maintaining bonds. In human romantic partnerships, relationship satisfaction, previous experience of familial affection, and trust correlate positively with self-reports of how people groom one another—for example, how often they brush or play with someone else's hair or wipe away their tears (Nelson & Geher, 2007). The stage of the relationship is also important when it comes to the role of intensive touching and grooming (Emmers & Dindia, 1995). Indeed, different neural mechanisms may come into play during the initiation of an affiliative relationship and during its maintenance (Depue & Morrone-Strupinsky, 2005). People who reported themselves as being more anxious also reported more frequent grooming behavior, suggesting that people with more anxious personality traits may also tend to seek more secure bonds through social touch behavior.

Even in a nonmammal species, tactile stimulation has been found to have effects on behavior resembling that of the social modulation of fear. In zebrafish (*Danio rerio*), lateral line stimulation (stimulation of the tactile sensors by a water current) can abolish hiding behavior after exposure to a fear-inducing pheromone, with effects comparable to swimming alongside familiar conspecifics in the same tank (Schirmer, Jesuthasan, & Mathuru, 2013). In humans, the contact pressure of holding hands reduces the anxiety posed by an impending threat (Coan et al., 2006).

CONCLUSION

We are at the cusp of an exciting new revolution in the way affective touch is understood and studied, especially with respect to its brain bases. Affective touch, such as gentle pressure or a caress, carries emotional and social significance. The discovery of CT afferents suggests that the role of affective touch may be so distinct from other forms of touch as to constitute a special neural pathway from the skin to the brain. The brain networks engaged by affective, social touch process stimulus information (predominantly in the insula and also in the somatosensory areas on the pariental operculum) and integrate it with other social information (involving superior temporal sulcus) as well as with reward- and decision-making networks that guide behavior (involving orbitofrontal cortex). Future research will map these networks further, for example disentangling the precise functional roles of insula and SII. It will also probe the hypothesis that affective touch influences behavior by modulating efferent "outflow" pathways, such as autonomic systems that regulate heartbeat, breathing, and muscle readiness, in a way that promotes positive subjective experience and well-being.

REFERENCES

Ackerley, R., Backlund Wasling, H., Liljencrantz, J., Olausson, H., Johnson, R. D., & Wessberg, J. (2014). Human C-tactile afferents are tuned to the temperature of a skin-stroking caress. *Journal of Neuroscience, 34*, 2879–2883.

Ainsworth, M. D. S., Blehar, M. C., Waters, E., & Wall, S. (1978). *Patterns of attachment: A psychological study of the strange situation.* Hillsdale, NJ: Erlbaum.

Andrew, D. (2010). Quantitative characterization of low-threshold mechanoreceptor inputs to lamina I spinoparabrachial neurons in the rat. *Journal of Physiology, 588*, 117–124.

Atwood, M. (2000). *The Blind Assassin.*

Bennett, R. H., Bolling, D. Z., Anderson, L. C., Pelphrey, K. A., & Kaiser, M. D. (2014). fNIRS detects temporal lobe response to affective touch. *Social Cognitive and Affective Neuroscience, 9*, 470–476.

Bessou, P., Burgess, P. R., Perl, E. R., & Taylor, C. B. (1971). Dynamic properties of mechanoreceptors with unmyelinated (C) fibers. *Journal of Neurophysiology, 34*, 116–131.

Björnsdotter, M., Löken, L., Olausson, H., Vallbo, A., & Wessberg, J. (2009). Somatotopic organization of gentle touch processing in the posterior insular cortex. *Journal of Neuroscience, 29*, 9314–9320.

Bowlby, J. (1973). *Attachment and loss, Vol. 2. Separation: Anxiety and anger.* New York, NY: Basic Books

Brossard, L., & Decarie, T. (1968). Comparative reinforcing effects of eight stimulations on the smiling responses of infants. *Journal of Child Psychology and Psychiatry, 9*, 51–59.

Burgoon, J. K., Walther, J. B., & Baesler, E. J. (1992). Interpretations, evaluations, and consequences of interpersonal touch. *Human Communication Research, 19*, 237–263.

Cascio, C., McGlone, F., Folger, S., Tannan, V., Baranek, G., Pelphrey, K. A., & Essick, G. (2008). Tactile perception in adults with autism: A multidimensional psychophysical study. *Journal of Autism and Developmental Disorders, 38*, 127–137.

Cascio, C. J., Moana-Filho, E. J., Guest, S., Nebel, M. B., Weisner, J., Baranek, G. T., & Essick, G. K. (2012). Perceptual and neural response to affective tactile texture stimulation in adults with autism spectrum disorders. *Autism Research, 5*, 231–244.

Coan, J. A., Schaefer, H. S., & Davidson, R. J. (2006). Lending a hand: Social regulation of the neural response to threat. *Psychological Science, 17*, 1032–1039.

Cole, J. D., Bushnell, M. C., McGlone, F., Elam, M., Lamarre, Y., Vallbo, A. B., & Olausson, H. (2006). Unmyelinated tactile afferents underpin detection of low-force monofilaments. *Muscle Nerve, 34*, 105–107.

Craig, A. D. (1995). Distribution of brainstem projections from spinal lamina I neurons in the cat and the monkey. *Journal of Comparative Neurology, 361,* 225–248.

Craig, A. D. (2002). How do you feel? Interoception: The sense of the physiological condition of the body. *Nature Reviews Neuroscience, 3,* 655–666.

Crusco, A. H., & Wetzel, C. G. (1984). The Midas touch: The effects of interpersonal touch on restaurant tipping. *Personal Social Psychology Bulletin, 10,* 512–517.

Deen, B., Pitskel, N. B., & Pelphrey, K. A. (2011). Three systems of insular functional connectivity identified with cluster analysis. *Cerebral Cortex, 7,* 1498–1506.

Depue, R. A., & Morrone-Strupinsky, J. V. (2005). A neurobehavioral model of affiliative bonding: Implications for conceptualizing a human trait of affiliation. *Behavioral and Brain Sciences, 28,* 313–395.

Dunbar, R. I. (2010). The social role of touch in humans and primates: Behavioural function and neurobiological mechanisms. *Neuroscience and Biobehavioral Reviews, 34,* 260–268.

Ebisch, S. J., Ferri, F., Salone, A., Perrucci, M. G., D'Amico, L., Ferro, F. M., . . . Gallese, V. (2011). Differential involvement of somatosensory and interoceptive cortices during the observation of affective touch. *Journal of Cognitive Neuroscience, 23,* 1808–1822.

Einarsdottir, E., Carlsson, A., Minde, J., Toolanen, G., Svensson, O., Solders, G., . . . Holmberg, M. (2004). A mutation in the nerve growth factor beta gene (NGFB) causes loss of pain perception. *Human Molecular Genetics, 13,* 799–805.

Emmers, T. M., & Dindia, K. (1995). The effect of relational stage and intimacy on touch: An extension of Guerrero and Andersen. *Personal Relationships, 2,* 225–236.

Fisher, J. D., Rytting, M., & Heslin, R. (1976). Hands touching hands: Affective and evaluative effects of an interpersonal touch. *Sociometry, 39,* 416–421.

Gazzola, V., Spezio, M. L., Etzel, J. A., Castelli, F., Adolphs, R., & Keysers, C. (2012). Primary somatosensory cortex discriminates affective significance in social touch. *Proceedings of the National Academy of Science USA, 109,* E1657–1666.

Gordon, I., Voos, A. C., Bennett, R. H., Bolling, D. Z., Pelphrey, K. A., & Kaiser, M. D. (2011). Brain mechanisms for processing affective touch. *Human Brain Mapping, 34,* 914–922.

Harlow, H. F. (1958). The nature of love. *American Psychologist, 13,* 335–346.

Hertenstein, M. J., & Campos, J. J. (2001). Emotion regulation via maternal touch. *Infancy, 2,* 549–566.

Hertenstein, M. J., Verkamp, J. M., Kerestes, A. M., & Holmes, R. M. (2006a). The communicative functions of touch in humans, nonhuman primates, and rats: A review and synthesis of the empirical research. *Social Genetic Psychology Monographs, 132,* 5–94.

Hertenstein, M. J., Keltner, D., App, B., Bulleit, B. A., & Jaskolka, A. R. (2006b). Touch communicates distinct emotions. *Emotion, 6,* 528–533

Hornik, J (1992). Tactile stimulation and consumer response. *Journal of Consumer Research, 19,* 449–458.

Iggo, A. (1960). Cutaneous mechanoreceptors with afferent C fibres. *Journal of Physiology, 152,* 337–353.

Iggo, A., & Kornhuber, H. H. (1977). A quantitative study of C-mechanoreceptors in hairy skin of the cat. *Journal of Physiology, 271,* 549–565.

Joule, R. V., & Guégen, N. (2007). Touch, compliance, and awareness of tactile contact. *Perception and Motor Skills, 104*, 581–588.

Kleinke, C. L. (1977). Compliance to requests made by gazing and touching experimenters in field settings. *Journal of Experimental and Social Psychology, 13*, 218–223.

Krämer, H. H., Lundblad, L., Birklein, F., Linde, M., Karlsson, T., Elam, M., & Olausson, H. (2007). Activation of the cortical pain network by soft tactile stimulation after injection of sumatriptan. *Pain, 133*, 72–78.

Kress, I. U., Minati, L., Ferraro, S., & Critchley, H. D. (2011). Direct skin-to-skin versus indirect touch modulates neural responses to stroking versus tapping. *Neuroreport, 14*, 646–651.

Kurth, F., Zilles, K., Fox, P. T., Laird, A. R., & Eickhoff, S. B. (2010). A link between the systems: Functional differentiation and integration within the human insula revealed by meta- analysis. *Brain Structure and Function, 214*, 519–534.

Lindgren, L., Westling, G., Brulin, C., Lehtipalo, S., Andersson, M., & Nyberg, L. (2012). Pleasant human touch is represented in pregenual anterior cingulate cortex. *Neuroimage, 59*, 3427–3432.

Liu, Q., Vrontou, S., Rice, F. L., Zylka, M. J., Dong, X., & Anderson, D. J. (2007). Molecular genetic visualization of a rare subset of unmyelinated sensory neurons that may detect gentle touch. *Nature Neuroscience, 10*, 946–948.

Löken, L. S., Wessberg, J., Morrison, I., McGlone, F., & Olausson, H. (2009). Coding of pleasant touch by unmyelinated afferents in humans. *Nature Neuroscience, 5*, 547–548.

Lovero, K. L., Simmons, A. N., Aron, J. L., & Paulus, M. P. (2009). Anterior insular cortex anticipates impending stimulus significance. *Neuroimage, 45*, 976–983.

Menard, J. L., Champagne, D. L., & Meaney, M. J. (2004). Variations of maternal care differentially influence "fear" reactivity and regional patterns of cFos immunoreactivity in response to the shock-probe burying test. *Neuroscience, 129*, 297–308.

Minde, J., Andersson, T., Fulford, M., Aguirre, M., Nennesmo, I., & Remahl, I. N. (2009). A novel NGFB point mutation: A phenotype study of heterozygous patients. *Journal of Neurological and Neurosurgical Psychiatry, 80*, 188–195.

Minde, J., Toolanen, G., Andersson, T., Nennesmo, I., Remahl, I. N., & Svensson, O. (2004). Familial insensitivity to pain (HSAN V) and a mutation in the NGFB gene. A neurophysiological and pathological study. *Muscle Nerve, 30*, 752–760.

Morrison, I., Björnsdotter, M., & Olausson, H. (2011). Vicarious responses to social touch in posterior insular cortex are tuned to pleasant caressing speeds. *Journal of Neuroscience, 31*, 9554–9562.

Morrison, I., Löken, L. S., Minde, J., Wessberg, J., Perini, I., Nennesmo, I., & Olausson, H. (2011). Reduced C-afferent fibre density affects perceived pleasantness and empathy for touch. *Brain, 134*, 1116–1126.

Morrison, I., Löken, L. S., & Olausson, H. (2010). The skin as a social organ. *Experimental Brain Research, 204*, 305–314.

Morrison, India (in press). ALE meta-analysis reveals dissociable networks for affective and discriminatory aspects of touch. *Human Brain Mapping*.

Nelson, H., & Geher, G. (2007). Mutual grooming in human dyadic relationships: An ethological perspective. *Current Psychology, 26*, 121–140.

Nordin, M. (1990). Low-threshold mechanoreceptive and nociceptive units with unmyelinated (C) fibres in the human supraorbital nerve. *Journal of Physiology, 426,* 229–240.

Olausson, H., Lamarre, Y., Backlund, H., Morin, C., Wallin, B. G., Starck, G., et al. (2002). Unmyelinated tactile afferents signal touch and project to insular cortex. *Nature Neuroscience, 5,* 900–904.

Olausson, H., Wessberg, J., Morrison, I., McGlone, F., & Vallbo, Å. (2010). The neurophysiology of unmyelinated tactile afferents. *Neuroscience and Biobehavioral Reviews, 34,* 185–191.

Owens, N. C., Sartor, D. M., & Verberne, A. J. (1999). Medial prefrontal cortex depressor response: Role of the solitary tract nucleus in the rat. *Neuroscience* 89: 1331–1346.

Pelhez-Nogueras, M., Gewirtz, J. L., Field, T., Cigales, M., Malphurs, J., Clasky, S., & Sanchez, A. (1996). Infants' preference for touch stimulation in face-to-face interactions. *Journal of Applied Developmental Psychology, 17,* 19–21.

Perini, I., Björnsdottir, M., & Morrison, I. (2015). Seeking pleasant touch: Neural correlates of behavioral preferences for skin stroking. *Frontiers in Behavioral Neuroscience.* doi: 10.3389/fnbeh.2015.00008.

Porges, S. W. (2007). The polyvagal perspective. *Biological Psychiatry, 74,* 116–143.

Rubin, R. (1963). Maternal touch. *Nursing Outlook, 11,* 828–829.

Schirmer, A., Jesuthasan, S., & Mathuru, A. S. (2013). Tactile stimulation reduces fear in fish. *Frontiers in Behavioral Neuroscience, 7,* 167.

Sliz, D., Smith, A., Wiebking, C., Northoff, G., & Hayley, S. (2012). Neural correlates of a single- session massage treatment. *Brain Imaging and Behavior, 6,* 77–87.

Stack, D. M., & Muir, D. W. (1992). Adult tactile stimulation during face-to-face interactions modulates five-month-olds' affect and attention. *Child Development, 63,* 1509–1525.

Vallbo, Å., Olausson, H., Wessberg, J., & Norrsell, U. (1993). A system of unmyelinated afferents for innocuous mechanoreception in the human skin. *Brain Research, 628,* 301–304.

Voos, A. C., Pelphrey, K. A., & Kaiser, M. D. (2013). Autistic traits are associated with diminished neural response to affective touch. *Social Cognitive and Affective Neuroscience, 8,* 378–386.

Vrontou, S., Wong, A. M., Rau, K. K., Koerber, H. R., & Anderson, D. J. (2013). Genetic identification of C fibres that detect massage-like stroking of hairy skin in vivo. *Nature, 493,* 669–673.

Wessberg, J., Olausson, H., Fernstrom, K. W., & Vallbo, A. B. (2003). Receptive field properties of unmyelinated tactile afferents in the human skin. *Journal of Neurophysiology, 89,* 1567–1575.

Zotterman, Y. (1939). Touch, pain and tickling: An electrophysiological investigation on cutaneous sensory nerves. *Journal of Physiology, 95,* 1–28.

2

The Neural Correlates of Individual Variation in Paternal Nurturance

JAMES K. RILLING AND JENNIFER MASCARO ■

Considerable evidence suggests that sensitive parenting, defined as contingent, reciprocating responses to children, is associated with positive child outcomes, whereas insensitive parenting, as in neglect, abuse, or as is sometimes found with postpartum depression, is associated with poor developmental outcomes (Barrett & Fleming, 2011; Belsky et al., 2006; Feldman, 2007).Cross-fostering experiments in animals suggest that these associations may be direct and causal (Champagne & Meaney, 2001). Despite the importance of sensitive care for healthy child development, modern lifestyles often challenge the ability of parents to provide sensitive and sufficient caregiving. Humans are an alloparental species (Hrdy, 2009), meaning that although mothers are typically the primary caregiver, they usually receive help from fathers, grandmothers, sisters, brothers, older children, and so on. However, modern Western parents often live with their children in isolated nuclear families, removed from kin who might otherwise provide assistance. Moreover, the proportion of American women participating in the labor force has increased from 34% in 1950 to 58.6% in 2010, as reported by the US Department of Labor (2011; Toossi, 2002), suggesting that American mothers face increasing demands on their time that limit their availability for child care. These combined circumstances render fathers an essential source of allomaternal care. Yet despite this, paternal investment is highly variable among men, and father absence has increased precipitously over the last half of the 20th century (Cabrera, Tamis-LeMonda, Bradley, Hofferth, & Lamb, 2000). These facts highlight the need to identify factors that support positive paternal involvement. This chapter will begin by reviewing patterns of paternal care across animal species and across human cultures. It will then present evidence that paternal care contributes to positive developmental outcomes in children living in modern, Western societies. This will be followed by presentation of a theoretical framework for explaining variation in paternal care among men within a given society. Finally, we review our own and other published data on the biological and neural bases of paternal nurturance and its variability.

PATERNAL CARE ACROSS SPECIES

Although most mammalian fathers do *not* parent, paternal care tends to be found when it can improve offspring survival, when other mating opportunities are limited, and when paternity certainty is high (Woodroffe & Vincent, 1994). Paternal care is most common in three mammalian orders: rodents, primates, and canids. Among rodents, significant paternal care is found in California mice, Djungarian hamsters, Mongolian gerbils, and prairie voles, and this care contributes to pup survival (Dudley, 1974; Elwood, 1975; Gubernick & Teferi, 2000; Oliveras & Novak, 1986; Wynne-Edwards, 1987). Paternal care in these species includes grooming, carrying, and retrieving pups to the nest. Fathers also huddle with pups to keep them warm, and they assist in nest building. Male Djuangarian hamsters even assist with delivery of pups at birth (Jones & Wynne-Edwards, 2000). Among canids, male foxes and coyotes provision their young with meat (Gittleman, 1986). Many primate males protect their young, but more extensive paternal care is uncommon and is concentrated among New World monkeys. Titi and Owl monkey fathers carry their relatively large infants, allowing their female mates to conserve calories for lactation that will feed the infant. Males of these species also share food and play with infants, although older siblings may be the most common playmates (Wright, 1984). Owl and titi monkeys are considered biparental. However, humans are more similar to cooperative breeders who rely on an array of alloparental caregivers, not only the mother and father, to raise offspring (Hrdy, 2009). The classic primate examples are marmoset and tamarin monkeys. In both species, males carry twin infants most of the time, and they may also provision and groom offspring (Ingram, 1977; Tardif, Carson, & Gangaware, 1992). Among our closest living relatives, the great apes, paternal care is quite limited. The best example is probably the defense of offspring from infanticidal adult males among gorillas. Though certainly more developed than in great apes, human paternal care is highly variable across cultures.

PATERNAL CARE CROSS-CULTURALLY

Paternal care can take many forms, but it is often categorized as either direct or indirect care. Indirect paternal care, in the form of provisioning offspring with food or money, is common across many human cultures. Direct forms of paternal care, including holding, carrying, feeding, bathing, playing with, and teaching children, is far more variable cross-culturally. Among traditional, preindustrial societies, direct paternal care is most common in hunter-gatherers. Direct paternal care is next most common in horticulturalists and agriculturalists, and least common among pastoralists (Konner, 2010). Cross-cultural comparisons also reveal that direct paternal care is more common in societies where men do not engage in military activities, where they mate monogamously rather than polygynously, and where the mother's subsistence workload is high (Katz & Konner, 1981). Grandmothers are another important source of allomaternal care across a wide range of societies, and there often seems to be a trade-off between paternal and grandmaternal care. That is, fathers will do more when grandmothers do less and vice-versa.

Fathers tend to be less involved with infants than with older children. Aka pygmy fathers do more infant caregiving than fathers in any other known society. However, even among the Aka, infants are held by mothers far more (51%) than they are held by fathers (22%) (Hewlett, 1991). Limited parental involvement in infancy could be partially attributable to the father's inability to breastfeed, as well as hormonal influences that bias mothers toward and fathers away from infant care. Oxytocin released at parturition and during breastfeeding may facilitate rapid mother–infant bonding (Kendrick, 2000; Pedersen, Ascher, Monroe, & Prange, 1982) and also decrease hostility in response to infant crying (Bakermans-Kranenburg, van Ijzendoorn, Riem, Tops, & Alink, 2012; Naber, van Ijzendoorn, Deschamps, van Engeland, & Bakermans-Kranenburg, 2010). Although both mothers and fathers experience a small increase in baseline OT across infant development (Gordon, Zagoory-Sharon, Leckman, & Feldman, 2010), fathers do not experience the additional OT exposure that mothers do during nursing and at parturition. In addition, men have higher testosterone levels, which could contribute to unregulated aggressive impulses (Bos, Panksepp, Bluthe, & van Honk, 2012; Carre, McCormick, & Hariri, 2011), as well as limited empathy for infants (Fleming, Corter, Stallings, & Steiner, 2002; van Honk et al., 2011). This might explain why men are more likely to commit infanticide in response to inconsolable infant crying (Brewster et al., 1998). The fact that testosterone decreases when men become fathers is consistent with its antagonistic effects on infant care that are mitigated by the decrease.

As children get older, fathers have more opportunity to get involved with physical play and with teaching children how to become competent adults of their society. In traditional human societies, fathers tend to be more involved in the care of sons than in the care of daughters, presumably because it is their responsibility to teach boys gender-specific skills (e.g., hunting and fighting) (Gray & Anderson, 2010).

PATERNAL CARE AND CHILD DEVELOPMENT

Survival

Among a sample of over 217,000 infants born in 1989–1990 to women who were residents of Georgia, the risk of infant mortality was 2.3 times higher among infants of mothers not listing a father on the birth certificate compared with those who did list a father on the birth certificate (Gaudino et al., 1999). This study suggests that fathers may still play a role in infant survival in modern, economically developed societies like ours.

Psychosocial Development

Father involvement is associated with improved social functioning in childhood and adulthood, better educational outcomes, less aggressive behavior, lower incidence of delinquency and criminality, and decreased psychological morbidity (Sarkadi, Kristiansson, Oberklaid, & Bremberg, 2008). Paternal involvement and closeness has also been linked with greater altruism and generosity (Rutherford & Mussen, 1968) in children and greater empathic concern in adults (Koestner, Franz, & Weinberger, 1990).

Despite the importance of men being present in their children's lives, fathers also have the potential to harm infants through physical abuse. The first 2–4 months of infancy is a time when infants are particularly at risk from paternal abuse (Barr, Trent, & Cross, 2006). Shaken baby syndrome peaks during this interval (Barr et al., 2006) and men are disproportionately responsible (Starling, Holden, & Jenny, 1995). The peak of abuse closely follows the peak of infant crying at 5 weeks of age, suggesting that infant crying may contribute to paternal abuse and infanticide (Barr et al., 2006). Indeed, one study found that 5.6% of parents reported having smothered, slapped, or shaken their baby at least once because of its crying (Reijneveld, van der Wal, Brugman, Sing, & Verloove-Vanhorick, 2004), and case reports show that inconsolable infant crying can provoke fatal abuse (Krugman, 1983). The fact that men rate cry stimuli as more aversive than women do (Zeifman, 2003) may partially explain their higher rates of infanticide. The challenge that all parents face is to respond to this potentially aversive stimulus with sensitivity and compassion rather than frustration.

THEORETICAL PERSPECTIVES ON VARIATION IN PATERNAL NURTURANCE

Why do some men choose to not be involved in raising their children? According to a branch of evolutionary theory known as life history theory, organisms have a finite amount of energy and resources that they allocate toward the competing demands of growth, maintenance, parenting, and mating (Lack, 1954). Effort devoted to one category cannot be used for another. Evolution is expected to have optimized species' allocations among these categories so as to maximize reproductive success. Although originally proposed as an explanation for cross-species diversity in life history strategies, the theory may also have utility in explaining within-species variation (Figueredo et al., 2006).

If energy devoted to growth and maintenance is held constant, the theory predicts that men face a trade-off between investments in mating and parenting. It predicts that men will invest in whichever of these yields the greatest payoff in terms of reproductive success. The following factors would be expected to increase the allocation of resources to parenting: (1) circumstances in which paternal care would improve a child's survival or improve a child's developmental outcomes and "mate value," (2) high paternity certainty, (3) limited mating opportunities outside the pair-bond, and (4) limited availability of alloparental assistance.

THE NEURAL BASES OF PATERNAL NURTURANCE

Nonhuman Research

Research into the neurobiology of human paternal care is limited to noninvasive techniques such as neuroimaging, measurement of peripheral hormone levels, and most recently, pharmacological studies (e.g., intranasal OT administration). On the other hand, research with nonhuman animals enables more detailed study, including neurochemical receptor distributions (immunocytochemistry and autoradiography), neurochemical concentrations (microdialysis), and behavioral consequences of experimental lesions. Although human parenting and its neural substrates may differ in important ways from that found in nonhuman animals, nonhuman studies have led to the development of comprehensive models that provide a rich source of hypotheses for human studies. Given the primacy of mothers in parenting, the neurobiology of maternal care has been studied to a far greater extent than has the neurobiology of paternal care. However, paternal behavior may have evolved from preexisting neural systems that were already in place to support maternal behavior (Wynne-Edwards & Reburn, 2000), and so the extensive body of nonhuman animal research on the neurobiology of maternal care may be relevant to understanding paternal care.

Numan (2007) argues that adult female rats have separate systems motivating approach and avoidance of offspring, and that maternal behavior emerges when the former exceeds the latter. The medial preoptic area (MPOA) is a critical node that both activates the mesolimbic dopamine (approach) system and inhibits an avoidance circuit that runs from the medial amygdala through the anterior hypothalamic nucleus to the periaqueductal gray of the midbrain. In both male and nulliparous female rats, several days of habituation to pups are required to suppress the avoidance system to the point where parental behavior is exhibited. However, pregnancy-related hormones like prolactin and estrogen augment MPOA function so that maternal behavior emerges at parturition. Oxytocin (OT) facilitates parental behavior through actions at MPOA (Pedersen, Caldwell, Walker, Ayers, & Mason, 1994) but also acts at each node of the mesolimbic dopamine (DA) system (ventral tegmental area [VTA] and nucleus accumbens [NA]) to facilitate DA release in the NA (Numan & Stolzenberg, 2009). Given the role of the mesolimbic DA system in reward processing, OT may augment the reward value of offspring. The mesolimbic DA system is more active in rat mothers that lick and groom their offspring more frequently and are presumably more nurturing (Champagne, Diorio, Sharma, & Meaney, 2001). Intriguingly, high licking and grooming rat dams have more OT receptors in MPOA (Champagne et al., 2001; Francis, Champagne, & Meaney, 2000), and female prairie voles with more OT receptors in the NA are more likely to exhibit spontaneous alloparental care in the absence of pregnancy (Olazabal & Young, 2006).

Is Numan's model of maternal care relevant to paternal care? Studies in California mice support this possibility because MPOA lesions inhibit paternal behavior, and pup exposure increases Fos-like immunoreactivity in the MPOA in new fathers but not in other males (de Jong, Chauke, Harris, & Saltzman, 2009). Furthermore, OT receptor antagonists can interfere with paternal behavior in male prairie voles (Bales, Kim, Lewis-Reese, & Sue Carter, 2004). However, paternal behavior also has its own dedicated neural circuitry in some species, and this circuitry involves vasopressin (AVP). For example,

AVP injections into the lateral septum elicit paternal behavior in male prairie voles (Wang, Ferris, & De Vries, 1994), and AVP-immunoreactive staining in BNST terminals predicts paternal behavior in California mice (Bester-Meredith & Marler, 2003). In male prairie voles, pup exposure increases activity of PVN neurons stained for either OT or AVP (Kenkel et al., 2012). Studies in marmoset monkeys additionally implicate structures outside the limbic system. Marmoset fathers have increased V1a vasopressin receptor density as well as increased dendritic spine density on neurons in prefrontal cortex (Kozorovitskiy, Hughes, Lee, & Gould, 2006).

Human Research

PAST RESEARCH

As with nonhuman studies, most studies on the neurobiology of human parental care have been conducted on mothers. There are only a few published studies with fathers (Kuo, Carp, Light, & Grewen, 2012; Seifritz et al., 2003; Wittfoth-Schardt et al., 2012). The first showed that, compared with nonfathers, fathers have a stronger response to infant cries in both the insula and the amygdala (Seifritz et al., 2003). A second imaged fathers as they viewed videos of their own and unknown infants sitting in an infant carrier with neutral expressions. Viewing own infant videos was associated with stronger activation in the thalamus, as well as putative mirror neuron regions, including the inferior parietal and inferior frontal cortex (Kuo et al., 2012). Thus, fathers may have been empathizing with their own infants to a greater degree than the unknown infants. The third study imaged 19 fathers of 3- to 6-year-old children as they viewed pictures of their own child, a familiar child, and an unfamiliar child, both after intranasal OT administration as well as after intranasal placebo administration. In the placebo condition, viewing the own child was associated with activation in regions linked with empathy (inferior frontal gyrus, anterior insula) and approach-related motivation or reward (medial orbitofrontal cortex, VTA, globus pallidus) (Wittfoth-Schardt et al., 2012). As discussed earlier, rodent studies would predict OT to enhance activation in the DA reward system in response to offspring cues; however, OT instead suppressed activation within the globus pallidus. These results are difficult to interpret in the context of the existing nonhuman animal literature, and it will be important to see them replicated.

Collectively, there is evidence that both mothers and fathers activate components of the mesolimbic DA system when viewing pictures of their own children, and that plasma OT levels in mothers are positively correlated with this response (Atzil, Hendler, & Feldman, 2011; Bartels & Zeki, 2004; Strathearn, Fonagy, Amico, & Montague, 2009). This result is consistent with Numan's model in which OT augments the reward value offspring, which may in turn motivate responsive caregiving. Although describing the parental neural response to infant stimuli has merit, a few studies have extended this approach to investigate how these responses might relate to real-world parenting. For example, maternal functional magnetic resonance imaging (fMRI) responses have been linked with maternal sensitivity and intrusiveness in free play inter- actions with infants (Musser, Kaiser-Laurent, & Ablow, 2012). Only one prior study has attempted to relate paternal fMRI activity to paternal behavior out- side the scanner (Kuo et al., 2012).

PRESENT RESEARCH
Variation in Paternal Neural Responses to Own Child Pictures

We have imaged 60 fathers of 1- to 3-year-old children as they view pictures of their own children, unknown children, and unknown adults displaying happy, sad, and neutral expressions in a standard fMRI block paradigm. Viewing pic- tures of one's own child compared to an unknown adult robustly activated the ventral tegmental area (Mascaro et al., 2013), the source of the mesolimbic DA projections that are postulated to mediate the motivation to approach and nurture offspring (Numan, 2007) (Figure 2.1a).

Fathers and their partners also completed a battery of measures to assess level of paternal investment in their children. All fathers completed ques- tionnaires that measure warmth or nurturance, as well as parental respon- sibility or level of instrumental support. Paternal warmth or nurturance was measured using a modified version of the Block Child Rearing Practices Report (Rickel & Biasatti, 1982), consisting of 28 Likert scale questions regarding child care beliefs, including both restrictiveness and nurturing subscales. Instrumental support was measured using a scale developed by our colleague Sherryl Goodman at Emory University, which asks the parent to designate who has primary responsibility for 24 tasks along a five-point scale, ranging from 1 (*mother almost always*) to 5 (*father almost always*). Responsibility is defined for the parent as remembering, planning, and scheduling the task. Higher scores indicate a higher degree of paternal responsibility.

Mothers and fathers show strong agreement of responses on the parental responsibility scale ($r = .70, p < .001$). Importantly, more involved fathers show a stronger response to their own child's face in the VTA (Figure 2.1b). We interpret these results to suggest that fathers who are more rewarded by their child's appearance are more involved in their care, perhaps because the child's appearance positively reinforces caregiving. Alternatively, fathers who spend

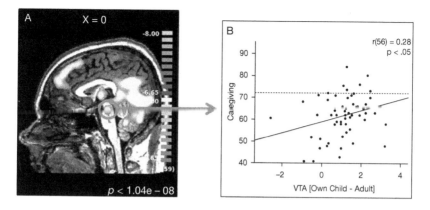

Figure 2.1 (A) Brain regions in color are more active when fathers view pictures of their own child than when they view pictures of an adult of the same sex and ethnicity. (B) Activation within the midbrain, which encompasses brain reward circuitry, is positively correlated with a measure of the father's involvement in day-to-day caregiving of the child. A shows the main effect of the contrast [Own Child—Adult] for all emotions combined, Bonferroni-corrected $p < .001$, uncorrected $p < 1.04$ e-08. A region of interest in the midbrain was determined by identifying the voxel with peak activity and including all activated voxels within 10 voxels of that peak in the X, Y, and Z direction. B plots paternal responsibility versus beta contrast values [Own Child—Adult] from functionally derived midbrain region of interest. The dotted red line indicates the score (72) at which mothers and fathers are equally responsible for their child's daily care. VTA, ventral tegmental area.

more time with their children may come to find the child more rewarding by virtue of the stronger bond they develop.

Collectively, these results suggest that Numan's model of the neurobiology of rat maternal care may be relevant to paternal care in humans. However, an important next step will be to image fathers following pretreatment with intranasal OT to determine if OT augments activity in the reward system pathways when viewing pictures of children.

Variation in Paternal Neural Responses to Own Child Cry Stimuli

In addition to imaging the paternal neural response to child pictures, we have also imaged $n = 36$ fathers as they listen to infant cry stimuli. We used cry stimuli from two unknown infants. Two types of control stimuli were synthesized for each cry. For one control, an emotionally neutral baby vocalization was created to match the duration, intensity, spectral content, and amplitude envelope of the cry stimulus. The second control was a pure tone that preserved the mean fundamental frequency and amplitude envelope of the cry. Figure 2.2a shows the contrast between cry and tone control stimuli. Activation is observed in bilateral anterior insula (AI), a region strongly implicated in empathic respond-ing, at a conservative statistical threshold. Our data also show that fathers who are more restrictive in their parenting style, as assessed by the Block Child Rearing Practices report, have less AI activation (Figure 2.2b). Restrictive par-ents score high on questions such as *"I teach my child to keep control of his or her feelings at all times"* and *"I believe that scolding and criticism make a child improve."* We suspect restrictive parents are often less empathic and this may be reflected in their attenuated AI response to infant cry stimuli. One might expect more empathic fathers to be more involved in the instrumental care of their children, and so one might predict a positive correlation between the anterior insula response to cry stimuli and our parental responsibility mea-sure. However, the relationship instead follows an inverted u-shaped trajec-tory in which parental responsibility initially increases with increasing insula activation, reaches a maximum at intermediate levels, and decreases thereafter (Figure 2.2c). We suggest that very high levels of anterior insula activity might represent the phenomenon known as "empathic overarousal," in which one empathizes with another's pain to such a great extent that one becomes mired in personal distress, resulting in reduced motivation to help. Thus, there may be an optimal level of anterior insula responsiveness that facilitates paternal involvement in instrumental care of young children (Mascaro et al., 2014).

The dotted red line indicates the score (72) at which mothers and fathers are equally responsible for their child's daily care.

FUTURE RESEARCH

These investigations barely scratch the surface of constructing an understand-ing of the biological bases of paternal care. There is much more to be done.

One interesting question is to what extent does the quality of paternal care depend on characteristics of the father versus characteristics of the child? We tend to think that good fathers produce happy and healthy children, but the opposite could be true. Perhaps healthy, attractive, engaging children are more effective at eliciting paternal nurturance. Future research should sys-tematically investigate the influence of characteristics of both the child and the father on paternal behavior. Characteristics of the child that should be considered include age, sex, attractiveness (or "cuteness"), growth percentiles, care-eliciting behaviors, illness frequency, and so on. Fathers tend to be more involved as children get older, and in some societies, they are more involved in raising boys than girls. It will be interesting to examine how a father's neural response to children varies as a function of the child's sex or age. Characteristics of the father that should be considered include upbringing, attachment security, hormone levels, physical attractiveness, mating effort, and brain function.

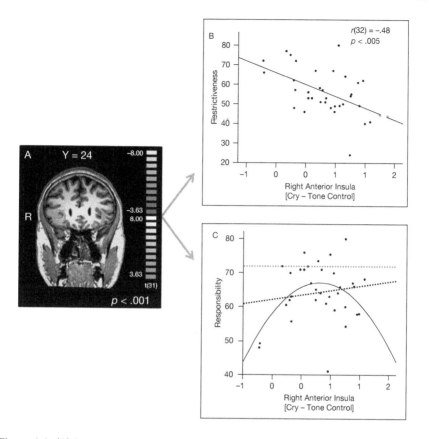

Figure 2.2 (A) Brain regions in color are more active when fathers listen to infant cries than when they listen to an auditory tone control stimulus. (B) Activation within the anterior insula is negatively correlated with restrictiveness. (C) Paternal responsibility is highest at moderate levels of anterior insula activation. *A* shows main effect of the contrast [Cry—Tone Control] thresholded at $p < .001$, uncorrected. The anterior insula region of interest was generated by identifying the local maximum of activity within the anterior insula (AI) and including all activated voxels within 10 voxels of the peak in the X, Y, and Z direction; *B* plots restrictiveness versus beta contrast values [Cry—Tone Control] from functionally derived right anterior insula ROI; *C* plots responsibility versus beta contrast values [Cry—Tone Control] from functionally derived right anterior insula region of interest. Linear and quadratic fits are indicated by the dotted and solid black lines, respectively. Only the quadratic fit is significant ($F(29) = 5.52, p < .01$ for quadratic vs. $r(30) = .09, p = .61$ for linear).

Although recent studies have investigated the role of OT in human paternal care, no studies have examined a potential role for AVP. Yet AVP is very strongly implicated in paternal care in both rodents and primates. Future studies should investigate the potential role of AVP in human fatherhood.

Interventions should be developed for abusive fathers and fathers with postpartum depression. Given that infant crying is a common trigger for paternal abuse, fathers should be educated about infant crying. One ongoing program (the PURPLE Crying program) teaches parents that inconsolable infant crying is normal, that it does not reflect bad parenting, that it is understandably frustrating, and that its frequency peaks around 5 weeks of age and decreases thereafter (Barr, 2012). Meditation interventions have shown promise for reducing stress and negative affect in new moms, and it may be an effective intervention for decreasing aggression and increasing compassion in fathers (Duncan & Bardacke, 2010). Pharmacological interventions are also possible. Given that OT is known to decrease parental hostility, intranasal OT may be an effective intervention for at-risk fathers. Neuroimaging could be used to evaluate the likely effectiveness of these interventions.

Fathers are just one of many alloparents that help raise human children. We also need to study grandparents and older siblings who help care for children. And we need to study day care and foster care workers who, despite the best intentions, may have limited empathy and compassion to partition among the many children in their care. It is also critical that we study step-parents, given the very high rates of child abuse in this population (Daly & Wilson, 1988).

CONCLUSION

Our research has identified neural correlates of direct paternal caregiving, including a larger VTA response to pictures of their own child's face and intermediate responses of the anterior insula to infant crying. Longitudinal studies are needed to establish the direction of causality behind these associations. If such studies establish that brain activity causes paternal involvement, then pharmacological (e.g., intranasal OT) and behavioral (e.g., PURPLE) interventions aimed at improving paternal care can be evaluated for their likely effectiveness using brain imaging.

REFERENCES

Atzil, S., Hendler, T., & Feldman, R. (2011). Specifying the neurobiological basis of human attachment: Brain, hormones, and behavior in synchronous and intrusive mothers. *Neuropsychopharmacology*, 36(13), 2603–2615.

Bakermans-Kranenburg, M. J., van Ijzendoorn, M. H., Riem, M. M., Tops, M., & Alink, L. R. (2012). Oxytocin decreases handgrip force in reaction to infant crying in females without harsh parenting experiences. *Social Cognitive and Affective Neuroscience*, 7(8), 951–957.

Bales, K. L., Kim, A. J., Lewis-Reese, A. D., & Sue Carter, C. (2004). Both oxytocin and vasopressin may influence alloparental behavior in male prairie voles. *Hormones and Behavior, 45*(5), 354–361.

Barr, R. G. (2012). Preventing abusive head trauma resulting from a failure of normal interaction between infants and their caregivers. *Proceedings of the National Academy of Sciences USA, 109*(Suppl. 2), 17294–17301.

Barr, R. G., Trent, R. B., & Cross, J. (2006). Age-related incidence curve of hospitalized shaken baby syndrome cases: Convergent evidence for crying as a trigger to shaking. *Child Abuse and Neglect, 30*(1), 7–16.

Barrett, J., & Fleming, A. S. (2011). Annual research review: All mothers are not created equal: Neural and psychobiological perspectives on mothering and the importance of individual differences. *Journal of Child Psychology and Psychiatry, 52*(4), 368–397.

Bartels, A., & Zeki, S. (2004). The neural correlates of maternal and romantic love. *Neuroimage, 21*(3), 1155–1166.

Belsky, J., Booth-LaForce, C. L., Bradley, R., Brownell, C. A., Campbell, S. B., Clarke-Stewart, K. A., . . . Weinraub, M. (2006). Infant-mother attachment classification: Risk and protection in relation to changing maternal caregiving quality. *Developmental Psychology, 42*(1), 38–58.

Bester-Meredith, J. K., & Marler, C. A. (2003). Vasopressin and the transmission of paternal behavior across generations in mated, cross-fostered Peromyscus mice. *Behavioral Neuroscience, 117*(3), 455–463.

Bos, P. A., Panksepp, J., Bluthe, R. M., & van Honk, J. (2012). Acute effects of steroid hormones and neuropeptides on human social-emotional behavior: A review of single administration studies. *Frontiers in Neuroendocrinology, 33*(1), 17–35.

Brewster, A. L., Nelson, J. P., Hymel, K. P., Colby, D. R., Lucas, D. R., McCanne, T. R., & Milner, J. S. (1998). Victim, perpetrator, family, and incident characteristics of 32 infant maltreatment deaths in the United States Air Force. *Child Abuse and Neglect, 22*(2), 91–101.

Cabrera, N. J., Tamis-LeMonda, C. S., Bradley, R. H., Hofferth, S., & Lamb, M. E. (2000). Fatherhood in the twenty-first century. *Child Development, 71*(1), 127–136.

Carre, J. M., McCormick, C. M., & Hariri, A. R. (2011). The social neuroendocrinology of human aggression. [Review]. *Psychoneuroendocrinology, 36*(7), 935–944.

Champagne, F., Diorio, J., Sharma, S., & Meaney, M. J. (2001). Naturally occurring variations in maternal behavior in the rat are associated with differences in estrogen-inducible central oxytocin receptors. *Proceedings of the National Academy of Sciences USA, 98*(22), 12736–12741.

Champagne, F., & Meaney, M. J. (2001). Like mother, like daughter: Evidence for non-genomic transmission of parental behavior and stress responsivity. *Progress in Brain Research, 133*, 287–302.

Daly, M., & Wilson, M. (1988). *Homicide.* New York, NY: Aldine de Gruyter.

de Jong, T. R., Chauke, M., Harris, B. N., & Saltzman, W. (2009). From here to paternity: Neural correlates of the onset of paternal behavior in California mice (Peromyscus californicus). *Hormones and Behavior, 56*(2), 220–231.

Dudley, D. (1974). Paternal behavior in the California mouse, Peromyscus californicus. *Behavioral Biology, 11*(2), 247–252.

Duncan, L. G., & Bardacke, N. (2010). Mindfulness-based childbirth and parenting education: Promoting family mindfulness during the perinatal period. *Journal of Child and Family Studies, 19*(2), 190–202.

Elwood, R. W. (1975). Paternal and maternal-behavior in Mongolian gerbil. *Animal Behaviour, 23*(Nov), 766–772.

Feldman, R. (2007). Parent-infant synchrony and the construction of shared timing; physiological precursors, developmental outcomes, and risk conditions. *Journal of Child Psychology and Psychiatry, 48*(3–4), 329–354.

Figueredo, A. J., Vasquez, G., Brumbach, B. H., Schneider, S. M. R., Sefcek, J. A., Tal, I. R., . . . Jacobs, W. J. (2006). Consilience and life history theory: From genes to brain to reproductive strategy. *Developmental Review, 26*(2), 243–275.

Fleming, A. S., Corter, C., Stallings, J., & Steiner, M. (2002). Testosterone and prolactin are associated with emotional responses to infant cries in new fathers. *Hormones and Behavior, 42*(4), 399–413.

Francis, D. D., Champagne, F. C., & Meaney, M. J. (2000). Variations in maternal behaviour are associated with differences in oxytocin receptor levels in the rat. *Journal of Neuroendocrinology, 12*(12), 1145–1148.

Gaudino, J. A., Jr., Jenkins, B., & Rochat, R. W. (1999). No fathers' names: a risk factor for infant mortality in the State of Georgia, USA. *Soc Sci Med, 48*(2), 253–265.

Gittleman, J. L. (1986). Carnivore life-history patterns—Allometric, phylogenetic, and ecological associations. *American Naturalist, 127*(6), 744–771.

Gordon, I., Zagoory-Sharon, O., Leckman, J. F., & Feldman, R. (2010). Oxytocin and the development of parenting in humans. *Biological Psychiatry, 68*(4), 377–382.

Gray, P. B., & Anderson, K. G. (2010). *Fatherhood: Evolution and human paternal behavior.* Cambridge, MA: Harvard University Press.

Gubernick, D. J., & Teferi, T. (2000). Adaptive significance of male parental care in a monogamous mammal. *Proceedings of the Royal Society B: Biological Sciences, 267*(1439), 147–150.

Hewlett, B. S. (1991). *Intimate fathers: The nature and context of Aka Pygmy paternal infant care.* Ann Arbor: University of Michigan.

Hrdy, S. B. (2009). *Mothers and others.* Cambridge, MA: Harvard University Press.

Ingram, J. C. (1977). Interactions between parents and infants, and development of independence in common marmoset (Callithrix-Jacchus). *Animal Behaviour, 25*(4), 811–812.

Jones, J. S., & Wynne-Edwards, K. E. (2000). Paternal hamsters mechanically assist the delivery, consume amniotic fluid and placenta, remove fetal membranes, and provide parental care during the birth process. *Hormones and Behavior, 37*(2), 116–125.

Katz, M. M., & Konner, M. J. (1981). The role of the father: An anthropological perspective. In M. E. Lamb (Ed.), *The role of the father in child development* (pp. 155–186). New York, NY: Wiley.

Kendrick, K. M. (2000). Oxytocin, motherhood and bonding. *Experimental Physiology, 85*, 111S–124S.

Kenkel, W. M., Paredes, J., Yee, J. R., Pournajafi-Nazarloo, H., Bales, K. L., & Carter, C. S. (2012). Neuroendocrine and behavioural responses to exposure to an infant in male prairie voles. *Journal of Neuroendocrinol, 24*(6), 874–886.

Koestner, R., Franz, C., & Weinberger, J. (1990). The family origins of empathic concern: A 26-year longitudinal study. *Journal of Personality and Social Psychology*, *58*(4), 709–717.

Konner, M. J. (2010). *The evolution of childhood: Relationships, emotion, mind.* Cambridge, MA: Harvard University Press.

Kozorovitskiy, Y., Hughes, M., Lee, K., & Gould, E. (2006). Fatherhood affects dendritic spines and vasopressin V1a receptors in the primate prefrontal cortex. *Nature Neuroscience*, *9*(9), 1094–1095.

Krugman, R. D. (1983). Fatal child abuse: Analysis of 24 cases. *Pediatrician*, *12*(1), 68–72.

Kuo, P. X., Carp, J., Light, K. C., & Grewen, K. M. (2012). Neural responses to infants linked with behavioral interactions and testosterone in fathers. *Biological Psychiatry*, *91*(2), 302–306.

Lack, D. (1954). *The natural regulation of animal numbers.* Oxford, UK: Clarendon Press.

Mascaro, J. S., Hackett, P. D., & Rilling, J. K. (2013). Testicular volume is inversely correlated with nurturing-related brain activity in human fathers. *Proc Natl Acad Sci U S A*, *110*(39), 15746–15751.

Mascaro, J. S., Hackett, P. D., Gouzoules, H., Lori, A., & Rilling, J. K. (2014). Behavioral and genetic correlates of the neural response to infant crying among human fathers. *Soc Cogn Affect Neurosci*, *9*(11), 1704–1712.

Musser, E. D., Kaiser-Laurent, H., & Ablow, J. C. (2012). The neural correlates of maternal sensitivity: An fMRI study. *Developmental Cognitive Neuroscience*, *2*(4), 428–436.

Naber, F., van Ijzendoorn, M. H., Deschamps, P., van Engeland, H., & Bakermans-Kranenburg, M. J. (2010). Intranasal oxytocin increases fathers' observed responsiveness during play with their children: A double-blind within-subject experiment. *Psychoneuroendocrinology*, *35*(10), 1583–1586.

Numan, M. (2007). Motivational systems and the neural circuitry of maternal behavior in the rat. *Developmental Psychobiology*, *49*(1), 12–21.

Numan, M., & Stolzenberg, D. S. (2009). Medial preoptic area interactions with dopamine neural systems in the control of the onset and maintenance of maternal behavior in rats. *Frontiers in Neuroendocrinology*, *30*(1), 46–64.

Olazabal, D. E., & Young, L. J. (2006). Oxytocin receptors in the nucleus accumbens facilitate spontaneous\ maternal behavior in adult female prairie voles. *Neuroscience*, *141*(2), 559–568.

Oliveras, D., & Novak, M. (1986). A comparison of paternal behavior in the meadow vole Microtus-pennsylvanicus, the pine vole Microtus-pinetorum and the prairie vole Microtus-ochrogaster. *Animal Behaviour*, *34*, 519–526.

Pedersen, C. A., Ascher, J. A., Monroe, Y. L., & Prange, A. J., Jr. (1982). Oxytocin induces maternal behavior in virgin female rats. *Science*, *216*(4546), 648–650.

Pedersen, C. A., Caldwell, J. D., Walker, C., Ayers, G., & Mason, G. A. (1994). Oxytocin activates the postpartum onset of rat maternal behavior in the ventral tegmental and medial preoptic areas. *Behavioral and Brain Sciences*, *108*(6), 1163–1171.

Reijneveld, S. A., van der Wal, M. F., Brugman, E., Sing, R. A., & Verloove-Vanhorick, S. P. (2004). Infant crying and abuse. *Lancet*, *364*(9442), 1340–1342.

Rickel, A. U., & Biasatti, L. L. (1982). Modification of the block child rearing practices report. *Journal of Clinical Psychology, 38*(1), 129–134.

Rutherford, E., & Mussen, P. H. (1968). Generosity in nusery school boys. *Child Development, 39*, 755–765.

Sarkadi, A., Kristiansson, R., Oberklaid, F., & Bremberg, S. (2008). Fathers' involvement and children's developmental outcomes: A systematic review of longitudinal studies. *Acta Paediatrica, 97*(2), 153–158.

Seifritz, E., Esposito, F., Neuhoff, J. G., Luthi, A., Mustovic, H., Dammann, G., . . . Di Salle, F. (2003). Differential sex-independent amygdala response to infant crying and laughing in parents versus nonparents. *Biological Psychiatry, 54*(12), 1367–1375.

Starling, S. P., Holden, J. R., & Jenny, C. (1995). Abusive head trauma: The relationship of perpetrators to their victims. *Pediatrics, 95*(2), 259–262.

Strathearn, L., Fonagy, P., Amico, J., & Montague, P. R. (2009). Adult attachment predicts maternal brain and oxytocin response to infant cues. *Neuropsychopharmacology, 34*(13), 2655–2666.

Tardif, S. D., Carson, R. L., & Gangaware, B. L. (1992). Infant-care behavior of nonreproductive helpers in a communal-care primate, the cotton-top tamarin (Saguinusoedipus). *Ethology, 92*(2), 155–167.

Toossi, M. (2002). A century of change: The US labor force, 1950-2050. *Monthly Labor Review, 125*(5), 15–28.

US Department of Labor. (2011). *Women's employment during the recovery.*

van Honk, J., Schutter, D. J., Bos, P. A., Kruijt, A. W., Lentjes, E. G., & Baron-Cohen, S. (2011). Testosterone administration impairs cognitive empathy in women depending on second-to-fourth digit ratio. *Proceedings of the National Academy USA, 108*(8), 3448–3452.

Wang, Z., Ferris, C. F., & De Vries, G. J. (1994). Role of septal vasopressin innervation in paternal behavior in prairie voles (Microtus ochrogaster). *Proceedings of the National Academy of Sciences USA, 91*(1), 400–404.

Wittfoth-Schardt, D., Grunding, J., Wittfoth, M., Lanfermann, H., Heinrichs, M., Domes, G., . . . Waller, C. (2012). Oxytocin modulates neural reactivity to children's faces as a function of social salience. *Neuropsychopharmacology, 37*(8), 1799–1807.

Woodroffe, R., & Vincent, A. (1994). Mother's little helpers: Patterns of male care in mammals. *Trends in Ecology and Evolution, 9*(8), 294–297.

Wright, P. C. (1984). Biparental care in Aotus trivirgatus and Callicebus moloch. In M. F. Small (Ed.), *Female primates: Studies by women primatologists* (pp. 59–75). New York, NY: Liss.

Wynne-Edwards, K. E. (1987). Evidence for obligate monogamy in the Djungarian hamster, Phodopus campbelli: pup survival under different parenting conditions. *Behavioral Ecology and Sociobiology, 20*, 427–437.

Wynne-Edwards, K. E., & Reburn, C. J. (2000). Behavioral endocrinology of mammalian fatherhood. *Trends in Ecology and Evolution, 15*(11), 464–468.

Zeifman, D. M. (2003). Predicting adult responses to infant distress: Adult characteristics associated with perceptions, emotional reactions, and timing of intervention. *Infant Mental Health Journal, 24*(6), 597–612.

3

Toward a Neuroscience of Social Resonance

THALIA WHEATLEY AND BEAU SIEVERS ■

Far from static, the world constantly teems with events unfolding across multiple timescales. Some of these events are imperceptibly slow, like the creation of geological landscapes; others are imperceptibly fast, like the beating of a hummingbird's wings. Between these extremes sits a dynamic range for which humans are exquisitely tuned—the range of social communication. Here, a lingering touch, a wistful stare, or a crack in one's voice can communicate as much as the most gifted novelist. Being finely tuned to these dynamics is a benchmark of social intelligence.

The subtlety of dynamic social communication is even more remarkable when considering the mind of a perceiver. How is it that a touch lasting *a fraction of a second too long* is even noticed amid everything else? How do we separate meaning from noise? And how does the brain translate perceived dynamics into immediate and appropriate responses that forge social bonds? These questions remain poorly understood due, in part, to a field-wide reliance on static visual stimuli (e.g., face photographs). Recently, however, a spate of papers, special issues, and symposia has signaled a sea change. Neuroscientists are beginning to push toward more ecologically valid, dynamic approaches in order to understand the unfolding rhythms of social thought and behavior. Here we discuss several pioneering studies that are shaping this exciting new direction: the neuroscience of social resonance. First we approach the concept of social resonance from the perspective of an individual perceiving brain; then we expand outward to examine resonance between social brains.

PERCEPTUAL RESONANCE

Before we can begin to understand social resonance between brains, we must understand how the individual human brain perceives social signals. Neuroscientists investigating dynamic social perception have concentrated primarily on one of two senses: vision or audition, and on one realm of social communication: emotional expression. In this section, we summarize this literature and provide a unifying theory that suggests why emotional expressions are so rapidly and effectively perceived.

Hearing Emotion

The ability to hear emotion in a person's voice is taken for granted, but losing that ability (aprosodia) can have devastating social consequences. A recent meta-analysis found that schizophrenic patients were more than one standard deviation below the mean of healthy controls in recognizing emotional tone of voice cues. The impairment was so large that the authors concluded that aprosodia "was one of the most pervasive disturbances in schizophrenia that may contribute to social isolation" (Hoekert, Kahn, Pijnenborg, & Aleman, 2007, p. 135). Impairments in the production and processing of prosody have also been observed in autism and Parkinson's disease, despite the ability to discriminate pitch and nonspeech sounds normally (Gervais et al., 2004; Pell, 1996). These dissociations led Pell to suggest that the impairments lie at the stage of linking "specific acoustic parameters of stimuli" to social meaning. If so, aprosodic patients should also have difficulty understanding emotion in music, as music conveys emotion via acoustic configurations (Juslin & Laukka, 2003). Consistent with this conclusion, amusia, the inability to produce and/or appreciate music, is often comorbid with aprosodia, suggesting that they rely on overlapping perceptual or cognitive processes (Patel et al., 1998). In healthy participants, recognizing emotional voice and music has been localized to the mid-posterior extent of the right superior temporal cortex (Beaucousin et al., 2007; Grandjean et al., 2005; Kraemer, Macrae, Green, & Kelley, 2005; Steinbeis & Koelsch, 2008). Perhaps surprisingly, this region of cortex is most often associated with the *visual* perception of biological motion.

Seeing Emotion

Though we take for granted that for something to be seen as "social" it must be alive, it is possible to infer social information even in the absence of living form.

For example, Heider and Simmel (1944) demonstrated that complex social intentions and emotions, even personalities and genders, could be deciphered from the motion trajectories of simple shapes. It is also possible to extract social information from the movement of actors' joints illuminated by a handful of lights and filmed in a dark room (Johansson, 1973). A static snapshot of these lights (called "point light") looks like randomly distributed bright dots on a black background, but, set in motion, the dots become immediately recognizable as human movement. Point-light stimuli have been used with great effect to show that movement can convey gender, emotion, even personality (Atkinson, Dittrich, Gemmell, & Young, 2004; Clarke, Bradshaw, Field, Hampson, & Rose, 2005; Heberlein, Adolphs, Tranel, & Damasio, 2004; Pollick, Lestou, Ryu, & Cho, 2002). Dynamic stimuli such as these are critical for a complete understanding of social information processing and are known to engage a different neural pathway than static, structural features (Haxby, Hoffman, & Gobbini, 2000). Thus, the ability to process emotion in static images may not translate to equivalent ability to process emotion from visual motion cues. Indeed, while children on the autism spectrum may learn to recognize a frown in a photograph, they are relatively impaired in decoding dynamic social cues in real time (Hobson, 1986). Conversely, patients with bilateral amygdala damage may not be able to recognize fear in a picture of a face but are nonetheless unimpaired when fear is displayed in a moving body (Atkinson, Heberlein, & Adolphs, 2007). This suggests that recognizing emotion from motion may recruit more dissociable neural pathways than recognizing emotion from static form.

Neuroimaging studies, using a variety of methods and stimuli, have converged on the right superior temporal cortex (STC) as a key region in the perception and imagery of biological motion (Allison, Puce, & McCarthy, 2000; Beauchamp, Lee, Haxby, & Martin, 2002; Grossman, Battelli, & Pascual-Leone, 2005; Pavlova, Lutzenberger, Sokolov, & Birbaumer, 2004; Wheatley, Milleville, & Martin, 2007). Importantly, the right STC seems particularly tuned to social meaning conveyed by motion (Bonda, Petrides, Ostry, & Evans, 1996; Martin & Weisberg, 2005), and those with compromised functioning in this region (e.g., autism) are less accurate at decoding emotional compared to neutral point light actors (Boddaert et al., 2003; Dakin & Frith, 2005). Collectively, this research suggests that the same region that is important for *hearing emotion* also underlies the ability to *see emotion*.

The "Shared Structure" Hypothesis

The fact that auditory and visual motion activate the same cortices suggests that these stimuli share low-level features. Indeed, this idea of low-level correspondence dates back at least to 1929 when Wolfgang Köhler asked people to assign the labels "Takete" and "Baluma" to two shapes—one spiky and one rounded (see Figure 3.1). Participants in his study assigned "Takete" to the spiky shape and "Baluma" to the rounded shape. This assignment was replicated by Holland and Wertheimer (1964) and by other researchers using different labels in different regions around the world: "Takete" and "Maluma" (Köhler, 1947); "Takete" and "Uloomo" (Davis, 1961); "Tuhkeetee" and "Maaboomaa" (Maurer, Pathman, & Mondloch, 2006); "Taakootaa" and "Muhbeemee" (Nielsen & Rendall, 2011); and "Kiki" and "Bouba" (Ramachandran & Hubbard, 2001).

One favored explanation is that the spiky shape has high spatial frequency information (angular features) that maps onto the high temporal frequencies associated with the aspirated consonant "k" in words like "Kiki" and "Takete." The rounded shape, in contrast, shares low-frequency information with words like "Bouba" and "Maluma." Effects such as these suggest a fundamental efficiency in the processing of sensory input across modalities; that is, like goes with like.

This theory of dynamic correspondence across sensory domains is supported by a diverse literature. First, patients with aprosodia and amusia

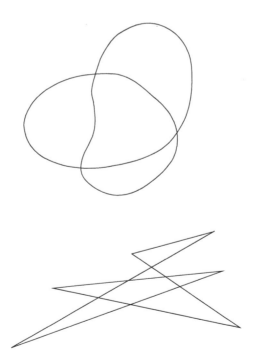

Figure 3.1 Kohler's (1929) "Maluma" and "Takete" shapes, from top to bottom.

have correlated deficits in recognizing gestures and facial expressions (Ross & Mesalum, 1979). Second, auditory and motion displays activate the same cortical region, as discussed earlier (right superior temporal cortex). This has resulted in claims that right STC is involved in music (Zatorre & Krumhansl, 2002), prosody (Beaucousin et al., 2007; Grandjean et al., 2005), and biological motion (Allison et al., 2000; Beauchamp et al., 2002; Pelphrey, Morris, Michelich, Allison, & McCarthy, 2005). Indeed, this region is physically well positioned to support multisensory perception. Because of the need to minimize axonal length, one would expect such an area to lie in close proximity to both auditory and visual input areas as the STC does.

THE COMMUNICATIVE IMPORTANCE OF PERCEPTUAL RESONANCE

Shared dynamics in multisensory perception would enable a kind of perceptual resonance. This resonance would be especially important for communication because it would increase the number of channels by which a communication can be perceived (redundancy) as well as the strength of the communicative signal (amplification).

Redundancy

Across the animal kingdom, evolved purposeful communication tends to be multimodal. Ethologists refer to this communication as "signals" in contrast to "cues" that are nonpurposeful artifacts of behavior. David Huron (2012) provides the following examples. The rattle of a rattlesnake is a signal—a specific, purposeful communication to warn. In contrast, the buzzing of a mosquito is a cue—an artifact of rapidly flapping insect wings. Both sounds portend the possibility of attack, but only the rattle is a purposeful communication intended to alert the perceiver. Signals, but not cues, tend to exhibit redundancy across multiple sensory channels—all the better to ensure communicative success. In the case of the rattlesnake's rattle, the signals are not only auditory but visual as well: The rattling tail raises up so it can be in full view of anyone looking.

Human communicative displays tend to be multimodal as well. We carry anger in our voices as well as our body language. Even facial expressions seem to have acoustic correlates. A smile, for example, draws the lips back across the teeth, thereby changing the acoustic properties of the mouth cavity and elevating vocal pitch. This leads the linguist John Ohala to conclude that the smile is actually a visualization of an acoustical display (high pitch)—both signaling friendliness (Ohala, 1994). High pitch is also associated with visual elevation (Parkinson, Kohler, Sievers, & Wheatley, 2012) and, correspondingly, the visual display of raising one's eyebrows. People tend to raise their eyebrows while singing a high note and lower their eyebrows while singing a low note (Huron, Dahl, & Johnson, 2009). Although prosodic expression has been studied extensively, these studies suggest that prosodic signals are accompanied by visual displays—even potentially nonfunctional ones—consistent with the ethological theory of purposeful signaling.

Amplification

Increasing the number of channels for communication increases the likelihood that the communication will be perceived, but the strength of that signal depends on whether those multimodal signals are mutually reinforcing. Imagine that *moving* angrily and *shouting* angrily each contributed similar, reinforcing dynamics in the mind of a perceiver (e.g., they produced similarly fast, downward, and irregularly spaced perceptual inputs). A shared dynamic structure would ensure not only redundancy across channels but a reinforced signal: a "double dose" to lift the signal out of the noise.

EVIDENCE FOR A "SHARED STRUCTURE" OF EMOTIONAL EXPRESSION

Universal Crossmodal Expressions of Emotion

Consistent with mutually reinforcing dynamics, emotions tend to be expressed the same way in music and movement. This correspondence is reflected in everyday language: In English we talk about how music "moves" us and describe movement and music in similar ways—for example, both happy-sounding music and the gait of a happy person are described as "upbeat" and "bouncy." We recently demonstrated that this correspondence runs deeper than metaphor. We wrote a computer program that allowed experimental participants to create examples of music or animated movement based on five parameters controlled by slider bars: rate, jitter, dissonance/spikiness, ratio of upward to downward movements, and ratio of big to small movements (Sievers, Polansky, Casey, & Wheatley, 2013; see Figure 3.2) Participants were split into two groups; one group only heard music, and the other only saw an animation of a bouncing ball. As the participants moved the slider bars, the

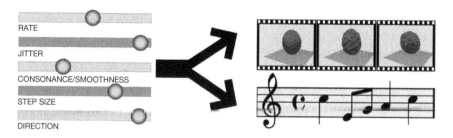

Figure 3.2 Participants manipulated five slider bars corresponding to five dynamic features to create either animations or musical clips that expressed different emotions.

music or animation changed in real time to match the participant's choices. Participants were asked to express each of five emotions—happy, angry, peaceful, sad, and, scared—using the program. In this way, the different modalities of music and movement could be directly compared.

We ran two versions of this experiment: the first in the United States, and the second in Lʼak, a remote tribal village in rural northeastern Cambodia. Across both cultures, participants were consistent about how they made each of the emotions. Angry, for example, was fast, dissonant/spiky, and downward for both the US and Cambodian participants. Moreover, this consistency was crossmodal as well: Participants made angry music and movement the same way. Each emotion had a particular dynamic signature that was the same across modalities and across cultures.

Shared Structure, Shared Hardware

Any automatic perceptual correspondence, as in the shared structure between music and movement, suggests an underlying neural correspondence. Fujioka et al. (2012), Janata et al. (2003), and Zatorre et al. (2007) have shown shared neural machinery for timekeeping and sequence learning. Similarly, the comorbidity of aprosodia and amusia discussed earlier (Patel et al. 1998) suggests there is some shared neural machinery for processing the dynamics of both speech and melody.[1] There are indications of further connections between music and motor processing: The deceleration of a runner coming to a stop tends to match the final ritard at the end of a musical performance (Friberg & Sundberg, 1999); musical tempi tend to match common biological rhythms of the human body (van Noorden & Moelents, 1999; Iyer, 2002); and people tend to sync their gait with the music they listen to (Styns, van Noorden, Moelants, & Leman, 2007).

Dehaene and Cohen (2007) suggest that neural representations of music "recycle" evolutionarily older representations of pitch, rhythm, and timbre.

We think this explanation can be pushed a level deeper: Representations of pitch, rhythm, and timbre recycle neural machinery evolved for spatiotemporal perception and action such as sequence learning, speech, and movement.

Multimodal correspondence at the neural level would explain how we perceive emotion across perceptual boundaries, and why information from one modality can increase the power of a signal in another. When neural representations are truly shared, no active mapping process is necessary to compare one domain to another, and thus there is little to no temporal overhead. Returning to the ethological distinction between *signals* and *cues*, the multimodal nature of many signals—such as the shaking and sounding of the rattlesnake's tail—is evolved to take advantage of the raw speed at which crossmodal neural signals are processed. In complex social contexts, emotional signals can have the same priority as the rattlesnake's tail. Failing to miss an emotional signal or cue can mean falling to the bottom of the social hierarchy and missing an opportunity to pass along one's genetic material—or worse. Clearly, crossmodal social processing needs to be as efficient as possible.

In true social communication, perception is only half of the story. Flourishing in a dynamic social world means not only perceiving social signals but also responding appropriately. Only by turning perception into action can we hope to respond in ways that forge meaningful social connection.

SOCIAL RESONANCE

Resonance Within Brains: The Perception-Production Circuit

The neural link between perception and (motor) production was first researched in the context of speech. In 1861, the French surgeon Paul Broca heard of a patient named Leborgne who could understand speech perfectly well but could not speak. Upon the patient's death, Broca performed an autopsy that revealed damage to the left posterior inferior frontal gyrus. Subsequently, he identified 12 more patients with similar neural injury and corresponding speech production difficulties. Around a decade later, the German neurologist Karl Wernicke noted a converse impairment. He observed that patients with injuries to the posterior section of the left superior temporal gyrus could speak perfectly well but had problems perceiving and interpreting speech. These two regions, known as Broca and Wernicke's areas, comprise one of the most famous "double dissociations" in neuroscience. Rather than a single faculty for all of speech processing, Broca's area underpins production but not perception and Wernicke's area underpins perception but not production.

Since the seminal work of Karl Wernicke and Paul Broca, scientists have postulated that one or more white matter tracts—the myelinated conduits that enable information flow—must connect these two gray matter regions. A candidate white matter tract was identified: the superior longitudinal fasciculus (SLF; see Figure 3.3), which not only connects Broca's and Wernicke's areas in the left but a second SLF connects homologous regions in the right hemisphere as well.

The right SLF is associated with melodic and fine-grained auditory pitch processing (Halwani, Loui, Rüber, & Schlaug, 2011; Loui, Alsop, & Schlaug, 2009; Loui, Li, Hohmann, & Schlaug, 2011; Loui, Li, & Schlaug, 2011). This tract is impoverished in tone-deaf individuals and comparatively robust in individuals with absolute pitch (Loui et al., 2009; Loui, Li, Hohmann, & Schlaug, 2011) and in those better able to learn pitch patterns (Loui, Li, & Schlaug, 2011). Thus, the SLF links temporo-parietal areas involved in pitch perception with inferior frontal areas implicated in pitch production (Loui et al., 2009).

How do these perception-production circuits relate to dynamic social intelligence? Quite simply, any meaningful social dialogue requires "give and take"—the ability to perceive social signals in real time and produce appropriate social signals in return (Chartrand & Bargh, 1999). Emotional empathy, in particular, is hypothesized to require rapid and automatic transference between perception and production cortices, evincing a near zero-lag between *seeing* a person's pain and *feeling* it. Functional magnetic resonance imaging (fMRI)

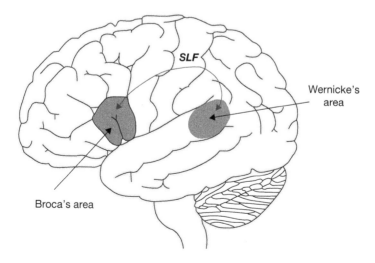

Figure 3.3 The superior longitudinal fasciculus (SLF) forms a myelinated conduit between Broca's area and Wernicke's area.

activation while viewing emotional expressions is consistent with the end-points of the right SLF (Leslie, Johnson-Frey, & Grafton, 2004; Schmahmann & Pandya, 2006), and higher responses to social stimuli in these regions correspond to higher empathic concern (Kaplan & Iacoboni, 2006; Pfeifer, Iacoboni, Mazziotta, & Dapretto, 2008; Schulte-Rüther, Markowitsch, Fink, & Piefke, 2007). Enhanced anatomical connectivity between areas involved in the perception and expression of emotion could suggest that emotional empathy might heighten affective responses to others' emotional expressions (Dimberg, Thunberg, & Elmehed, 2000; Sonnby-Borgström, 2002) and/or speed and clarify the perception of social cues, particularly in ambiguous contexts. Thus, enhanced anatomical coupling between areas involved in emotional perception and expression may enable more efficient communication between these areas when predicting social cues as they unfold in real time (Blakemore & Frith, 2005; Kilner, Friston, & Frith, 2007; Wilson & Knoblich, 2005).

Parkinson and Wheatley (2012) tested a potential link between SLF connectivity and empathy directly by assessing white matter (WM) structural correlates of empathic concern, a subscale of the Interpersonal Reactivity Index (IRI; Davis, 1980). They found that empathic concern was positively correlated with fractional anisotropic (FA) values in several WM tracts, including the SLF bilaterally, most extensively in the right hemisphere (see Figure 3.4). Fractional anisotropy comprises a general marker of axonal integrity. Larger FA values can reflect increased myelination, increased axonal coherence, and/or increased axonal caliber (Beaulieu 2002)—white matter features that enable efficient transference of information.

Emotional empathy appears to rely on rapid, privileged communication between perception and production regions—a kind of within-brain neural resonance. However, rich social communication requires an additional kind of resonance—one that happens *between* brains.

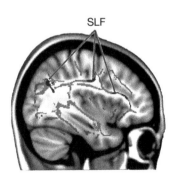

Figure 3.4 FA values correlated with emotional empathy in the superior longitudinal fasciculus (SLF). Dark clusters indicate significance.

Resonance Between Brains: Interpersonal Synchrony

Successful social interaction depends on interpersonal fluency. Semin and Cacioppo posit that interaction, done right, is a synchronous dance that allows individuals to "get on the same page" by granting "simultaneous partial mutual access to internal states" (Semin, 2007, p. 631). As Semin makes clear, this synchrony is not simply at the level of overt actions but is also manifest neurally (Semin, 2007). For example, an observer's motor cortex "resonates" in phase with the actions of the person being observed (Fadiga, Craighero, & Olivier, 2005; Gangitano, Mottaghy, & Pascual-Leone, 2001). While this resonance may lead to synchronous motor behavior at times, Baldissera and colleagues suggest that an inhibitory mechanism in the spinal cord prevents "underthreshold" neural synchrony from resulting in constant action mimicry (Baldissera, Cavallari, Craighero, & Fadiga, 2001).

In one sense, between-brain neural synchrony is merely a description of two brains processing information in the same way at the same time. However, this simultaneity likely confers an important evolutionary advantage: neural efficiency. The brain is a very metabolically expensive organ. Neural synchrony presumably allows the brain to consolidate two informational streams in one. This may be one reason why great conversation feels effortless whereas conversations requiring constant updating of what the other person is thinking feel like hard work. Mental connection is colloquially described as "sharing a mind" or "being on the same wavelength." Although poetic, these turns of phrases may contain a literal truth. By representing two streams of information as one, the brain blurs the boundary between self and other (Wheatley, Kang, Parkinson, & Looser, 2012).

Despite inhibitory mechanisms to thwart constant action mimicry (Baldissera et al., 2001), neural synchrony likely increases the probability of behavioral synchrony. It is quite common, for example, for one conversational partner to mimic the posture of the other. Although this synchrony is not required for mutual understanding, its occurrence has powerful effects on affiliation. Those who synchronize motorically report greater liking for their movement partners (Bernieri, 1988; Ramseyer & Tschacher, 2011), stronger ties to community (McNeill, 1995, as cited in Wiltermuth & Heath, 2009), and are perceived as a single social unit (Lakens, 2010; Marsh, Johnston, Richardson, & Schmidt, 2009; Wiltermuth & Heath, 2009). In addition to rapport, synchrony also increases the likelihood of prosocial behavior (Valdesolo & DeSteno, 2011).

Behavioral synchrony does not have to arise naturally to be effective. Artificially created synchrony—whether due to the cadence of a military march or the conditions of a laboratory experiment—yields similar effects, as long as people are naïve to the contrivance (Lakens & Stel, 2011). Wiltermuth and Heath (2009) found that synchronous physical activity among strangers leads them to act more cohesively. In one of their studies, strangers sang and waved cups in time to "O Canada," the Canadian national anthem, while sitting in a group. By having the people wear headphones, the experimenters could manipulate whether the people in each group were listening to the track at the same time or at different times. Groups who sang and moved synchronously performed more cooperatively in a subsequent task, felt more connected with, and trusted their group members more than groups who had earlier performed the song asynchronously. Similarly, Hove and Risen (2009) found that participants who tapped a computer screen in synchrony with the experimenter rated her as more "likeable" at the end of the experiment. As one might imagine, inhibiting physical synchrony has the predicted opposite effect. When synchrony is inhibited, people rate interactions less positively (Marsh, Richardson, & Schmidt, 2009).

In short, resonance—whether within or between brains—is a marker of fluency. This fluency can be described as a kind of neural "flow" (Csíkszentmihályi, 1990) or "oneness," which presumably has its own reward signal distinguishable from other known pleasures (e.g., food, sex). One candidate reward signal, oxytocin, has been associated with affiliation in multiple species (Wheatley et al., 2012). In humans, at least, this pleasure is almost palpable whenever large groups converge on a shared purpose. As moral psychologist Jonathan Haidt put it, "People need to lose themselves occasionally by becoming part of an emergent social organism in order to reach the highest levels of human flourishing" (Haidt, Seder, & Kesebir, 2008, p. 133). It is hardly surprising, therefore, that music is central to large, ritualistic gatherings from sporting events to political rallies and, of course, rock concerts. Turning a thousand strangers into a single, emergent social organism requires a strong signal upon which to entrain.

CONCLUSION

"Man is by nature a social animal" (Aristotle, trans. 1986), and as such, our lives are governed by our relationships, which are in turn embedded in rich and complex social networks. Thriving as a social animal means forging connections by accurately perceiving the social signals of others and responding appropriately in return. Recent scientific discoveries suggest that high social intelligence requires a number of neural efficiencies. In the current chapter we have highlighted three such neural efficiencies, each of which can be described in terms of resonance.

First, we described how human social perception relies on the real-time, shared encoding of dynamics across perceptual systems in the brain (e.g. vision, audition). We suggest that this crossmodal perceptual resonance increases the likelihood of detecting social signals. Second, we showed that resonance across the perception-production neural circuit predicts emotional empathy—the ability to translate perceived social signals into one's own motor and affective responses automatically. Finally, we highlighted a number of recent studies investigating resonance between brains in the form of neural and behavioral synchrony. Synchrony between people confers its own neural efficiency by allowing the brain to follow a shared informational stream rather than two. This resonance happens naturally when two people—presumably tuned to the same internal rhythms—seem to "click." However, human innovation appears to have found a way to reverse-engineer resonance. By creating synchrony artificially—such as with a simple musical beat—humans can effect large-scale group synchrony, even with strangers.

The ability to resonate information across perceptual maps, over perception-production circuits, and between brains affords a dynamic and hyper-connected social world. Scientists are just beginning to elucidate these processes and how they may interact with and build upon each other. As a new direction for psychology and neuroscience, the science of social resonance promises a deeper understanding of how we connect, relate and thrive as a social species.

NOTE

1. Zatorre and colleagues (2012) have shown both shared and dissociable pitch representations for prosody and melody: a coarse contour representation shared by both domains, and a fine pitch representation unique to music. Here we are referring to the total dynamics of speech and melody, not just pitch; while some neural systems for processing speech and music are dissociable, some of them are certainly shared.

REFERENCES

Allison, T., Puce, A., & McCarthy, G. (2000). Social perception from visual cues: Role of the STS region. *Trends in Cognitive Sciences, 4*, 267–278.

Aristotle (1986). In W. D. Ross (Ed. & Trans.), *Politica* (p. 1253) Oxford, UK: Oxford University Press.

Atkinson, A. P., Dittrich, W. H., Gemmell, A. J., & Young, A. W. (2004). Emotion perception from dynamic and static body expressions in point-light and full-light displays. *Perception, 33*, 717–746.

Atkinson, A. P., Heberlein, A. S., & Adolphs, R. (2007). Spared ability to recognize fear from static and moving whole-body cues following bilateral amygdala damage, *Neuropsychologia, 45*, 2772–2782.

Baldissera, F., Cavallari, P., Craighero, L., & Fadiga, L. (2001). Modulation of spinal excitability during observation of hand actions in humans. *European Journal of Neuroscience, 13*, 190–194.

Beauchamp, M. S., Lee, K. E., Haxby, J. V., & Martin, A. (2002). Parallel visual motion processing streams for manipulable objects and human movements. *Neuron, 34*, 149–159.

Beaucousin, V., Lacheret, A., Turbelin, M., Morel, M., Mazoyer, B., & Tzourio-Mazoyer, N. (2007). fMRI study of emotional speech comprehension. *Cerebral Cortex, 17*, 339–352.

Beaulieu, C. (2002). The basis of anisotropic water diffusion in the nervous system—A technical review. *NMR in Biomedicine, 15*, 435–455.

Bernieri, F. J. (1988). Coordinated movement and rapport in teacher-student interactions. *Journal of Nonverbal Behavior, 12*, 120–138.

Blakemore, S. J., & Frith, C. (2005). The role of motor contagion in the prediction of action. *Neuropsychologia. 43*, 260–267.

Boddaert, N., Belin, P., Chabane, N., Poline, J. B., Barthelemy, C., Mouren-Simeoni, M. C., . . . Zilbovicius, M. (2003). Perception of complex sounds: Abnormal pattern of cortical activation in autism. *American Journal of Psychiatry, 160*, 2057–2060.

Bonda, E., Petrides, M., Ostry, D., & Evans, A., (1996). Specific involvement of human parietal systems and the amygdala in the perception of biological motion. *Journal of Neuroscience, 16*, 3737–3744

Chartrand, T. L., & Bargh, J. A. (1999). The chameleon effect: The perception-behavior link and social interaction. *Journal of Personality and Social Psychology, 76*, 893–910.

Clarke, T. J., Bradshaw, M. F., Field, D. T., Hampson, S. E., & Rose, D. (2005). The perception of emotion from body movement in point-light displays of interpersonal dialogue. *Perception, 34*, 1171–1180.

Csikszentmihalyi, M. (1990). *Flow: The psychology of optimal experience.* New York, NY: Harper & Row.

Dakin, S., & Frith, U. (2005). Vagaries of visual perception in autism. *Neuron, 48*, 497–507.

Davis, M. H. (1980). A multidimensional approach to individual differences in empathy. *JSAS Catalog of Selected Documents in Psychology, 10*, 85.

Davis, R. (1961). The fitness of names to drawings. A cross-cultural study in Tanganyika. *British Journal of Psychology, 52*, 259–268.

Dehaene, S., & Cohen, L. (2007). Cultural recycling of cortical maps. *Neuron, 56*, 384–398.

Dimberg, U., Thunberg, M., & Elmehed, K. (2000). Unconscious facial reactions to emotional facial expressions. *Psychological Science, 11*, 86–89.

Fadiga, L., Craighero, L., & Olivier, E. (2005). Human motor cortex excitability during the perception of others' action. *Current Opinion in Neurobiology, 15*, 213–218.

Friberg, A., & Sundberg, J. (1999). Does music performance allude to locomotion? A model of final ritardandi derived from measurements of stopping runners. *Journal of the Acoustical Society of America, 105*, 1469–1484.

Fujioka, T., Trainor, L. J., Large, E.W., & Ross, B. (2012). Internalized timing of isochronous sounds is represented in neuromagnetic β oscillations. *Journal of Neuroscience, 32*, 1791–1802.

Gangitano, M., Mottaghy, F. M., & Pascual-Leone, A. (2001). Phase-specific modulation of cortical motor output during movement observation. *Cognitive Neuroscience and Neuropsychology, 12*, 1489–1492.

Gervais, H., Belin, P., Boddaert, N., Leboyer, M., Coez, A., Staello, I., ... Zilbovicius, M. (2004). Abnormal cortical voice processing in autism. *Nature Neuroscience, 7*, 801–802.

Grafton, S. T., & Hamilton, A. F. (2007). Evidence for a distributed hierarchy of action representation in the brain. *Human Motor Sciences, 26*, 590–616.

Grandjean, D., Sander, D., Pourtois, G., Schwartz, S., Seghier, M. L., Scherer, K. R., & Vuilleumier, P. (2005). The voices of wrath: Brain responses to angry prosody in meaningless speech. *Nature Neuroscience, 8*, 145–146.

Grossman, E. D., Battelli, L., & Pascual-Leone, A. (2005). Repetitive TMS over posterior STS disrupts perception of biological motion. *Vision Research, 45*, 2847–2853.

Haidt, J., Seder, J. P., & Kesebir, S. (2008). Hive psychology, happiness, and public policy. In E. A. Posner & C. R. Sunstein (Eds.), *Law and happiness* (pp. 133–156). Chicago, IL: University of Chicago Press.

Halwani, G. F., Loui, P., Rüber, T., & Schlaug, G. (2011). Effects of practice and experience on the arcuate fasciculus: Comparing singers, instrumentalists, and non-musicians. *Frontiers in Psychology, 2*, 156.

Haxby, J. V., Hoffman, E. A., & Gobbini, M. I. (2000). The distributed human neural system for face perception. *Trends in Cognitive Science, 4*, 223–233.

Heberlein, A. S., Adolphs, R., Tranel, D., & Damasio, H. (2004). Cortical regions for judgments of emotions and personality traits from point-light walkers. *Journal of Cognitive Neuroscience, 16*, 1143–1158.

Heider, F., & Simmel, M. (1944). An experimental study of apparent behavior. *American Journal of Psychology, 57*, 243–259.

Hobson, R. P. (1986). The autistic child's appraisal of expressions of emotion. *Journal of Child Psychology and Psychiatry, and Allied Disciplines, 27*, 321–342.

Hoekert, M., Kahn, R. S., Pijnenborg, M., & Aleman, A. (2007). Impaired recognition and expression of emotional prosody in schizophrenia: Review and meta-analysis. *Schizophrenia Research, 96*, 135–145.

Holland, M. K., & Wertheimer, M. (1964). Some physiognomic aspects of naming, or, maluma and takete revisited. *Perceptual and Motor Skills, 19*, 111–117.

Hove, M. J., & Risen, J. L. (2009). It's all in the timing: Interpersonal synchrony increases affiliation. *Social Cognition, 27*, 949–961.

Huron, D. (2012). *Understanding music-related emotion: Lessons from ethology.* Paper presented at the 12th International Conference on Music Perception and Cognition, Greece.

Iyer, V. (2002). Embodied mind, situated cognition, and expressive microtiming in African-American music. *Music Perception, 19*(3), 387–414.

Janata, P., & Grafton, S. T. (2003). Swinging in the brain: Shared neural substrates for behaviors related to sequencing and music. *Nature Neuroscience, 6*, 682–687.

Johansson, G. (1973). Visual perception of biological motion and a model for its analysis. *Perception and Psychophysics, 14,* 201–211.

Juslin, P. N., & Laukka, P. (2003). Emotional expression in speech and music. *Annals of the New York Academy of Sciences, 1000,* 279–282.

Kaplan, J. T., & Iacoboni, M. (2006). Getting a grip on other minds: Mirror neurons, intention understanding, and cognitive empathy. *Social Neuroscience, 1,* 175–183.

Kilner, J. M., Friston, K. J., & Frith, C. D. (2007). Predictive coding: An account of the mirror neuron system. *Cognitive Processes, 8,* 159–166.

Köhler, W. (1929). *Gestalt psychology.* New York, NY: Liveright.

Köhler, W. (1947). *Gestalt psychology* (2nd. ed.). New York, NY: Liveright.

Kraemer, D. J. M., Macrae, C. N., Green, A. E., & Kelley, W. M. (2005). The sound of silence: Spontaneous musical imagery activates auditory cortex. *Nature, 434,* 158.

Lakens, D. (2010). Movement synchrony and perceived entitativity. *Journal of Experimental Social Psychology, 46,* 701–708.

Lakens, D., & Stel, M. (2011). If they move in sync, they must feel in sync: Movement synchrony leads to attributions of rapport and entitativity. *Social Cognition, 29,* 1–14.

Leslie, K. R., Johnson-Frey, S. H., & Grafton, S. T. (2004). Functional imaging of face and hand imitation: Towards a motor theory of empathy. *NeuroImage, 21,* 601–607.

Loui, P., Alsop, D., & Schlaug, G. (2009). Tone deafness: A new disconnection syndrome? *Journal of Neuroscience, 29,* 10215–10220.

Loui, P., Li, H. C., Hohmann, A., & Schlaug, G. (2011). Enhanced cortical connectivity in absolute pitch musicians: A model for local hyperconnectivity. *Journal of Cognitive Neuroscience, 23,* 1015–1026.

Loui, P., Li, H. C., & Schlaug, G. (2011). White matter integrity in right hemisphere predicts pitch-related grammar learning. *Neuroimage, 55,* 500–507.

Marsh, K. L., Richardson, M. J., & Schmidt, R. C. (2009). Social connection through joint action and interpersonal coordination. *Topics in Cognitive Science, 1,* 320–339.

Martin, A., & Weisberg, J. (2003). Neural foundations for understanding social and mechanical concepts. *Cognitive Neuropsychology, 20,* 575–587.

Maurer, D., Pathman, T., & Mondloch, C. J. (2006). The shape of boubas: Sound–shape correspondences in toddlers and adults. *Developmental Science, 9,* 316–322.

McNeill, W. H. (1995). *Keeping together in time: Dance and drill in human history.* Cambridge, MA: Harvard University Press.

Nielsen, A., & Rendall, D. (2011). The sound of round: Evaluating the sound-symbolic role of consonants in the classic Takete-Maluma phenomenon. *Canadian Journal of Experimental Psychology, 65,* 115.

Ohala, J. (1994). The frequency code underlies the sound-symbolic use of voice pitch. In L. Hinton, J. Nichols, & J. Ohala (Eds.), *Sound symbolism* (pp. 325–347). Cambridge, UK: Cambridge University Press.

Parkinson, C., & Wheatley, T. (2012). Relating anatomical and social connectivity: White matter microstructure predicts emotional empathy. *Cerebral Cortex, 24,* 614–625.

Parkinson, C., Kohler, P. J., Sievers, B. R., & Wheatley, T. (2012). Associations between auditory pitch and visual elevation do not depend on language: Evidence from a remote population. *Perception, 41,* 854–861.

Patel, A. D., Peretz, I., Tramo, M., & Labreque, R. (1998). Processing prosodic and musical patterns: A neuropsychological investigation. *Brain and Language, 61*, 123–144.

Pavlova, M., Lutzenberger, W., Sokolov, A., & Birbaumer, N. (2004). Dissociable cortical processing of recognizable and non-recognizable biological movement: Analyzing gamma MEG activity. *Cerebral Cortex, 14*, 181–188.

Pell, M. D. (1996). On the receptive prosodic loss in Parkinson's. *Cortex, 32*, 693–704.

Pelphrey, K. A., Morris, J. P., Michelich, C. R., Allison, T., & McCarthy, G. (2005). Functional anatomy of biological motion perception in posterior temporal cortex: An fMRI study of eye, mouth and hand movements. *Cerebral Cortex, 15*, 1866–1876.

Pfeifer, J. H., Iacoboni, M., Mazziotta, J. C., & Dapretto, M. (2008). Mirroring others' emotions relates to empathy and interpersonal competence in children. *Neuroimage, 39*, 2076–2085.

Pollick, F. E., Lestou, V., Ryu, J., & Cho, S. B. (2002). Estimating the efficiency of recognizing gender and affect from biological motion. *Vision Research, 42*, 2345–2355.

Ramachandran, V. S., & Hubbard, E. M. (2001). Synaesthesia—A window into perception, thought and language. *Journal of Consciousness Studies, 8*, 3–34.

Ramseyer, F., & Tschacher, W. (2011). Nonverbal synchrony in psychotherapy: Coordinated body movement reflects relationship quality and outcome. *Journal of Consulting and Clinical Psychology, 79*, 284–295.

Ross, R., & Mesalum, M. (1979). Dominant language functions of the right hemisphere. *Archives of Neurology, 36*, 144–148.

Schmahmann, J. D., & Pandya, D. N. (2006). *Fiber pathways of the brain*. Oxford, UK: Oxford University Press.

Schulte-Rüther, M., Markowitsch, H. J., Fink, G. R., & Piefke, M. (2007). Mirror neuron and theory of mind mechanisms involved in face-to-face interactions: A functional magnetic resonance imaging approach to empathy. *Journal of Cognitive Neuroscience, 19*, 1354–1372.

Semin, G. R. (2007). Grounding communication: Synchrony. In A. W. Kruglanski & E. T. Higgins (Eds.), *Social psychology: Handbook of basic principles* (2nd ed., pp. 630–649). New York, NY: Guilford Press.

Sievers, B., Polansky, L., Casey, M., & Wheatley, T. (2013). Music and movement share a dynamic structure that supports universal expressions of emotion. *Proceedings of the National Academy of Sciences USA, 110*, 70–75.

Sonnby-Borgström, M. (2002). Automatic mimicry reactions as related to differences in emotional empathy. *Scandanavian Journal of Psychology, 43*, 433–443.

Steinbeis, N., & Koelsch, S. (2008). Comparing the processing of music and language meaning using EEG and fMRI provides evidence for similar and distinct neural representations. *PLoS One, 3*, e2226.

Styns, F., van Noorden, L., Moelants, D., & Leman, M. (2007). Walking on music. *Human Movement Science, 26*, 769–785.

Valdesolo, P., & DeSteno, D. (2011). Synchrony and the social tuning of compassion. *Emotion, 11*, 262–266.

van Noorden, L., & Moelants, D. (1999). Resonance in the perception of musical pulse. *Journal of New Music Research, 28*, 43–66.

Wheatley, T., Kang, O., Parkinson, C., & Looser, C.E. (2012). From mind perception to mental connection: Synchrony as a mechanism for social understanding. *Social Psychology and Personality Compass, 6*, 589–606.

Wheatley, T., Milleville, S. C., & Martin, A. (2007). Understanding animate agents: Distinct roles for the social network and mirror system. *Psychological Science, 18*, 469–474.

Wilson, M., & Knoblich, G. (2005). The case for motor involvement in perceiving conspecifics. *Psychological Bulletin, 131*, 460–473.

Wiltermuth, S. S., & Heath, C. (2009). Synchrony and cooperation. *Psychological Science, 20*, 1–5.

Zatorre, R. J., & Baum, S. R. (2012). Musical melody and speech intonation: Singing a different tune. *PLoS Biology, 10*:e1001372.

Zatorre, R. J., Chen, J. L., & Penhune, V. B. (2007). When the brain plays music: auditory–motor interactions in music perception and production. *Nature Reviews Neuroscience, 8*, 547–558.

Zatorre, R. J., Halpern, A. R., Perry, D. W., Meyer, E., & Evans, A. C. (1996). Hearing in the mind's ear: A PET investigation of musical imagery and perception. *Journal of Cognitive Neuroscience, 8*, 29–46.

Zatorre, R. J., & Krumhansl, C. L. (2002). Neuroscience mental models and musical minds. *Science, 298*, 2138–2139.

PART II

Altruism

4

Prosociality as a Form of Reward Seeking

JAMIL ZAKI AND JASON P. MITCHELL ■

Humans, relative to many other animals, are weak, slow, small, and frustratingly incapable of useful behaviors such as flying or breathing underwater. And yet we have unequivocally won the cross-species competition for global domination. This is not because any of us alone is a particularly impressive specimen, but rather because of our ability to act collectively, through cooperation and coordination. Myriad human actions—from organizing a hunting party to building a suspension bridge—rely on such cooperation. Cooperation, in turn, is undergirded by individuals' willingness to act in the best interest of their group, oftentimes at a cost to the individual herself. Such acts—including helping, sharing resources with, and providing information to others—constitute *prosocial behavior*, broadly construed (Batson, 2011; Tomasello, 2009).[1]

Classically, prosociality has proved an ill fit for standard models of human behavior, especially in economics and evolutionary theory. This is because both of these fields explicitly posit that people should act in their own best interest, maximizing outcomes for themselves and not worrying about the welfare of others. An individual who sacrifices for others violates these rules. Darwin (1871) himself noted that such sacrifice would reduce individuals' evolutionary fitness, because "he who was ready to sacrifice his life . . . rather than betray his comrades, would often leave no offspring to inherit his noble nature" (p. 130). Economists similarly viewed prosocial decision making as an "anomaly" that challenged standard models of individuals as rational maximizers (Camerer & Thaler, 1995).

Theoretical advances have since resolved this so-called problem of prosociality. Evolutionary theorists have demonstrated ways in which prosociality could prove adaptive, including kin selection (an individual who sacrifices for her relatives proliferates her genes effectively; Hamilton, 1964) and reciprocity (prosocial individuals benefit from others paying back favors in kind; Axelrod & Hamilton, 1981; Trivers, 1971). Here, however, we will not focus on these *ultimate* reasons that prosociality might have evolved over a glacial timescale, but rather on the *proximate* mechanisms that cause individuals to act prosocially at a given moment.

Over the centuries, economists, philosophers, and psychologists have nominated several such proximate mechanisms (Smith, 1790/2002). Broadly speaking, these can be divided into two categories: *extrinsic* and *intrinsic* sources of prosociality. Extrinsic models focus on the instrumental or strategic use of prosocial behaviors to obtain a valued personal end, such as social status (Harbaugh, 1998) or the reduction of personal distress produced by others' suffering (Cialdini & Kenrick, 1976). On this view, prosociality is a social analogue of executive control tasks such as the delay of gratification (Mischel, Shoda, & Rodriguez, 1989): Individuals suppress their true preferences, such as preferences for immediate rewards or selfish actions and act in opposition to these preferences, for instance by waiting or acting prosocially, in order to cultivate more important gains, such as larger, later rewards or high social status, down the road (Stevens & Hauser, 2004).

By contrast, *intrinsic* models suggest that individuals place irreducible value on prosocial outcomes, such as fairness and cooperation (Becker, 1974; Bolton & Ockenfels, 2000; Fehr & Schmidt, 1999). On this nobler view, prosocial acts reflect individuals' deep-seated preferences, and prosocial acts are ends unto themselves, as opposed to means for achieving personal goals (Batson & Shaw, 1991). Multiple lines of research have provided behavioral evidence for the intrinsic value of prosocial outcomes. For instance, economists have demonstrated that individuals' choices reflect stable preferences for social outcomes such as equity (Loewenstein, Thompson, & Bazerman, 1989) and "efficiency" (maximizing the gains of an entire group, as opposed to one's self; see Charness & Rabin, 2002). Furthermore, people's willingness to spend money to "buy" prosocial outcomes—for instance, by donating money to others—can be modeled in a manner similar to willingness to pay for personal goods (Andreoni & Miller, 2002). Similarly, Batson and colleagues have demonstrated several cases in which individuals appear motivated to help others even when other personal goals (e.g., reducing discomfort, accruing positive reputation) are removed (Batson et al., 1988, 1991; Coke & Batson, 1978), suggesting that people indeed experience an irreducible desire to improve others' well-being.

PROSOCIALITY AS REWARD SEEKING

Prosociality is almost certainly supported by both extrinsic and intrinsic motives, but extant theoretical models often fail to specify the psychological roots of these motives. That is, which cognitive and emotional states underlie individuals' desires to help others? Understanding prosociality at this level of analysis is critical to characterizing the structure of prosocial motives, as well as understanding exactly why these motives vary across social contexts.

Here we address this issue, focusing exclusively on the states underlying *intrinsic* prosocial motives (i.e., our "deeper" valuation of others' well-being). One intriguing and parsimonious prediction is that—as opposed to building a motivational system specific to prosociality—nature instead allowed prosocial motivation to "piggyback" on a much older psychological system designed to guide goal-related behavior. Specifically, *prosocial outcomes may be experienced as a reward, akin to food, shelter, and sex.* If this is the case, then prosocial behaviors—aimed at producing such outcomes—would reflect the same motivational states that support other reward-seeking behaviors, such as foraging and dating.

Behavioral data from economics and psychology provide initial evidence for a reward-seeking model of prosociality (Andreoni & Miller, 2002; Smith, Keating, & Stotland, 1989). However, behavior alone leaves unclear the extent to which the reward associated with prosocial behavior resembles other, personal forms of reward. Luckily, cognitive neuroscience provides a basis for answering this question. This is because neuroscientists, over the past two decades, have robustly and consistently tied the experience of reward to the engagement of a set of brain regions comprising the brain's mesolimbic dopaminergic system. In particular, activity in the ventral striatum (VS) and ventromedial prefrontal cortex (vMPFC) tracks the reward value with which organisms imbue events and outcomes (O'Doherty, Dayan, Friston, Critchley, & Dolan, 2003; Schultz, 2002; Schultz, Dayan, & Montague, 1997), and activity in these regions further predicts value-based decision making, for instance between two potentially rewarding actions (Montague & Berns, 2002; Rangel & Hare, 2010; Rushworth, Noonan, Boorman, Walton, & Behrens, 2011).[2] Interestingly, VS and vMPFC activity tracks the reward value of multiple, seemingly incommensurable outcomes, including food (Grabenhorst & Rolls, 2011; Small, Zatorre, Dagher, Evans, & Jones-Gotman, 2001), water (de Araujo, Kringelbach, Rolls, & McGlone, 2003), money (Knutson, Taylor, Kaufman, Peterson, & Glover, 2005), commercial goods and branding (Knutson, Rick, Wimmer, Prelec, & Loewenstein, 2007; McClure et al., 2004), and beautiful faces (Cloutier, Heatherton, Whalen, & Kelley, 2008; Zaki, Schirmer, & Mitchell, 2011). Broadly, these data suggest that *activity in this system represents a broad, domain general neural marker of subjective value.*

This neuroscientific literature provides a clear and simple test of the reward-seeking model of prosociality: To the extent that this model is correct, prosocial outcomes should engage the same dopaminergic targets as other forms of reward. As it turns out, neuroscientists have produced several such demonstrations (see Fehr & Camerer, 2007 for a review of some of this work). For instance, observing others reciprocate a cooperative gesture engages both VS and vMPFC (Rilling et al., 2002; Tabibnia, Satpute, & Lieberman, 2008), as does punishing unfair behavior (de Quervain et al., 2004; Seymour, Singer, & Dolan, 2007) and observing a charity or other individual receive monetary rewards (Harbaugh, Mayr, & Burghart, 2007; Mobbs et al., 2009).

Although these data are compelling, most examinations of brain activity in response to prosocial outcomes focus on cases in which individuals passively view such outcomes, as opposed to making decisions between acting prosocially or selfishly. Furthermore, early neuroimaging studies of prosocial reward largely examined cases in which prosocial outcomes (e.g., watching others cooperate) produce no cost for participants. By contrast, many everyday prosocial gestures involve incurring nontrivial personal cost or discomfort. Finally, even the few neuroscientific studies that have examined costly prosocial decision making (Dawes et al., 2012; Hare, Camerer, Knoepfle, & Rangel, 2010) have focused exclusively on sharing material resources (e.g., money), whereas prosocial behavior applies equally well to other domains. For instance, individuals commonly choose to share information with each (e.g., through pedagogy). Such teaching and informing form an important, but underevaluated, cornerstone of human prosociality (Warneken & Tomasello, 2009).

Here, we briefly describe a program of research aimed at broadening a reward-seeking model of prosociality in three ways. First, we examined whether costly prosocial decision making produces activity in regions associated with subjective reward. Second, we tested whether a single area of vMPFC tracks both personal and vicarious reward, a prediction consistent with the idea that these two classes of reward are truly isomorphic. Third, we examined the extent to which similar neural mechanisms underlie a separate type of prosociality: information sharing.

The Subjective Value of Costly Prosocial Choices

In a first study, participants briefly met a confederate (hereafter: the "receiver") whom they believed was another participant in a two-person study on impression formation. Through an ostensibly random—but actually fixed—randomization, participants were assigned to be scanned by fMRI while the receiver completed other tasks outside the scanner. While being scanned,

participants completed an economic choice task that they had not discussed with the receiver. This task comprised a variant of the *dictator game*
(cf. Hoffman, McCabe, & Smith, 1996): Participants made a series of binary
choices between allocating a given amount of money to themselves or allocating an amount of money to the receiver.

Two critical features of this task are worth mentioning. First, the amounts of
money available to each "player" in the dictator game varied across trials, such
that sometimes the participant stood to gain more than the receiver, and sometimes the receiver stood to gain more than the participant. Thus, in order to opti-
mally benefit the pair of players—and uphold a prosocial norm related to fairness
that economists term "efficiency" (Charness & Rabin, 2002)—participants should
give to whomever (themselves or the receiver) stood to gain the most. This created four types of possible choices, determined by two dimensions: whether the
participant acted in a *self-serving* or *generous* way (by giving to themselves or to
the receiver, respectively) and in a *fair* or *unfair* way (by giving to the person who
stood to gain more or to the person who stood to gain less, respectively).

Second, true to its name, the dictator game is designed to give power to
one member of a dyad: in this case, the participant. Unlike other economic
games, the receiver here had no recourse to punish participants for acting selfishly. Dictator games feature this design in order to isolate participants' "true"
preferences for giving to others, independent of extrinsic social pressures. To
further reduce such pressures, we told participants that receivers would not
even be aware that participants were playing the dictator game. Instead, the
receiver would simply receive an additional payment for the study. This lack
of information was meant to further reduce social pressures for participants
to give (Eckel & Grossman, 1996; Hoffman, McCabe, Shachat, & Smith, 1994).

Despite the reduced social pressure produced by this design, participants
nonetheless acted generously a substantial amount of the time, especially
when generous choices were also fair (i.e., when the receiver stood more to
gain than the participant). In fact, participants gave away over 20% of the total
money available over the course of the session. Although consistent with prior
work in this literature (Engel, 2011), giving in such dictator games constitutes a remarkable violation of economic models of self-interested rationality
(Camerer & Thaler, 1995). Did our participants' giving reflect their experience of reward when upholding prosocial norms? To answer this question, we
examined brain activity while participants made different forms of choices.
Our data were strongly consistent with a reward-seeking account of prosociality: When making fair, as compared to unfair, decisions, participants engaged
a subregion of vMPFC broadly associated with the experience of subjective
value, suggesting that they imbue this class of prosocial decision with value
(see Figure 4.1 and Zaki & Mitchell, 2011). Remarkably, vMPFC responded

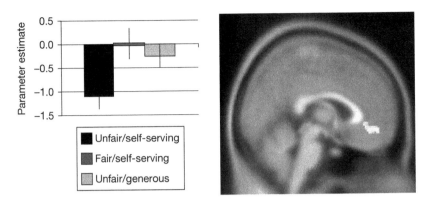

Figure 4.1 Activity in the ventromedial prefrontal cortex (vMPFC) is sensitive to prosocial rewards, not monetary gain. When participants chose to take small amounts of money rather than donate larger amounts to another person, vMPFC activity was significantly deactivated (leftmost bar), suggesting that participants experienced reduced subjective value when acting selfishly. In contrast, the vMPFC did not differentiate between receiving and donating money, so long as participants' choice was fair (center and rightmost bars).

more strongly to the upholding of prosocial norms than to the experience of personal reward. Specifically, this region demonstrating similar levels of activity during all fair choices, regardless of whether these choices were self-serving or generous. By contrast, vMPFC demonstrated a strong negative deflection when participants made self-serving, unfair choices, even though these choices resulted in monetary gain for participants. This is consistent with the intriguing idea that prosocial norms are not only experienced as rewarding, but that their reward value can "overwrite" the value of material gain.

Isomorphism Between Self- and Other-Oriented Reward

Even if prosocial behaviors are experienced as rewarding, this leaves unclear what the *source* of such reward might be. At least two possibilities come to mind. First, individuals may enjoy the *action* of engaging in prosocial behavior, a phenomenon often referred to as a hedonic "warm glow" of giving (Andreoni, 1990; Waytz & Zaki, submitted). Second, people may experience reward based on prosocial *outcomes*, such as the vicarious joy one experiences while watching others receive prizes or display positive emotion (Harbaugh et al., 2007; Mobbs et al., 2009; Zaki & Ochsner, 2012). Evidence supports both of these accounts, but two critical, interrelated questions remained unanswered. First, does the reward value of prosocial outcomes, such as vicariously experiencing others' reward, predict prosocial action? And second, are personal and vicarious reward represented through isomorphic—or functionally overlapping—cognitive and affective processes?

In our further analysis of our dictator game, we sought to answer this question by combining techniques from economics and neurophysiology. Specifically, economists have long argued that individuals often make choices between seemingly incommensurable outcomes (for instance, between a product and the money it would cost to buy that product) by reducing these outcomes to a "common currency" of subjective value, or how much each outcome is worth to that individual (Cabanac, 1992; Godel, 1938). More recently, neuroscientists have revealed that this common value currency tightly tracks activity in vMPFC in response to different classes of rewards (e.g., money vs. food; see Levy & Glimcher, 2011).

We sought to test the predictions that (1) vMPFC likewise tracks the common value currency of both personal and vicarious reward, and (2) this common value signal predicts self-serving and generous decision making. To do so, we capitalized on another feature of our dictator game: The amounts individuals could allocate to themselves or the receiver were related by a set of *other:self ratios*. For instance, a participant might choose between allocating $3 to the receiver versus $2 to herself (a 1.5:1.0 other:self ratio), or between allocating $1 to the receiver versus $2 to herself (a 0.5:1 other:self ratio). These ratios allowed us to estimate individuals' preferences for rewards allocated to themselves, as compared to the receiver (see also Andreoni & Miller, 2002; Padoa-Schioppa & Assad, 2006, 2008, for other uses of similar techniques). Briefly, we modeled the proportion of prosocial choices (allocations to the receiver) that participants made at each other:self ratio. We used this information to estimate each participant's *interpersonal indifference ratio*; that is, the other:self ratio at which a participant would be equally likely to allocate money to himself or to another person.

The group average indifference ratio was ~1.25:1.00 (demarcated by the dotted line in Figure 4.2), indicating that—on average—participants placed equal value on receiving $1.00 and allowing another person to receive $1.25. However, not all participants were equally prosocial; instead, indifference ratios varied widely across our sample. We used each participant's indifference ratio to estimate a common value currency across self- and other-oriented reward. Specifically, we modeled the reward value we believed each participant would experience when receiving money herself and watching the receiver win money, on *a single scale*. For instance, if a participant's choices indicated a 2:1 other:self indifference ratio, we would expect her to experience the same reward value when observing $2 given to the receiver and $1 given to herself.

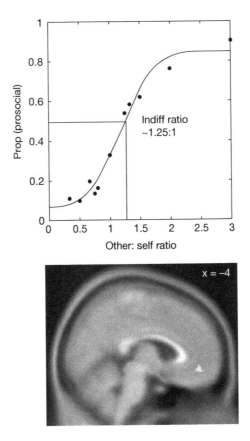

Figure 4.2 Other/self indifference ratios estimated based on prosocial choice patterns at each other:self reward ratio. Overall, participants appeared to value their own outcomes about 1.25 times as much as those of another person. Indifference ratios further predicted activity in the ventromedial prefrontal cortex.

We used this information to model brain activity during separate trials in which participants watched passively while they or the receiver won varying amounts of money. Specifically, we isolated brain activity representing the subjective value associated with *both* self and other gains. Even though we searched for such activity across the whole brain, only vMPFC reflected this common value currency (see Figure 4.2 and Zaki, Lopez, & Mitchell, 2013).

These findings add depth to a reward-seeking account of prosociality. First, they suggest that personal and vicarious rewards are indeed processed through a common currency—both instantiated in vMPFC—suggesting that viewing others receive rewards "feels" very much like the reward we experience following personal positive events. Second, this vicarious experience of others' rewards tightly tracks individuals' prosocial decision making, suggesting that the enjoyment of others' well-being factors heavily into the calculus associated with generous versus self-serving action.

The Value of Helping Others by Sharing Information

The foregoing evidence suggests that people value sharing material resources with others, but they leave unexplored whether the experience of reward also drives other forms of prosociality. For instance, people often help each other by sharing needed information (e.g., giving directions to strangers or tutoring fellow students). Such sharing is ubiquitous, begins early in life (Liszkowski, Carpenter, & Tomasello, 2007), and forms the basis of interpersonal communication (Clark, 1996; Tomasello, 2008a). Furthermore, such sharing is absent in our closest evolutionary relatives, such as great apes (Tomasello, 2008b; Warneken & Tomasello, 2009), suggesting the desire to share information is uniquely human.

Does our proclivity to share helpful information with others reflect a form of reward seeking? If that were the case, we would expect information sharing to exhibit behavioral and neural properties associated with other forms of reward. Behaviorally, we might expect individuals to sacrifice other valuable resources in order to share information with others. Neurally, we would predict that opportunities to helpfully inform others, like sharing monetary resources, should produce engagement in targets of the dopaminergic system.

To test this behavioral prediction, we adapted a "willingness to pay" paradigm developed by Deaner et al. (2005) to examine whether individuals indeed give up resources to inform others. Participants (hereafter: "teachers") played a game in which they saw an array of four cards and learned which was the "correct" one to choose on a given trial. They were then given the opportunity to teach this correct answer to another participant (hereafter: the "learner") or to keep the answer private while the learner guessed. Two things about this game bear noting. First, it was quite minimalistic: There were no rules determining the "correct" answer on a given trial, no prizes given for guessing the correct answer, and teachers were told that learners would not know whether information about the right answer had been delivered by the teacher or by the experimenter.

Second, choices to share or not share information were each paired with small nonzero sums of money. For instance, on a given trial, teachers might choose between taking $0.03 and sharing the correct answer with the learner, or taking $0.01 and not sharing the answer; these amounts vary independently from $0.01 to $0.04. This paradigm allows for a very straightforward measure of preferences: If teachers equally value sharing and not sharing information,

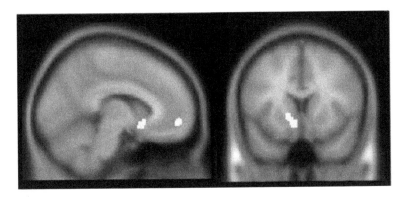

Figure 4.3 When individuals find out that they have the opportunity to prosocially inform another participant about the correct answer on a task, they engage the ventromedial prefrontal cortex and the ventral striatum.

they should choose whichever option is associated with the larger monetary gain. However, this is not how our teachers behaved. Instead, they opted to share information ~70% of the time, even when it was costly to them. In fact, teachers sacrificed ~25% of total possible earnings during this task in order to helpfully inform learners, suggesting that they indeed value chances to share information.

To provide converging neural evidence for a reward-seeking view of informing, we scanned a separate group of "teachers" with fMRI while they learned the correct answer to a card game and either shared or did not share this information with learners. However, in this version of the task, teachers did not elect to share or not share information; instead, they were simply told on each trial whether or not they would inform the learner about the correct answer. Interestingly, opportunities to share information with others engaged both the vMPFC and VS (see Figure 4.3 and Tamir, Zaki, & Mitchell, in press), the same regions involved in reward processing observed in our earlier studies. These results build on earlier findings (Tamir & Mitchell, 2011) to suggest that individuals value opportunities to help others by sharing information, and they represent this value in the same neural system associated with prosociality and reward processing more broadly.

A COMMON CURRENCY FOR GIVING AND TAKING

Although prosocial behavior once puzzled theorists across the natural and social sciences, scientists have since identified multiple key forces that support humans' tendencies to help each other. Our research joins a groundswell of interdisciplinary evidence to strongly suggest that prosociality often reflects a form of *reward seeking* (Fehr & Camerer, 2007; Zaki & Mitchell, 2013). Specifically, the work reviewed here demonstrates that prosocial behaviors and outcomes—including (1) prosocially sharing resources, (2) watching others receive rewards, and (3) prosocially sharing information—produce patterns of behavior and neural activity similar to those that mirror those associated with receiving and pursuing personal rewards such as food, water, and sex. This view provides a compelling and parsimonious mechanism by which people might be motivated to help others: Psychologically speaking, such helping often serves as its own reward. A reward-seeking model also suggests that cooperative social behaviors, rather than relying on dedicated psychological processes, may have their roots in evolutionarily old motivational systems that govern other forms of reward seeking such as foraging, hunting, and mating.

It is worth noting that although reward seeking likely plays a role in some prosocial behaviors, it is by no means the only mechanism that supports helping. Specifically, a reward-seeking model may better explain *intrinsically* motivated prosocial behaviors (those reflecting "true" preferences for others' well-being), but not *extrinsically* motivated prosocial acts. When pursuing such extrinsic motives, individuals might not find prosocial actions rewarding, but strategically carry them out nonetheless in hopes of later gaining from them. We might expect such strategic prosocial acts—instead of engaging neural structures associated with reward—would rely on brain activity associated with controlled behaviors such as delaying gratification or inhibiting instinctual responding. Indeed, a small but growing number of studies have documented such cases. For instance, acting prosocially under the threat of sanction (Spitzer, Fischbacher, Herrnberger, Gron, & Fehr, 2007) and making decisions to uphold a prosocial social norm (Baumgartner, Knoch, Hotz, Eisenegger, & Fehr, 2011) both engage lateral prefrontal regions typically associated with exerting such control. Together, this work suggests that outwardly similar prosocial decisions can be supported by very different psychological mechanisms of reward seeking or control. Future work should focus on examining the situational and interpersonal factors that "toggle" prosocial behavior between these mechanisms.

A reward-seeking model of prosocial behavior provides new predictions about the structure of human prosociality. For instance, this model suggests that prosocial behavior should follow the same "rules" as other forms of reward seeking. Classic models of value and reward from psychology (Rescorla & Wagner, 1972), physiology (Schultz, 2002), and computer science (Sutton & Barto, 1998) provide several examples of such rules. For instance, the value of a reward (e.g., a piece of chocolate) rapidly declines when an individual has recently experienced that reward already (*satiety*) or when the reward will not occur for a while (*temporal discounting*). To the extent that prosocial outcomes are rewards like any other, they should demonstrate similar properties.

Finally, a reward-seeking model of prosociality might strike some readers as disheartening. At least since Kant (1785/2002), theorists have drawn a bright line between "pure" and "impure" forms of altruism. Specifically, an altruistic act that produces a gain for the actor (including a subjective sense of well-being) cannot be construed as truly other oriented. On this view, a reward-seeking model reduces the lion's share of human prosociality to an impure status, and it removes some of the specialness of altruism, because it suggests that both giving (prosocially) and taking (selfishly) rely on the same broad value system.

We feel strongly that a reward-seeking model, instead, speaks to a profound feature of our species. Our work, along with that of others, strongly suggests that humans' central motivational system responds not only to our own well-being but also to the well-being of others. This suggests that even our "selfish" reward mechanisms are tuned to upholding prosocial norms, and that our species may indeed be built for prosociality.

NOTES

1. The more common term "altruism" refers to a subset of prosocial behaviors that come at a cost to prosocial actors.
2. Importantly, VS and vMPFC play distinct, but complementary roles in reward processing: The VS encodes "prediction errors," or discrepancies between rewards an organism receives and what it expected, whereas vMPFC tracks the overall value of outcomes and actions. Roughly speaking, VS allows organisms to learn new information about reward value, whereas vMPFC integrates over multiple sources of information to compute reward value in the service of decision making. A closer discussion of this system is outside the scope of this chapter, but we refer readers to Glimcher (2011), Rangel and Hare (2010), and Rushworth et al. (2011).

REFERENCES

Andreoni, J. (1990). Impure altruism and donations to public goods: a theory of warm-glow giving. *The Economic Journal, 100*, 464–477.

Andreoni, J., & Miller, J. (2002). Giving according to GARP: An experimental study of rationality and altruism. *Econometrica, 70*(2), 737–753.

Axelrod, R., & Hamilton, W. D. (1981). The evolution of cooperation. *Science, 211,* 1390–1396.

Batson, C. D. (2011). *Altruism in humans.* New York, NY: Oxford University Press.

Batson, C. D., Batson, J. G., Slingsby, J. K., Harrell, K. L., Peekna, H. M., & Todd, R. M. (1991). Empathic joy and the empathy-altruism hypothesis. *Journal of Personality and Social Psychology*, *61*(3), 413–426.

Batson, C. D., Dyck, J. L., Brandt, J. R., Batson, J. G., Powell, A. L., McMaster, M. R., & Griffit, C. (1988). Five studies testing two new egoistic alternatives to the empathy-altruism hypothesis. *Journal of Personality and Social Psychology*, *55*(1), 52–77.

Batson, C. D., & Shaw, L. (1991). Evidence for altruism: Toward a pluralism of prosocial motives. *Psychological Inquiry*, *2*(2), 107–122.

Baumgartner, T., Knoch, D., Hotz, P., Eisenegger, C., & Fehr, E. (2011). Dorsolateral and ventromedial prefrontal cortex orchestrate normative choice. *Nature Neuroscience*, *14*(11), 1468–1474.

Becker, G. (1974). *A theory of social interactions*. Cambridge, MA: National Bureau of Economic Research.

Bolton, G., & Ockenfels, A. (2000). ERC: A theory of equity, reciprocity, and competition. *American Economic Review*, *90*(1), 166–193.

Cabanac, M. (1992). Pleasure: The common currency. *Journal of Theoretical Biology*, *155*(2), 173–200.

Camerer, C., & Thaler, R. H. (1995). Anomalies: Ultimatums, dictators and manners. *Journal of Economic Perspectives*, *9*(2), 209–219.

Charness, G., & Rabin, M. (2002). Understanding social preferences with simple tests. *Quarterly Journal of Economics*, *117*(3), 817–869.

Cialdini, R. B., & Kenrick, D. T. (1976). Altruism as hedonism: A social development perspective on the relationship of negative mood state and helping. *Journal of Personality and Social Psychology*, *34*(5), 907.

Clark, H. H. (1996). *Using language*. Cambridge, UK: Cambridge University Press.

Cloutier, J., Heatherton, T. F., Whalen, P. J., & Kelley, W. M. (2008). Are attractive people rewarding? Sex differences in the neural substrates of facial attractiveness. *Journal of Cognitive Neuroscience*, *20*(6), 941–951.

Coke, J. S., & Batson, C. D. (1978). Empathic mediation of helping: A two stage model. *Journal of Personality and Social Psychology*, *36*, 752–766.

Darwin, C. (1871). *The descent of man, and selection in relation to sex*. London, UK: John Murray.

Dawes, C. T., Loewen, P. J., Schreiber, D., Simmons, A. N., Flagan, T., McElreath, R., ... Paulus, M. P. (2012). Neural basis of egalitarian behavior. *Proceedings of the National Academy of Sciences USA*, *109*(17), 6479–6483.

de Araujo, I. E., Kringelbach, M. L., Rolls, E. T., & McGlone, F. (2003). Human cortical responses to water in the mouth, and the effects of thirst. *Journal of Neurophysiology*, *90*(3), 1865–1876.

de Quervain, D. J., Fischbacher, U., Treyer, V., Schellhammer, M., Schnyder, U., Buck, A., & Fehr, E. (2004). The neural basis of altruistic punishment. *Science*, *305*(5688), 1254–1258.

Deaner, R. O., Khera, A. V., & Platt, M. L. (2005). Monkeys pay per view: Adaptive valuation of social images by rhesus macaques. *Current biology*, *15*(6), 543–548.

Eckel, C., & Grossman, P. (1996). Altruism in anonymous dictator games. *Games and Economic Behavior*, *16*(2), 181–191.

Engel, J. (2011). Dictator games: A meta study. *Experimental Economics*, *14*, 583–610.

Fehr, E., & Camerer, C. F. (2007). Social neuroeconomics: The neural circuitry of social preferences. *Trends in Cognitive Sciences, 11*(10), 419–427.

Fehr, E., & Schmidt, K. (1999). A theory of fairness, competition, and cooperation. *Quarterly Journal of Economics, 114*(3), 817–868.

Glimcher, P. W. (2011). Understanding dopamine and reinforcement learning: The dopamine reward prediction error hypothesis. *Proceedings of the National Academy of Sciences USA, 108*(Suppl. 3), 15647–15654.

Godel, K. (1938). The consistency of the axiom of choice and of the generalized continuum-hypothesis. *Proceedings of the National Academy of Sciences USA, 24*(12), 556–557.

Grabenhorst, F., & Rolls, E. T. (2011). Value, pleasure and choice in the ventral prefrontal cortex. *Trends in Cognitive Sciences, 15*(2), 56–67.

Hamilton, W. D. (1964). The genetical evolution of social behaviour. I. *Journal of Theoretical Biology, 7*(1), 1–16.

Harbaugh, W. T. (1998). What do donations buy? A model of philanthropy based on prestige and warm glow. *Journal of Public Economics, 67*(2), 269–284.

Harbaugh, W. T., Mayr, U., & Burghart, D. R. (2007). Neural responses to taxation and voluntary giving reveal motives for charitable donations. *Science, 316*(5831), 1622–1625.

Hare, T. A., Camerer, C. F., Knoepfle, D. T., & Rangel, A. (2010). Value computations in ventral medial prefrontal cortex during charitable decision making incorporate input from regions involved in social cognition. *Journal of Neuroscience, 30*(2), 583–590.

Hoffman, E., McCabe, K., Shachat, K., & Smith, V. (1994). Preferences, property rights and anonymity in bargaining games. *Games and Economic Behavior, 7*, 346–380.

Hoffman, E., McCabe, K., & Smith, V. L. (1996). Social distance and other-regarding behavior in dictator games. *American Economic Review, 86*(3), 653–660.

Kant, I. (2002). *Groundwork of the metaphysics of morals.* New Haven, CT: Yale University Press. (Originally published in 1785).

Knutson, B., Rick, S., Wimmer, G. E., Prelec, D., & Loewenstein, G. (2007). Neural predictors of purchases. *Neuron, 53*(1), 147–156.

Knutson, B., Taylor, J., Kaufman, M., Peterson, R., & Glover, G. (2005). Distributed neural representation of expected value. *Journal of Neuroscience, 25*(19), 4806–4812.

Levy, D. J., & Glimcher, P. W. (2011). Comparing apples and oranges: Using reward-specific and reward-general subjective value representation in the brain. *Journal of Neuroscience, 31*(41), 14693–14707.

Liszkowski, U., Carpenter, M., & Tomasello, M. (2007). Pointing out new news, old news, and absent referents at 12 months of age. *Developmental Science, 10*(2), F1–F7.

Loewenstein, G. F., Thompson, L., & Bazerman, M. H. (1989). Social utility and decision making in interpersonal contexts. *Journal of Personality and Social Psychology, 57*(3), 426.

McClure, S. M., Li, J., Tomlin, D., Cypert, K. S., Montague, L. M., & Montague, P. R. (2004). Neural correlates of behavioral preference for culturally familiar drinks. *Neuron, 44*(2), 379–387.

Mischel, W., Shoda, Y., & Rodriguez, M. (1989). Delay of gratification in children. *Science, 244*(4907), 933.

Mobbs, D., Yu, R., Meyer, M., Passamonti, L., Seymour, B., Calder, A. J., . . . Dalgleish, T. (2009). A key role for similarity in vicarious reward. *Science, 324*(5929), 900.

Montague, P. R., & Berns, G. S. (2002). Neural economics and the biological substrates of valuation. *Neuron, 36*(2), 265–284.

O'Doherty, J. P., Dayan, P., Friston, K., Critchley, H., & Dolan, R. J. (2003). Temporal difference models and reward-related learning in the human brain. *Neuron, 38*(2), 329–337.

Padoa-Schioppa, C., & Assad, J. A. (2006). Neurons in the orbitofrontal cortex encode economic value. *Nature, 441*(7090), 223–226.

Padoa-Schioppa, C., & Assad, J. A. (2008). The representation of economic value in the orbitofrontal cortex is invariant for changes of menu. *Nature Neuroscience, 11*(1), 95–102.

Rangel, A., & Hare, T. (2010). Neural computations associated with goal-directed choice. *Current Opinion in Neurobiology, 20*(2), 262–270.

Rescorla, R., & Wagner, A. (1972). A theory of pavlovian conditioning: Variations in the effectiveness of reinforcement and nonreinforcement. In A. Black & W. Prokasy (Eds.), *Classical conditioning II: Current research and theory* (pp. xx–xx). New York, NY: Appleton-Century-Crofts.

Rilling, J., Gutman, D., Zeh, T., Pagnoni, G., Berns, G., & Kilts, C. (2002). A neural basis for social cooperation. *Neuron, 35*(2), 395–405.

Rushworth, M. F. S., Noonan, M. A. P., Boorman, E. D., Walton, M. E., & Behrens, T. E. (2011). Frontal cortex and reward-guided learning and decision-making. *Neuron, 70*(6), 1054–1069.

Schultz, W. (2002). Getting formal with dopamine and reward. *Neuron, 36*(2), 241–263.

Schultz, W., Dayan, P., & Montague, P. R. (1997). A neural substrate of prediction and reward. *Science, 275*(5306), 1593–1599.

Seymour, B., Singer, T., & Dolan, R. (2007). The neurobiology of punishment. *Nature Reviews Neuroscience, 8*(4), 300–311.

Small, D. M., Zatorre, R. J., Dagher, A., Evans, A. C., & Jones-Gotman, M. (2001). Changes in brain activity related to eating chocolate: From pleasure to aversion. *Brain, 124*(Pt. 9), 1720–1733.

Smith, A. (2002). *The theory of moral sentiments.* Cambridge, UK: Cambridge University Press. (Originally published in 1790).

Smith, K. D., Keating, J. P., & Stotland, E. (1989). Altruism reconsidered: The effect of denying feedback on a victim's status to empathic witnesses. *Journal of Personality and Social Psychology, 57*(4), 641.

Spitzer, M., Fischbacher, U., Herrnberger, B., Gron, G., & Fehr, E. (2007). The neural signature of social norm compliance. *Neuron, 56*(1), 185–196.

Stevens, J. R., & Hauser, M. D. (2004). Why be nice? Psychological constraints on the evolution of cooperation. *Trends in Cognitive Sciences, 8*(2), 60–65.

Sutton, R. S., & Barto, A. G. (1998). *Reinforcement learning: An introduction.* Cambridge, MA: MIT Press.

Tabibnia, G., Satpute, A. B., & Lieberman, M. D. (2008). The sunny side of fairness: Preference for fairness activates reward circuitry (and disregarding unfairness activates self-control circuitry). *Psychological Science, 19*(4), 339–347.

Tamir, D., & Mitchell, J. (2011). Disclosing information about the self is intrinsically rewarding. *Proceedings of the National Academy of Sciences USA, 109*(21), 8038–8043.

Tamir, D., Zaki, J., & Mitchell, J. P. (in press). Informing others is associated with behavioral and neural signatures of value. *Journal of Experimental Psychology: General.*

Tomasello, M. (2008a). *Origins of human communication.* Cambridge, MA: MIT Press.

Tomasello, M. (2008b). Why don't apes point? *Trends in Linguistic Studies, 197,* 375.

Tomasello, M. (2009). *Why we cooperate.* Cambridge, MA: MIT Press.

Trivers, R. (1971). The evolution of reciprocal altruism. *Quarterly Review of Biology, 46,* 35–57.

Warneken, F., & Tomasello, M. (2009). Varieties of altruism in children and chimpanzees. *Trends in Cognitive Sciences, 13*(9), 397–402.

Zaki, J., Lopez, G., & Mitchell, J. (2013). Activity in ventromedial prefrontal cortex covaries with revealed social preferences: Evidence for person-invariant value. *Social Cognitive and Affective Neuroscience, 9*(4), 464–469.

Zaki, J., & Mitchell, J. (2011). Equitable decision making is associated with neural markers of subjective value. *Proceedings of the National Academy of Sciences USA, 108*(49), 19761–19766.

Zaki, J., & Mitchell, J. P. (2013). Intuitive prosociality. *Current Directions in Psychological Sciences, 22*(6), 466–470.

Zaki, J., & Ochsner, K. (2012). The neuroscience of empathy: Progress, pitfalls, and promise. *Nature Neuroscience, 15*(5), 675–680.

Zaki, J., Schirmer, J., & Mitchell, J. (2011). Social influence modulates the neural computation of value. *Psychological Science, 22*(7), 894–900.

5

Is Human Prosocial Behavior Unique?

Insights and New Questions From Nonhuman Primates

LINDSEY A. DRAYTON AND LAURIE R. SANTOS ∎

For centuries, thinkers from a number of disciplines have assumed that human psychology is—at its core—deeply selfish. Economists using models of utility maximization and rational choice have long assumed that people are inherently self-interested and thus should spend most of their time maximizing their own personal wealth and resources. Evolutionary biologists have long held a similar assumption, presuming that humans and other organisms are built to maximize their own selfish reproductive needs. Under this view, human psychology should be largely concerned with accumulating goods associated with survival and reproduction. Although the idea that human beings are deeply self-interested fits squarely with both economic and biological theory, this assumption contradicts most people's experience with actual human interactions. Indeed, across all cultures, people are shockingly *less* self-interested than economic and evolutionary models seem to assume. People regularly behave in ways that systematically violate their own self-interest. Many of these deviations from self-interest involve cases in which people forego a personal payoff in order to do nice things for others. From pausing to hold the elevator for a stranger to donating money to help disaster victims, we humans engage in a number of behaviors that reduce our own welfare in order to benefit others. Such widespread prosocial acts have led social scientists to argue that humans possess what have come to be known as *other-regarding preferences*, namely preferences for maximizing other people's welfare in addition to our own.

Why do people prefer to sacrifice their own wealth and time in order to benefit others' welfare? Recent research in the field of positive psychology suggests a provocative yet remarkably intuitive answer: *We're nice to others because it feels good.* A growing body of empirical evidence suggests that prosocial actions are intrinsically rewarding (Andreoni, 1990; Lyubomirsky, King, & Diener, 2005; Seligman, 2002). People feel a sense of satisfaction when others experience positive outcomes (Singer & Fehr, 2005) and report more positive well-being after engaging in prosocial actions such as giving to charity or volunteering (e.g., Thoits & Hewitt, 2001). Indeed, recent empirical work suggests that spending money on others increases one's personal well-being more than spending money on oneself (Dunn, Aknin, & Norton, 2008). Taken together, this work suggests that we humans may prefer taking costs to make others feel good because doing so has the counterintuitive effect of making us feel good too.

In the last few years, research in the field of positive neuroscience has gained better insight into why being nice to others feels so good—actions that benefit others seem to recruit some of the same neural systems as actions that benefit the self (Fehr & Camerer, 2007; Chapter 4, this volume). In a landmark paper, Moll et al. (2006) observed that making charitable monetary donations seemed to activate mesolimbic reward systems, the same regions that are activated when people experience selfishly rewarding events like winning money (Knutson, Adams, Fong, & Hommer, 2001; O'Doherty, Kringelbach, Rolls, Hornak, & Andrews, 2001) or eating delicious food (O'Doherty, Deichmann, Critchley, & Dolan, 2002; for similar results see Harbaugh, Mayr, & Burghart, 2007; Zaki & Mitchell, 2011). Similarly, work in positive neuroscience has revealed that when paying a cost to punish norm violators, participants recruit neural areas associated with anticipated monetary rewards, even though the participants' own money is being lost rather than gained (de Quervain et al., 2004). Finally, Tabibnia, Satpute, and Lieberman (2008) observed that reward regions responded more to gaining a monetary payoff when that payoff represented a fair share of an allotment than when it represented an unfair offer. In this way, our tendency to prefer prosocial behaviors to purely selfish behaviors may be mediated by the neural regions that represent reward contingencies. Specifically, these regions may respond more strongly when we engage in acts that help others compared to those that help only ourselves. Furthermore, these positive neuroscience studies suggest that this preference is rooted in some pretty basic neurocircuitry—the neural regions that represent reward contingencies across a variety of mammalian species. Our ancient mammalian reward systems may thus be wired to respond when rewarding events happen to others (see also Chang, Winecoff, & Platt, 2011).

THE EVOLUTIONARY ORIGINS
OF SOCIAL PREFERENCES

The fact that human prosocial preferences are encoded in reward circuitry that is evolutionarily ancient raises an important question about the evolution of these preferences: If human other-regarding preferences rely on relatively evolutionarily ancient neural circuitry, then is it possible that similar social preferences exist in our distant evolutionary relatives as well? Are humans the only species that cares about others' rewards? Or do our close evolutionary relatives—the extant nonhuman primates (hereafter, just primates)—show similar other-regarding preferences?

Our goal in this chapter is to explore these questions about the evolutionary origins of human prosociality. Specifically, we will review what primate researchers have learned in the last decade about the other-regarding preferences of our closest living relatives. Just as social scientists have developed empirical techniques for tapping into human social preferences, so too have primate researchers established empirical methods for testing such preferences in other primate species. Although these empirical tasks have given primate cognition researchers new insights into primates' tendencies to help and donate resources to others, they have also given rise to some controversy about what—if any—other-regarding tendencies primates actually possess (see reviews in de Waal, 2008; Silk & House, 2012; Warneken & Tomasello, 2009). Here, we review primates' performance in these experimental tasks, pointing out areas where there are still open questions in the field. After reviewing this new body of work on primates' prosocial preferences, we will argue that results from our own positive neuroscience project as well as results from other labs have demonstrated two clear cases where primates' social preferences may differ markedly from those of our own species. We will then discuss what these two differences mean for future studies investigating the neural mechanisms underlying human social behavior.

EXPLORING THE NATURE OF PRIMATE
SOCIAL PREFERENCES

Human prosociality is undoubtedly unique in many respects—no other species runs marathons to raise money for charities, engages in formal pedagogical instruction, and works to preserve the environment for strangers in future generations. Nevertheless, despite obvious differences, it is clear that primates naturally act in ways that benefit others in some contexts (see review in de Waal, 2008). One often-cited naturalistic example of primates' concern for others occurs in the aftermath of aggression. Primates from a variety of species will perform friendly behaviors toward another individual who was just part of a conflict (Aureli, Cords, & van Schaik, 2002). In one of the first studies of these post-aggression behaviors, de Waal and van Roosmalen (1979) observed that chimpanzees who had recently engaged in a fight would increase social contact with one another after the altercation, often grooming, embracing, or kissing each other shortly thereafter. This type of postconflict reunion, referred to as reconciliation, has now been documented in many different primate species (for a review, see Aureli et al., 2002). Some primates, specifically great apes, also engage in third-party consolation, in which individuals who were merely bystanders to the original aggressive situation seek out victims in order to give their support (e.g., Cordoni, Palagi, & Tarli, 2006; de Waal & Roosmalen 1979; Palagi, Cordoni, Borgognini, & Tarli, 2006). Such behaviors have been interpreted as evidence for a prosocial motivation to console victims of aggression (de Waal, 2008).

These cases of consolation suggest that primates are—at least in some cases—motivated to act in ways that make other conspecifics feel better. Unfortunately, although such naturalistic cases provide compelling hints that primates are concerned with other individuals' outcomes, it is rather tricky to compare such naturalistic behaviors with the sorts of measures used to test other-regarding preferences in humans. For this reason, primate researchers have recently begun developing experimental tests of primates' other-regarding tendencies that match tasks developed for humans (for a review of such human tasks, see Camerer, 2003). The goal of these new experimental approaches is to both advance our understanding of the cognitive factors that promote and hinder the expression of prosociality across primates and to address the question of whether such preferences in primates are similar to the other-regarding preferences observed in humans.

DO PRIMATES SHOW OTHER-REGARDING PREFERENCES IN EXPERIMENTAL TASKS?

Primate Instrumental Helping Tasks

One experimental task developed to test primates' prosocial preferences involves setting up cases in which primate participants have the opportunity to help another recipient reach a particular goal (e.g., Barnes, Hill, Langer, Martinez, & Santos, 2008; Drayton & Santos, 2014a; Skerry, Sheskin, & Santos, 2011; Warneken & Tomasello, 2006; Warneken, Hare, Melis, Hanus, & Tomasello, 2007; Yamamoto, Humle, & Tanaka, 2012). In one classic study, Warneken and Tomasello (2006) presented chimpanzees with situations in which a human experimenter appeared to have trouble achieving a certain goal, such as trying to get an out-of-reach object. Even though the chimpanzees were never rewarded for helping, they tended to help the humans achieve their goal at relatively high rates. Capuchin monkeys in our own lab also show high rates of helping human experimenters on this task, at least in cases in which they are given a reward for helping (Barnes et al., 2008). Finally, chimpanzees and bonobos are willing to help a conspecific obtain out-of-reach food items by unlocking a door that leads to the desired food (Hare & Kwetuenda, 2010; Warneken et al., 2007). In these helping studies, primates often (though not always, see Skerry et al., 2011) are willing to take small costs to perform actions that help others complete their goals.

Primate Donation Games

In an attempt to better compare primates' other-regarding preferences with those of adult humans tested on experimental economic tasks, primate cognition researchers have also developed a set of experimental "donation" methods in which primate subjects have the option to donate food to another conspecific. In a typical study (e.g., Silk et al., 2005), the actor primate can pull one of two tools: One gives him and a recipient a desirable piece of food, whereas the other gives the actor the same desirable piece of food but a smaller piece of food (or no food) to the recipient. Note that in this set-up, the actor's own reward does not differ between the two choices, and thus a preference for one choice over the other can be interpreted as reflecting a desire for giving the partner a specific outcome. Primate actors can therefore do one of three things: They can choose to give the recipient the generous option, they can be mean and give the recipient the less valued option, or they can act totally indifferent to the other individual's rewards and just choose randomly.

The logic of this donation task is pretty straightforward, but the pattern of primates' performance on this task has been anything but. When researchers first tested chimpanzees on this task, they were surprised to learn that chimpanzees did not seem to care about other individuals' payoffs (Jensen, Hare, Call, & Tomasello, 2006; Silk et al., 2005; Vonk et al., 2008); chimpanzees who have now been tested across a number of labs tend to perform at chance on this task, failing to show any preference for the recipient's payoff (although see Horner, Carter, Suchak, and de Waal [2011] for at least one study showing generous performance in chimpanzees on a similar choice task). Although this pattern of indifferent performance in chimpanzees is mirrored in some other primate species, such as cotton-top tamarin monkeys (Cronin, Schroeder, Rothwell, Silk, & Snowdon, 2009; Stevens, 2010), several other primate species show more generous performance on donation tasks (Burkart, Fehr, Efferson, & van Schaik, 2007; de Waal, Leimgruber, & Greenberg, 2008; Lakshminarayanan & Santos, 2008;

Takimoto, Kuroshima, & Fujita, 2010). Capuchin monkeys—the species we worked with in our own lab—have consistently performed generously on dona-tion tasks, statistically choosing to give the best possible reward to the recipient (de Waal et al., 2008; Lakshminarayanan & Santos, 2008; Takimoto et al., 2010). However, as our new studies as part of this positive neuroscience project have revealed, even in capuchins the actual rates of generous donations are relatively low (e.g., around 60%) and sometimes inconsistent across tasks (see Drayton & Santos, 2014b) for a case in which capuchins fail to behave generously on a dona-tion task). Interestingly, there is also evidence that capuchins perform generously only in situations in which the recipient can see their generous actions. de Waal et al. (2008), for example, found that actor capuchins selectively chose the mean option when the recipient monkey could not easily see them, suggesting that capuchins care about others' payoffs only in cases where they stand to gain some reputational benefit (for similar results in human children, see Leimgruber, Shaw, Santos, & Olson, 2012). Finally, as part of our positive neuroscience project, we have observed that capuchins' generosity on donation tasks depends a lot on their own recent interactions with others. Leimgruber et al. (2014) allowed capuchins to first play the role of the recipient on the donation game before acting as the actor in this task (Figure 5.1). They found that monkeys who received the bad pay-off as a recipient were statistically more likely to give the same bad payoff when they played the role of an actor donating to a different monkey; in contrast, when capuchins first received a prosocial payoff, they were reliably more likely to give a generous prosocial reward to a third monkey. These results suggest that monkeys' prosocial behaviors may be more shaped by their recent interactions with other individuals than a general preference to behave prosocially.

When all these disparate primate donation tasks findings are considered together, it is somewhat difficult to know what to conclude about primates' prosocial motivations. Even when primates do show generous performance on these tasks, their performance is relatively fragile at best. From this set of find-ings, it seems that most primate species lack a consistent human-like motive to be generous across all donation situations, which is particularly surprising since being nice involves no cost during this set-up.

Conclusions From Primate Experimental Economic Tasks

The experimental studies of primates' prosocial motivations to date reveal a somewhat complicated pattern of performance in experimental donation and helping tasks. On the one hand, some primates tested in instrumental helping tasks are motivated to take small costs to help other individuals complete their goals (see also Warneken & Tomasello, 2009). On the other hand, primates

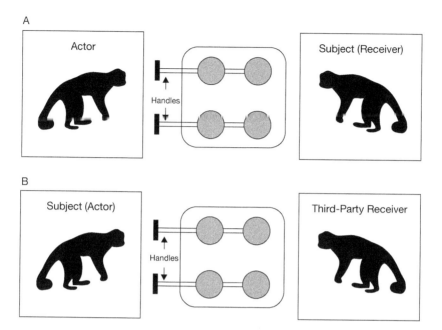

Figure 5.1 Schematic of testing set-up used in Leimgruber et al. (2014): (a) an actor monkey was given the opportunity to pull one of two handles. Pulling either handle delivered the same reward to the actor, but one of these handles delivered a good (prosocial) payoff to the subject and the other handle delivered a bad payoff; (b) the subject was then given the opportunity to choose whether to deliver a good or bad payoff to a third monkey. We found that subject monkeys tended to give the third monkey whatever they had received previously.

show relatively inconsistent prosociality when tested in food donation tasks, with few species showing consistently prosocial patterns across all studies (see Silk & House, 2012). In this way, primates do demonstrate some prosocial behaviors but fail to exhibit the sort of consistency regularly observed in the human species (e.g., Camerer & Thaler, 1995).

TWO POTENTIALLY HUMAN, UNIQUE SOCIAL MOTIVATIONS

Primates' inconsistent performance on the experimental tasks reviewed earlier makes it somewhat difficult to develop strong conclusions about the extent to which primates' prosocial preferences match the ones observed in the human species. However, more recent work using related experimental tasks has begun to suggest that primates may lack two salient aspects of human prosocial preferences.

Uniquely Human, Third-Party Punishment

The first domain in which primate preferences seem to differ from those of humans involves third-party situations. As both experimental and real-world examples attest, human prosocial behaviors often extend beyond cases of direct actions toward a recipient. Humans regularly take costly actions on behalf of unrelated individuals—we like to punish individuals who have behaved unfairly toward anonymous third parties (e.g., Fehr & Fischbacher, 2004) and to reward those who have done nice things to others we do not know (e.g., Almenberg, Dreber, Apicella, & Rand, 2011). Importantly, we are willing to prosocially reward and punish third-party individuals even in cases when we ourselves were not directly affected by these individuals' behaviors. In this way, humans seem to engage regularly in costly behaviors purely on behalf of other third parties. In addition, our species seems to exhibit these prosocial tendencies in third-party cases from early in life (Hamlin, Wynn, Bloom, & Mahajan, 2011), across all human cultures tested to date (Henrich et al., 2006), and fairly automatically (Rand, Greene, & Nowak, 2012).

Despite the widespread observation of third-party punishment and reward in the human species (Fehr & Fischbacher, 2004), there has been to date no experimental evidence that other primates care about what happens to other individuals in third-party situations. Riedl, Jensen, Call, and Tomasello (2012) developed an elegant experimental situation in which chimpanzees could punish those who stole food from others. In their set-up, subject chimpanzees had the opportunity to pull a heavy rope to open a trapdoor that dropped food that another conspecific was eating into an inaccessible location. The researchers then varied how that conspecific "thief" had obtained the food. In one case, the conspecific obtained the food by stealing it from the subject himself; in this case, Riedl et al. found that chimpanzees opened the trapdoor at high rates, ostensibly taking a small cost to punish an individual who had stolen food from them (see Jensen, Call, & Tomasello, 2007, for a similar result in chimpanzees, and Leimgruber, Rosati & Santos, 2015, for a similar result in capuchins). In contrast, when the thief had stolen the food from a third unrelated chimpanzee, subject chimpanzees tended not to release the trapdoor. Indeed, chimpanzees' rates of releasing the trapdoor in this third-party case were as low as a case in which there was no thief chimpanzee and no victim involved. As part of our positive neuroscience project, we have observed similar results in our own lab on a capuchin monkey test of third-party punishment (unpublished data). We allowed subject capuchins to watch how a second conspecific stooge monkey behaved toward an unrelated individual in a donation set-up. In some conditions, this stooge monkey behaved prosocially toward the third monkey, whereas in others he behaved selfishly, giving the smallest possible payoff. After witnessing the stooge monkey's behavior toward the third party, subjects then had a chance to donate food to the stooge. The question of interest was whether subjects would reward generous behavior and punish selfish behavior. Like chimpanzees, capuchins showed no evidence of third-party punishment—subjects did not donate differently to the stooge monkey based on his behavior toward a third party. Taken together, this work suggests that primates lack an important aspect of human prosocial preferences—in contrast to what is observed regularly in humans, primates' prosocial tendencies may not extend to third-party cases[1]; primates do not selectively punish or reward another conspecific except in cases in which they themselves were directly affected by that individual's behaviors.

Uniquely Human Advantageous Inequity Aversion

The second domain in which human prosocial preferences seem to obviously differ from those of other primates stems from situations of inequity. Much research has demonstrated that humans have a set of social preferences for avoiding cases in which rewards are distributed unevenly or unfairly across individuals. Overall, humans tend to be averse to inequity and will often take costs to ensure fair outcomes (Camerer & Thaler, 1995; Fehr & Schmidt, 1999). This aversion is perhaps unsurprising in cases of *disadvantageous inequity*, situations in which the individual in question receives less than is fair. However, people also show aversion to cases of *advantageous inequity*, situations in which they themselves benefit from having more than is fair. A number of experimental economic games have shown that people readily take costs to avoid having more than their fair share (Fehr & Schmidt, 1999). In this way, people tend to be almost as concerned that others' payoffs are fair as they are that their own payoffs are fair.

In the past few years, primate researchers have investigated whether other primates also share human-like preferences for avoiding inequity. In a famous study, Brosnan and de Waal (2003) argued that capuchins react negatively to cases of disadvantageous inequity. Brosnan and de Waal found that capuchins would stop performing a task if the reward they received (e.g., a low-valued cucumber) was less valuable than the reward given to a conspecific for performing a similar task (e.g., a high-valued grape). Although some researchers have failed to observe similar levels of inequity aversion in both capuchins (Dubreuil, Gentile, & Visalberghi, 2006; Silberberg, Crescimbene, Addessi, Anderson, & Visalberghi, 2009; Sheskin, Ashayeri, Skerry, & Santos, 2014) and other primates (Bräuer, Call, & Tomasello, 2006; but see Brosnan, Schiff, & de Waal, 2005), many have argued that primates do share human-like responses to cases of disadvantageous inequity (e.g., Brosnan, 2006). However, no research to date has shown that primates react negatively to cases of advantageous inequity, cases in which the subject gets unfairly more rewards than another individual. Indeed, Brosnan (2006) anecdotally noted that the stooge monkeys who received the high-valued rewards in her original experiment (Brosnan and de Waal, 2003) rarely rejected the higher valued reward when the subject monkeys received less. In fact, they sometimes preferred this advantageously inequitable situation:

> in several situations in which the subject rejected the cucumber slice, the partner would finish their grape and then reach through the mesh to take the subject's cucumber and eat it as well! Apparently to monkeys, cucumbers taste better if you have already had a grape. (Brosnan, 2006, p. 176)

To test more directly whether monkeys possess an aversion to advantageous inequity, we developed a test in which capuchin monkeys could choose between experimenters who had previously behaved either fairly or advantageously unfairly. Sheskin and colleagues (2014) first introduced capuchins to experimenters who provided either a fair payoff (one that was equal in value to that of a conspecific partner) or an advantageously unfair payoff (one that was better than the partner's). After being introduced to the behavior of these fair and unfair experimenters, subjects had the chance to obtain a high-valued reward from either the experimenter who had previously behaved fairly or the one who had previously behaved unfairly. Sheskin et al. found that monkeys performed at chance, failing to express a preference for the experimenter who behaved fairly over one who behaved advantageously unfairly[2]; monkeys basically ignored how the experimenter treated another conspecific so long as they themselves received a high-valued reward. In this way, monkeys' behavior seems to differ robustly from that of humans; humans are actively willing to take costs to avoid situations of advantageous inequity (e.g., Fehr & Schmidt, 1999), whereas monkeys seem indifferent to advantageous inequity situations even at no cost (Sheskin et al., under review).

CONCLUSION

Although other primates do behave prosocially in experimental tasks some of the time, overall primate prosociality seems to differ from that of humans in a few respects. First, primate prosocial preferences in experimental tasks seem relatively fragile. Second, other primates appear to critically lack two of the prosocial preferences observed widely in the human species—primates show no aversion to cases of advantageous inequity and are unwilling to take costs to punish others in third-party situations.

Taken together, the primate studies we have conducted and reviewed here suggest both important similarities and differences between human and non-human social preferences, ones that have valuable implications for neuroscientists interested in the neural basis of social preferences. On the one hand, these studies hint that primate reward systems may, like those of humans, be wired to respond to events that help others—at least under some circumstances. Future work using macaque neurophysiological techniques could potentially test these claims directly by employing the sorts of donation tasks reviewed earlier (for an example, see Chang, Gariepy, & Platt, 2013). On the other hand, the findings reviewed here suggest that reward processing in primate brains is likely to differ from humans in two critical respects. First, in contrast to humans (de Quervain et al., 2004), primates are unlikely to recruit neural areas associated with rewards when paying costs to punish others. Second, we predict that primates' reward regions will fail to respond less when primates receive unfairly high payoffs (e.g., Tabibnia et al., 2008; Zaki & Mitchell, 2011). In these two cases, we expect to find divergence in primate and human response patterns, with primate reward regions more tuned to selfish rather than prosocial rewards. Through experiments like these, neuroscientists could explore how differences in brain activity across species could potentially explain variation in the prosocial preferences observed across species.

NOTES

1. Note that some primatologists have argued that naturalistic cases of third-party policing (situations in which a dominant individual will intervene in a fight involving two unrelated individuals) may reflect cases of third-party punishment. However, many researchers have argued that these cases of naturalistic policing do not qualify as true examples of third-party punishment (see discussion in Riedl et al., 2012).
2. Monkeys in the Sheskin et al. (2014) study also failed to show a preference for a fair experimenter over one who behaved disadvantageously unfairly, again suggesting that primates' preference for equity may be fragile even in cases of disadvantageous inequity (see also Silk & House, 2012).

REFERENCES

Almenberg, J., Dreber, A., Apicella, C. L., & Rand, D. G. (2011). Third party reward and punishment: Group size, efficiency and public goods. In N. M. Palmetti & J. P. Russo (Eds.), *Psychology of punishment* (pp. 73–92). New York, NY: Nova Science.

Andreoni, J. (1990). Impure altruism and donations to public goods: A theory of warm-glow giving. *Economic Journal, 100,* 464–477.

Aureli, F., Cords, M., & van Schaik, C. P. (2002). Conflict resolution following aggression in gregarious animals: A predictive framework. *Animal Behaviour, 64,* 325–343.

Barnes, J. L., Hill, T., Langer, M., Martinez, M., & Santos, L. R. (2008). Helping behavior and regard for others in capuchin monkeys (*Cebus apella*). *Biology Letters, 4,* 638–640.

Bräuer, J., Call, J., & Tomasello, M. (2006). Are apes really inequity averse? *Proceedings of the Royal Society of London, Series B, 273,* 3123–3128.

Brosnan, S.F. (2006). Nonhuman species' reactions to inequity and their implications for fairness. *Social Justice Research, 19,* 153–185.

Brosnan, S. F., & de Waal, F. B. M. (2003). Monkeys reject unequal pay. *Nature, 425,* 297–299.

Brosnan, S. F., Schiff, H. C., & de Waal, F. B. M. (2005). Tolerance for inequity may increase with social closeness in chimpanzees. *Proceedings of the Royal Society of London, Series B, 272,* 253–258.

Burkart, J. M., Fehr, E., Efferson, C., & van Schaik, C. P. (2007). Other-regarding preferences in a non-human primate: Common marmosets provision food altruistically. *Proceedings of the National Academy of Sciences USA, 104,* 19762–19766.

Camerer, C. (2003). *Behavioral game theory.* Princeton, NJ: Princeton University Press.

Camerer, C. F., & Thaler, R. H. (1995). Anomalies: Dictators, ultimatums, and manners. *Journal of Economic Perspectives, 9,* 209–219.

Chang, S. W., Gariepy, J., & Platt, M. L. (2013). Neuronal reference frames for social decisions in primate frontal cortex. *Nature Neuroscience, 16,* 243–252.

Chang, S. W., Winecoff, A. A., & Platt, M. L. (2011). Vicarious reinforcement in rhesus macaques (*Macaca mulatta*). *Frontiers in Neuroscience, 5,* 27.

Cordoni, G., Palagi, E., & Tarli, S. (2006). Reconciliation and consolation in captive western gorillas. *International Journal of Primatology, 27,* 1365–1382.

Cronin, K. A., Schroeder, K. K., Rothwell, E. S., Silk, J. B., & Snowdon, C. T. (2009). Cooperatively breeding cottontop tamarins (*Saguinus oedipus*) do not donate rewards to their long-term mates. *Journal of Comparative Psychology, 123,* 231–241.

de Quervain, D. F., Fischbacher, U., Treyer, V., Schellhammer, M., Schnyder, U., Buck, A. & Fehr, E. (2004). The neural basis of altruistic punishment. *Science, 305,* 1254–1258.

de Waal, F. B. M. (2008). Putting the altruism back in altruism: The evolution of empathy. *Annual Review of Psychology, 59,* 279–300.

de Waal, F. B. M, Leimgruber, K., & Greenberg, A. R. (2008). Giving is self-rewarding for monkeys. *Proceedings of the National Academy of Sciences USA, 105,* 13685–13689.

de Waal, F. B. M., & van Roosmalen, A. (1979). Reconciliation and consolation among chimpanzees. *Behavioral Ecology and Sociobiology, 5,* 55–66.

Drayton, L. A., & Santos, L. R. (2014a). Capuchins' (*Cebus apella*) sensitivity to others' goal-directed actions in a helping context. *Animal Cognition, 17,* 689–700.

Drayton, L. A., & Santos, L. R. (2014b). Insights into intraspecies variation in primate prosocial behavior: Capuchins (*Cebus apella*) fail to show prosocial behavior on a touchscreen task. *Behavioral Sciences, 4,* 87–101.

Dubreuil, D., Gentile, M. S., & Visalberghi, E. (2006). Are capuchin monkeys (*Cebus apella*) inequity averse? *Proceedings of the Royal Society of London, Series B, 273,* 1223–1228.

Dunn, E. W., Aknin, L. B., & Norton, M. I. (2008). Spending money on others promotes happiness. *Science, 319*, 1687–1688.

Fehr, E., & Camerer, C. F. (2007). Social neuroeconomics: The neural circuitry of social preferences. *Trends in Cognitive Sciences, 11*, 419–427.

Fehr, E., & Fischbacher, U. (2004). Third-party punishment and social norms. *Evolution and Human Behavior, 25*, 63–87.

Fehr, E., & Schmidt, K. M. (1999). A theory of fairness, competition, and cooperation. *Quarterly Journal of Economics, 114*, 817–868.

Hamlin, J. K., Wynn, K., Bloom, P., & Mahajan, N. (2011). How infants and toddlers react to antisocial others. *Proceedings of the National Academy of Sciences USA, 108*, 19931–19936.

Harbaugh, W., Mayr, U., & Burghart, D. (2007). Neural responses to taxation and voluntary giving reveal motives for charitable donations. *Science, 316*, 1622–1625.

Hare, B., & Kwetuenda, S. (2010). Bonobos voluntarily share their own food with others. *Current Biology, 20*, R230–R231.

Henrich, J., McElreath, R., Barr, A., Ensminger, J., Barrett, C., Bolyanatz, A., . . . Ziker, J. (2006). Costly punishment across human societies. *Science, 312*, 1767–1770.

Horner, V., Carter, J. D., Suchak, M., & de Waal, F. B. M. (2011). Spontaneous prosocial choice by chimpanzees. *Proceedings of the National Academy of Sciences USA, 108*, 13847–13851.

Jensen, K., Call, J., & Tomasello, M. (2007). Chimpanzees are vengeful but not spiteful. *Proceedings of the National Academy of Sciences USA, 104*, 13046–13050.

Jensen, K., Hare, B., Call, J., & Tomasello, M. (2006). What's in it for me? Self-regard precludes altruism and spite in chimpanzees. *Proceedings of the Royal Society of London, Series B, 273*, 2013–2021.

Knutson, B., Adams, C. S., Fong, G. W., & Hommer, D. (2001). Anticipation of monetary reward selectively recruits nucleus accumbens. *Journal of Neuroscience, 21*, RC159.

Lakshminarayanan, V. R., & Santos, L. R. (2008). Capuchin monkeys are sensitive to others' welfare. *Current Biology, 18*, R999–1000.

Leimgruber, K. L., Rosati, A. G., & Santos, L. R. (2015). Capuchin monkeys punish those who have more. *Evolution and Human Behavior.* DOI: http://dx.doi.org/10.1016/j.evolhumbehav.2015.12.002

Leimgruber, K. L., Shaw, A., Santos, L. R., & Olson, K. R. (2012). Young children are more generous when others are aware of their actions. *PLoS ONE, 7*, e48292.

Leimgruber, K. L., Ward, A. F., Widness, J., Norton, M. I., Olson, K. R., Gray, K., & Santos, L. R. (2014). Give what you get: Capuchin monkeys (*Cebus apella*) and 4-year-old children pay forward positive and negative outcomes to conspecifics. *PLoS ONE, 9*, e87035.

Lyubomirsky, S., King, L. A., & Diener, E. (2005). The benefits of frequent positive affect. *Psychological Bulletin, 131*, 803–855.

Moll, J., Krueger, F., Zahn, R., Pardini, M., de Oliveira-Souza, R., & Grafman, J. (2006). Human fronto–mesolimbic networks guide decisions about charitable donation. *Proceedings of the National Academy of Sciences USA, 103*, 15623–15628.

O'Doherty, J., Deichmann, R., Critchley, H. D., & Dolan, R. J. (2002). Neural responses during anticipation of a primary taste reward. *Neuron, 33*, 815–826.

O'Doherty, J., Kringelbach, M. L., Rolls, E. T., Hornak, J., & Andrews, C. (2001). Abstract reward and punishment representations in the human orbitofrontal cortex. *Nature Neuroscience, 4,* 95–102.

Palagi, E., Cordoni, G., & Borgognini Tarli, S. (2006). Possible roles of consolation in captive chimpanzees (*Pan troglodytes*). *American Journal of Physical Anthropology, 129,* 105–111.

Rand, D. G., Greene, J. D., & Nowak, M. A. (2012). Spontaneous giving and calculated greed. *Nature, 489,* 427–430.

Riedl, K., Jensen, K., Call, J., & Tomasello, M. (2012). No third-party punishment in chimpanzees. *Proceedings of the National Academy of Sciences USA, 109,* 14824–14829.

Seligman, M. (2002). *Authentic happiness: Using the new positive psychology.* New York, NY: Free Press.

Sheskin, M., Ashayeri, K., Skerry, A., & Santos, L. (2014). Capuchin monkeys (*Cebus apella*) fail to show inequality aversion in a no-cost situation. *Evolution and Human Behavior, 35,* 80–88.

Silberberg, A., Crescimbene, L., Addessi, E., Anderson, J. R., & Visalberghi, E. (2009). Does inequity aversion depend on a frustration effect? A test with capuchin monkeys (*Cebus apella*). *Animal Cognition, 12,* 505–509.

Silk, J. B., Brosnan, S. F., Vonk, J., Henrich, J., Povinelli, D. J., Richardson, A. S., . . . Schapiro, S. J. (2005). Chimpanzees are indifferent to the welfare of unrelated group members. *Nature, 437,* 1357–1359.

Silk, J. B., & House, B. R. (2012). The phylogeny and ontogeny of prosocial behavior. In T. Shackelford & J. Vonk (Eds.), *The Oxford handbook of comparative evolutionary psychology* (pp. 381–397). New York, NY: Oxford University Press.

Singer, T., & Fehr, E. (2005). The neuroeconomics of mind reading and empathy. *American Economic Review, 95,* 340–345.

Skerry, A. E, Sheskin, M., & Santos, L. R. (2011). Capuchin monkeys are not prosocial in an instrumental helping task. *Animal Cognition, 14,* 647–654.

Stevens, J. R. (2010). Donor payoffs and other regarding preferences in cotton-top tamarins (*Saguinus oedipus*). *Animal Cognition, 13,* 663–670.

Tabibnia, G., Satpute, A. B., & Lieberman, M. D. (2008). The sunny side of fairness: Preference for fairness activates reward circuitry (and disregarding unfairness activates self-control circuitry). *Psychological Science, 19,* 339–347.

Takimoto, A., Kuroshima, H., & Fujta, K. (2010). Capuchin monkeys (*Cebus apella*) are sensitive to others' reward: An experimental analysis of food-choice for conspecifics. *Animal Cognition, 13,* 249–261.

Thoits, P. A., & Hewitt, L. N. (2001). Volunteering work and well-being. *Journal of Health Social Behavior, 42,* 115–131.

Vonk, J., Brosnan, S. F., Silk, J. B., Henrich, J., Richardson, A. S., Lambeth, S. P., . . . Povinelli, D. J. (2008). Chimpanzees do not take advantage of very low cost opportunities to deliver food to unrelated group members. *Animal Behaviour, 75,* 1757–1770.

Warneken, F., Hare, B., Melis, A. P., Hanus, D., & Tomasello, M. (2007). Spontaneous altruism by chimpanzees and young children. *PLoS Biology, 5,* e184.

Warneken, F., & Tomasello, M. (2006). Altruistic helping in human infants and young chimpanzees. *Science, 311,* 1301–1303.

Warneken, F., & Tomasello, M. (2009). Varieties of altruism in children and chimpanzees. *Trends in Cognitive Sciences, 13,* 397–402.

Yamamoto, S., Humle, T., & Tanaka, M. (2012). Chimpanzees' flexible targeted helping based on an understanding of conspecifics' goals. *Proceedings of the National Academy of Sciences USA, 108,* 3588–3592.

Zaki, J., & Mitchell, J. P. (2011). Equitable decision making is associated with neural markers of intrinsic value. *Proceedings of the National Academy of Sciences USA, 108,* 19761–19766.

6

When Feeling and Doing Diverge

Neural and Physiological Correlates of the Empathy–Altruism Divide

TONY W. BUCHANAN AND STEPHANIE D. PRESTON ■

Observing another individual in distress often elicits feelings of empathy and sympathy with a target, defined here as matching or resonating emotions *with* the target (empathy) and feelings of other-oriented compassion *for* the target (sympathy). While we can often imagine such states and situations in response to another's distress or need, do these feelings play a causal role in our decisions to help? Most existing research and theory assume that they do (Batson, 2011; de Waal, 2008; Eisenberg & Fabes, 1990; Preston & de Waal, 2002; Rapson, Hatfield, & Cacioppo, 1993). For example, perception-action models of empathy (PAM; Preston & de Waal, 2002), rooted in early philosophical models of sympathy (Hume, 1739-1740/1990; Lipps, 1903; Merleau-Ponty, 1962/1970) and perception-action concepts in motor psychology (Prinz, 1997), propose that our motivation to help derives from a basic nervous system design that maps the feelings perceived in others onto the observer's own substrates for feeling emotions. This nervous system design elegantly provides observers with access to another's state while simultaneously motivating them to help.

Considerable research already supports this view. For example, people often report feeling similar emotions in themselves that they observe in the target, and the observation of another individual in distress or pain can elicit physiological reactivity in the observer, which can even be linked to the observer's subsequent motivation to help (see review in Buchanan, Bagley, Stansfield, & Preston, 2012). Much of the existing neuroscientific work on this topic has focused on measures of the autonomic nervous system, skeletomuscular system, or indices of neural blood flow. Krebs (1975), for example, demonstrated many years ago that observers who reported feeling similar to confederates feigning pain and pleasure showed matching autonomic activity to them and donated more money to their similar partners, compared to dissimilar partners. Harrison and colleagues measured neural activity via functional magnetic resonance imaging and pupillary responses in individuals viewing images of sad faces. These observers showed changes in pupil size (controlled by the autonomic nervous system) that were correlated with the size of the pupil in the sad faces. They also observed changes in the level of activation in the brainstem region (hemodynamic changes reflective of neural blood flow) that controls pupillary function (Harrison, Singer, Rotshtein, Dolan, & Critchley, 2006). A large body of research has also documented overlapping neural activity associated with the first-person experience of pain and the observation of pain in others (see reviews in Decety & Jackson, 2006; Singer, 2006). Perceived pain in a conspecific mouse even produces the psychophysiological orienting response associated with empathic concern in humans (Chen, Panksepp, & Lahvis, 2009). Beyond pain, basic emotions such as fear, anger, and sadness have also shown to activate overlapping emotional, physiological, and neural responses when people imagine their own emotional experiences or try to imagine the experience of another person from within "their shoes" (Preston et al., 2007).

At the level of the underlying proximate mechanism, this empathic response has only rarely been clearly linked to helping in the immediate situation (see Krebs, 1975), but there are indications that the response correlates with trait measures of empathy (e.g., Singer et al., 2004), which have been shown to predict real-world or laboratory decisions to help (Davis, 1983a). More important, however, critics rightly point out that these more "automatic" views of empathy, which emphasize the degree to which people spontaneously activate personal representations of emotion when viewing those of the target, cannot explain why people so often do *not* help, sometimes even causing and enjoying others' distress (see commentary in Preston & de Waal, 2002, and Preston, 2013). Conversely, the most salient cases of heroic altruism in the national media almost always include explanations from the hero that she or he simply rushed in to help without even thinking—an instinct that is compatible with an automatic theory of empathy or altruism, but strangely lacks the subjective feelings like empathy and sympathy that have been so emphasized by experimental work on the empathy–altruism link (cf., Batson, 2011; Preston, 2013; Preston & Hofelich, 2012).

Taken together, an *empathy–altruism divide* exists in our behavior, theories, and research on the ways in which empathy does versus does not produce altruistic giving. In this chapter, we outline recent research and theory on how to reconcile these seemingly incongruous facts into a unified view of how observers represent and respond to others in need. We specifically outline more recent theoretical models that better explain how to integrate empathy and altruism, by focusing upon the necessity for emotional neural responses to understand others' plight as well as the physiological activation needed during active altruism that was previously overlooked. We also describe the results of our first studies to test this hypothesis, by examining the physiological resonance of the cortisol stress response between stressed targets and their observers.

NEW THEORETICAL APPROACHES TO BRIDGING THE EMPATHY–ALTRUISM DIVIDE

A Dynamic Systems View of Empathy

NEURAL VERSUS SUBJECTIVE SELF–OTHER OVERLAP

The first issue to address is the degree to which a perception-action mechanism implies that observers should *feel* the emotions of the observed target (for the detailed version of this argument, see Preston & Hofelich, 2012). Most assume that PAM models imply a direct correspondence between observation and feeling with the other. However, at the level of the proximate mechanism, observers are expected to only feel the target's state under particular conditions, which also only lead to helping under even more restricted conditions. In brief, a biological, dynamic-systems view assumes that all forms of empathy require self–other overlap at the level of the neural representation, which is the only automatic component in the model. Neural-level self–other overlap (that is, activating your personal representations for the target's state and situation) is absolutely required to accurately model and understand how the other feels. However, there are multiple reasons that this neural-level activation need not produce subjective feelings of empathy or sympathy in the observer or be accompanied by accurate understanding or aid. Activation of neural representations for the other's state can occur at a low level, below the threshold required to produce a downstream affective state that the observer would subjectively feel. The observer also may not have had a sufficiently similar past affective experience to that of the target, which would preclude understanding and accuracy, and limit the ability to generate a similar state. Even if the observer did feel a similar emotion to that of the target, these feelings can sometimes promote aid and sometimes inhibit aid (especially if they cause a self-focused state of distress). Therefore, complaints about how perception-action processes cannot be explanatory because people are not always walking around imitating others or feeling their emotions misunderstand the way that neural activity and subjective experience depart.

DISSOCIATING EMPATHY AND SYMPATHY

Having explained how one can observe another without feeling self–other overlap (due to the dissociation between neural and felt overlap), we next need to address when helping does and does not involve compassionate or sympathetic feelings toward the other—the emotions so prominently emphasized by the prosocial literature to date (see Batson, 1987; Batson, Early, & Salvarani, 1997; Batson & Shaw, 1991; Wispe, 1986). (Note that this sympathetic state of warm, tenderhearted, compassion is labeled "empathy" by Batson and colleagues (1987) and empathic or sympathetic concern by some others (e.g., Davis, 1983b; Zahn-Waxler & Radke-Yarrow, 1990).

At the level of the proximate mechanism, empathy (feeling *with* the other) does not compete with sympathy (feeling *for* the other). According to the PAM, neural self–other overlap occurs spontaneously during perception and can proceed to either empathy or sympathy, depending upon the conditions. However, testifying to the need for at least neural self–other overlap to experience sympathy, the most common method for inducing sympathy in the lab is to increase the perceived similarity between the target and observer or to instruct the observer to imagine how the target feels (Batson & Coke, 1981; Batson et al., 1997; Krebs, 1975). Thus, inducing greater self–other overlap assists in the process of generating sympathy for another's plight, as long as the observer does not begin to feel that she or he is the one in primary need.

WHEN IS SYMPATHY EVOKED?

Sympathy, in particular, appears to be evoked when the target is vulnerable, and it activates a nurturant response in the observer, like the tender feelings one has toward neonates or small animals (see Batson, 2011; de Waal, 2009; Preston, 2013). As such, it is not an accident that most sympathy and helping inductions involve children (e.g., Batson et al., 1988; Eisenberg et al., 1989, 1991; Toi & Batson, 1982). This surely reflects the evolution of sympathy as a tender emotion originating in the context of caregiving between mother and offspring (Batson, Lishner, Cook, & Sawyer, 2005; de Waal, 2008; Eibl-Eibesfeldt, 1971/1974; McDougall, 1908/1923; Schulkin, 2000). Because of this, the neural substrates of empathy should not overlap completely with sympathy or active altruism, because empathy need not engage the neural circuits for offspring care the same way that sympathy and altruism should (e.g., for nursing, retrieving, and huddling neonates; see caregiving view later). Additionally, sympathy requires the observer to have the time and distance to engage passively in reflection about how the target feels, without needing to act right away. For example, classic empathy–altruism paradigms require subjects to read or hear about targets after an accident or a loss, where their help is not needed right away but over the course of the coming months (Batson et al., 1988; Batson, O'Quin, Fultz, Vanderplas, & Isen, 1983; Eisenberg et al., 1989; Toi & Batson, 1982). In these cases, the target is vulnerable and has a serious need, but not an immediate one. The resulting tender feelings then can be subjectively appreciated by the passive observer, who then uses the feelings as affective inputs into his or her decision to help. Such cases contrast with those described later, when observers appear to help, even immediately, without first experiencing a sympathetic state.

The Caregiving View of Active Altruism

Helping Without Sympathy

Sometimes observers see a helpless and vulnerable target, but the danger and need are immediate (e.g., see Dovidio, Piliavin, Schroeder, & Penner, 2006; Latané, 1969). In such cases, the observer may act first, for example, rushing to pull a child out of a road or icy pond, only later reflecting upon their feelings. Because of the immediate response component, such aid can occur without the sustained, reflective feelings like sadness or sympathy (Dovidio et al., 2006). However, the PAM predicts that such automatic helping also requires preexisting representations in the observer for the appropriate behavioral response, which may explain why real-world heroes often report rushing into danger without thinking while those who do not help usually report not knowing what to do (Post, 2003).

The Requirement for Arousal and Activation

The urge to help an imperiled target may reflect an ancient neural system designed for offspring care, which has been extensively studied in rodents (see Brown, Brown, & Preston, 2011; Preston, 2013). As in rescue scenarios, rodent mothers must quickly retrieve their helpless and isolated newborns who have become separated from the nest. Dams are primed by perinatal hormones that motivate them to immediately retrieve these isolated and distressed pups, mediated by connections among the amygdala, hypothalamus, dopaminergic reward system, and downstream motor output systems (see Figure 6.1 from Preston, 2013; Lonstein & Morrell, 2007; Numan & Insel, 2003). This arrangement adaptively facilitates proximity with offspring, ensuring their safety and successful development. While the system evolved to ensure care in postpartum mothers, the response can also be elicited in nonmothers and males who are habituated to newborns. According to this "caregiving model of altruism" (Preston, 2013),

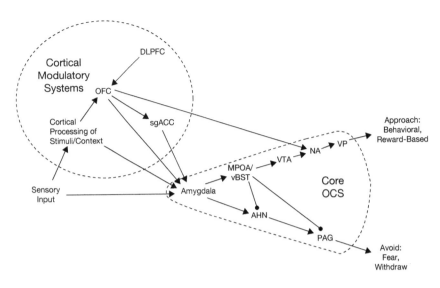

Figure 6.1 Major elements of the extended caregiving system. The major elements of
the rodent offspring care system (OCS) are retained in the more general caregiving
system in humans as core neural processes. The sensory input in the human caregiving
system is expected to be biased toward visual and auditory cues of distress, but the
core rodent offspring care system still exists in this expanded model, and olfactory
inputs likely still play an important role in maternal care, offspring recognition,
and bonding between kin and mates. The caregiving system augments the rodent
offspring care system with domain-general reward and decision processes in the
neocortex (particularly the prefrontal cortex), which augment caregiving to account
for the complexity of human altruistic responding. Note that only the most important
functional connections described in the text are included in the figure; known
connections among these areas and to other areas are not shown for simplicity.
AHN = anterior hypothalamus; PAG = periaqueductal gray; MPOA = medial preoptic
area of the hypothalamus; vBST = ventral bed of the stria terminalis; VTA = ventral
tegmental area; NAcc = nucleus accumbens; VP = ventral pallidum.
(From Preston, 2013; reprinted with permission.)

both empathy and active caregiving require the attention and understanding of
the observer, but only the caregiving response to an imperiled target requires
this motivating neurohormonal state and downstream response. The latter
requirements are not present in most scenarios and, thus, self–other overlap at
the neural level is considered necessary, but not sufficient, for active altruism.

Our subsequent experimental research has been particularly directed at this
aspect of the theoretical divide between empathy and altruism. The caregiving
model (Preston, 2013) makes many predictions in common with classic psychological models of prosocial behavior, particularly the assumption that empathy,
sympathy, and helping originate from behaviors originally designed to care

for related offspring. However, only the model by Preston (2013)—because it is rooted in the neuroscientific literature on expertise and offspring care—makes specific predictions about the role of one's ability to help in the particular need situation and the requirement for motor-autonomic activation to act quickly and effectively. Thus, the remainder of this chapter describes our initial experimental research conducted under the Positive Neuroscience project to demonstrate related key tenants of the PAM and caregiving model, particularly the role of motor-autonomic arousal and activation in the response to another's need.

NEW EXPERIMENTAL APPROACHES TO BRIDGE THE EMPATHY–ALTRUISM DIVIDE

The physiological stress response, as it has been studied in the biopsychology literature to date, is assumed to be designed to mobilize one's metabolic energy in situations of acute need (e.g., see Sapolsky, 2009; Sapolsky, Romero, & Munck, 2000). For example, when a male subordinate primate detects the presence of a dominant individual who is known to lash out at subordinates, a stress response may be activated in the observing subordinate that temporarily delays longer term processes like recovery and digestion while rendering him more capable of fighting or running away. Not only do physical threats activate the stress system, but psychological ones do as well, particularly in group-living animals like primates, including humans (Sapolsky, 1994). Thus, in human research, the most humane and reliable way to activate the stress system is to impose a psychological threat, for example in situations of uncontrollable social evaluation. In the current work we define stress as the perceived inability to cope with a challenge to well-being that includes motivated performance, uncontrollability, and social evaluation (after Mason, 1968).

There are many examples of situations in which we observe stress in others: a nervous public speaker, a harried coworker, or a waitstaff overloaded with customers during a busy lunch shift. These situations certainly make us feel bad for the individual under stress, but it is unknown whether such feelings reflect truly resonating forms of stress, in the sense that these feelings elicit the same physiological stress response in the observer as in the stressed target. It is likely that the observation of stress in a target will elicit simple arousal and bad feelings in an observer, but this is not the same as stress. The aforementioned characteristics of stress have a neurohormonal signature that includes activation of the hypothalamic-pituitary-adrenocortical (HPA) axis, which results in the release of cortisol (Dickerson & Kemeny, 2004). To demonstrate true empathic stress resonance between an observer and a target, the response of the observer must be the direct result of observing the target's response and must be similar in quality and proportion to the target's response (after McDougall, 1908/1923).

We first wanted to confirm, in keeping with the PAM, that physiological stress could resonate between individuals (Buchanan et al., 2012). We used the gold standard of laboratory stress in humans: the Trier Social Stress Test (TSST; Kirschbaum, Pirke, & Hellhammer, 1993). The TSST is a standardized laboratory task that reliably activates the HPA in participant speakers performing a speech and mental arithmetic before observing experimenters. A meta-analysis examining the efficacy of laboratory stressors demonstrated that the TSST includes all of the components that are most effective in eliciting a stress-induced cortisol response: motivated performance, uncontrollability, and social evaluation (Dickerson & Kemeny, 2004). In the typical TSST, physiological measures such as salivary alpha amylase (sAA; an index of autonomic function) and cortisol are collected from the person who undergoes the public speaking and mental arithmetic tasks before observing experimenters. In our "empathic TSST" (or eTSST), we collected sAA and cortisol from the observing experimenters (hereafter "observers") as well as the stressed speakers. This design allowed us to assess the physiological resonance of stress during an actual social situation. This is in contrast to most research in the area, which assesses resonance only indirectly by measuring physiology from one observer while viewing images of targets presumed to be in distress or confederates simulating pain or distress. To assess the role that trait empathy may play in the physiological resonance of stress, observers in our eTSST also completed the Interpersonal Reactivity Index (IRI; Davis, 1983b), a multidimensional trait empathy index with separate subscales for empathic concern, personal distress, perspective taking, and fantasy. Our results showed that observers did indeed produce resonant cortisol responses in response to viewing stressed speakers. The observers' cortisol responses were proportional to the responses of their paired speakers and were not affected by the sex of the observer or the speaker (e.g., male observers did not secrete more cortisol in response to female compared to male speakers). Furthermore, observers' trait empathic concern and perspective taking, assessed via the IRI (Davis, 1983b), were positively correlated with their cortisol and sAA responses (see Figure 6.2).

These findings provide the first evidence of empathic physiological resonance of the cortisol stress response (Buchanan et al., 2012). This response does not merely reflect a shared arousal between participants, as the cortisol response is not elicited by simple arousal (Lovallo et al., 1985; Lundberg & Frankenhaeuser, 1980), but requires combined feelings of uncontrollability and social evaluation (Dickerson & Kemeny, 2004). This resonance is particularly noteworthy given the difficulty in producing cortisol responses in

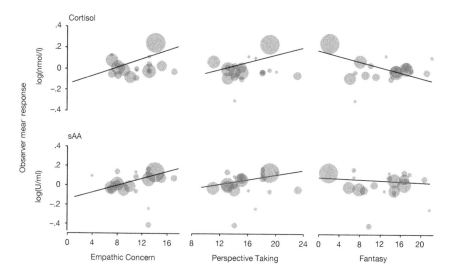

Figure 6.2 Weighted scatter plots showing associations between mean log-transformed observers' (N = 20) cortisol (top) and sAA (bottom) and trait measures of empathy from the Interpersonal Reactivity Index (IRI; see Davis, 1983b), including subscales for empathic concern (left), perspective taking (middle), and fantasy (right). Bubble sizes indicate the weight (number of observations: range 1 to 34), and trend lines indicate weighted correlations.

(From Buchanan, Bagley, Stansfield, and Preston, 2012; reprinted with permission.)

the laboratory (only 70% of TSST participants produce a cortisol response; Kirschbaum et al., 1993), and these responses are not reliably linked to observable behavior or self-reports of affect in the speakers (Abelson, 1989; Buchanan, al'Absi, & Lovallo, 1999). The "stress" signals from the speakers that the observers must have used to detect and resonate with their stress are currently uncertain but are being investigated. The PAM predicts that observers process a combination of signals such as speech patterns and nonverbal behavior from the stressed speaker, which are centrally processed by the observer, leading to the activation of a similar state in the observer. More empathic observers may show more physiological resonance with a speaker because they attend more closely to the speaker's behavior across channels (Hofelich & Preston, 2011). Future work will address the verbal and nonverbal cues from the speakers that may reliably lead to physiological resonance in observers as well as observer characteristics that predict greater reactivity.

It is also currently unknown whether this contagious or empathic stress response in observers of stress will predispose observers to help. The caregiving model predicts that observers who become contagiously activated by the immediate plight of the target should be more likely to help, but this is only for situations that require an immediate response that the observer can enact (Preston, 2013). In the TSST there is no obvious "response" that the observer could do to calm the target, other than maybe offering reassuring feedback. Moreover, stress physiology is generally more closely linked to antisocial, rather than prosocial behaviors (Miczek et al., 2007). However, other recent studies have shown that stress can lead to prosocial behaviors. For example, while males often exhibit a "fight-or-flight" response to stress, females may be better characterized by a more prosocial "tend and befriend" response (Preston, 2013; Taylor et al., 2000). Tending, meaning caring for offspring, and befriending, meaning connecting with conspecifics, together protects an organism's offspring and may help social groups collaborate group under stressful conditions. Preston (2013) extends this framework beyond females under stress to suggest a more general system that includes nonmothers (even males) to explain a host of findings that predict altruism during times of acute situation-related stress (i.e., emergencies). A recent empirical study provides support for the concept that stress can lead to prosocial behavior, even in males. In this study, healthy young men were exposed to a stressor (the TSST) or a non-stressful task, followed by a battery of tasks to assess prosocial and antisocial behaviors. The stress actually led to increased trust, trustworthiness, and sharing behavior, and no changes in punishment (an index of antisocial behavior) or nonsocial risk taking (von Dawans, Fischbacher, Kirschbaum, Fehr, & Heinrichs, 2012). These findings are counter to the notion that stressed men would automatically revert to an antisocial fight-or-flight behavior pattern and instead indicate that stress can promote prosocial behavior. The authors of the study suggest a potential role for oxytocin, which is released during stress (Pierrehumbert, Torrisi, Ansermet, Borghini, & Halfon, 2012; Pierrehumbert et al., 2010) and is known to increase social approach and prosocial behaviors (Carter, 1998; Insel & Young, 2001; Kosfeld, Heinrichs, Zak, Fischbacher, & Fehr, 2005), particularly in caregiving contexts (Preston, 2013; Taylor et al., 2000). Alternatively, stress could shift people's cooperative decision making from a deliberative to a more intuitive strategy, akin to the increased prosociality when people decide more quickly (Rand, Greene, & Nowak, 2012). Perhaps the pressure exerted by stress speeds up decisions regarding cooperation, resulting in a more intuitive decision to behave altruistically. In our research under the Positive Neuroscience project, we are extending this to the context of the secondary empathic stress in observers of the TSST in our eTSST paradigm. We aim to determine if either the speakers or the observers would act more prosocially after the speech, particularly when allowed to interact directly with one another. We will also assess any changes in emotion processing that may influence these results.

CONCLUSION

People have long been interested in the extent to which humans are essentially good or prosocial versus bad and self-serving, with plenty of evidence supporting at least some capacity for each. Research into the mammalian nervous system, particularly in group-living animals that provide extensive care for offspring, suggests that our system is at least designed to allow for the fairly spontaneous ability to feel with others' emotions, which, under the right conditions, can also motivate us to understand them, care about their plight, and feel motivated to help. In addition, the neural circuits that must have evolved primarily to support the care and protection of helpless neonates appear to be activated to nonkin in situations that mimic the needs of offspring. When other individuals are in immediate danger, distress, or need—particularly when they are vulnerable due to age, ability, or situation—the caregiving instinct appears to be activated, which can produce active aid without intervening feelings of empathy or sympathy. Of course, people may not help when they feel scared for their own safety or when they do not know how to respond, which similarly reflects a natural mammalian neural arrangement that opposes approach and avoidance mechanisms when it is adaptive. Much has already been learned at the intersection of psychology and neuroscience about the source for our (sometimes) astonishing capacity for good. However, there are still many mysteries to unravel. Future work needs to particularly focus on likely gender differences in the response to nurturant versus active or heroic need, the exact way in which glucocorticoid and oxytocin systems interact in the brain, and the multimodal cues that observers use to infer the stress or need of others. Through integrative research, which views human behavior through the lens of our evolved neural and psychological systems, we can understand why we are simultaneously capable of good and evil, finally permitting us to predict our variable response to need while shaping our future responses for the "greater good."

REFERENCES

Abelson, J. (1989). Cardiac and neuroendocrine responses to exposure therapy in height phobics: Desynchrony within the "physiological response system." *Behaviour Research and Therapy, 27*(5), 561.

Batson, C. D. (1987). Prosocial motivation: Is it ever truely altruistic? *Advances in Experimental Social Psychology, 20,* 65–122.

Batson, C. D. (2011). *Altruism in humans.* New York, NY: Oxford University Press.

Batson, C. D., & Coke, J. (1981). Empathy: A source of altruistic motivation for helping. In J. Rushton & R. Sorrentino (Eds.), *Altruism and helping behavior.* Hillsdale, NJ: Erlbaum.

Batson, C. D., Dyck, J. L., Brandt, J. R., Batson, J. G., Powell, A. L., McMaster, M. R., & Griffit, C. (1988). Five studies testing the new egoistic alternatives to the empathy-altruism hypothesis. *Journal of Personality and Social Psychology, 55*(1), 52–77. doi:10.1037/0022-3514.55.1.52

Batson, C. D., Early, S., & Salvarani, G. (1997). Perspective taking: Imagining how another feels versus imaging how you would feel. *Personality and Social Psychology Bulletin, 23*(7), 751758.

Batson, C. D., Fultz, J., & Schoenrade, P. A. (1987). Distress and empathy: Two qualitatively distinct vicarious emotions with different motivational consequences. *Journal of Personality, 55*(1), 19–39. doi:10.1111/j.1467-6494.1987.tb00426.x

Batson, C. D., Lishner, D. A., Cook, J., & Sawyer, S. (2005). Similarity and nurturance: Two possible sources of empathy for strangers. *Basic and Applied Social Psychology, 27*(1), 15–25. doi:10.1207/S15324834basp2701_2

Batson, C. D., O'Quin, K., Fultz, J., Vanderplas, M., & Isen, A. M. (1983). Influence of self-reported distress and empathy on egoistic versus altruistic motivation to help. *Journal of Personality and Social Psychology, 45*(3), 706–718.

Batson, C. D., & Shaw, L. (1991). Evidence for altruism: Toward a pluralism of prosocial motives. *Psychological Inquiry, 2*(2), 107–122.

Brown, S. L., Brown, R. M., & Preston, S. D. (2011). A model of human caregiving motivation. In S. L. Brown, R. M. Brown, & L. A. Penner (Eds.), *Moving beyond self interest: Perspectives from evolutionary biology, neuroscience, and the social sciences.* New York, NY: Oxford University Press.

Buchanan, T. W., al'Absi, M., & Lovallo, W. R. (1999). Cortisol fluctuates with increases and decreases in negative affect. *Psychoneuroendocrinology, 24*(2), 227–241.

Buchanan, T. W., Bagley, S. L., Stansfield, R. B., & Preston, S. D. (2012). The empathic, physiological resonance of stress. *Social Neuroscience, 7*(2), 191–201. doi:10.1080/17470919.2011.588723

Carter, C. S. (1998). Neuroendocrine perspectives on social attachment and love. *Psychoneuroendocrinology, 23*, 779–818.

Chen, Q., Panksepp, J. B., & Lahvis, G. P. (2009). Empathy is moderated by genetic background in mice. *PLoS One, 4*(2), e4387. doi:10.1371/journal.pone.0004387

Davis, M. H. (1983a). The effects of dispositional empathy on emotional reactions and helping: A multidimensional approach. *Journal of Personality, 51*(2), 167–184.

Davis, M. H. (1983b). Measuring individual differences in empathy: Evidence for a multidimensional approach. *Journal of Personality and Social Psychology, 44*(1), 113–126.

de Waal, F. B. M. (2008). Putting the altruism back into altruism: The evolution of empathy. *Annual Review of Psychology, 59*(1), 279–300. doi:10.1146/annurev.psych.59.103006.093625

Decety, J., & Jackson, P. L. (2006). A social-neuroscience perspective on empathy. *Current Directions in Psychological Science, 15*(2), 54–58. doi: 10.1111/j.0963-7214.2006.00406.x

Dickerson, S. S., & Kemeny, M. E. (2004). Acute stressors and cortisol responses: A theoretical integration and synthesis of laboratory research. *Psychological Bulletin, 130*, 355–391.

Dovidio, J. F., Piliavin, J. A., Schroeder, D. A., & Penner, L. A. (2006). *The social psychology of prosocial behavior*. Mahwah, NJ: Erlbaum.

Eibl-Eibesfeldt, I. (1971/1974). *Love and hate* (G. Strachan, Trans., 2nd ed.). New York, NY: Schocken Books.

Eisenberg, N., & Fabes, R. A. (1990). Empathy: Conceptualization, measurement, and relation to prosocial behavior. *Motivation and Emotion, 14*(2), 131–149. doi:10.1007/Bf00991640

Eisenberg, N., Fabes, R. A., Miller, P. A., Fultz, J., Shell, R., Mathy, R. M., & Reno, R. R. (1989). Relation of sympathy and personal distress to prosocial behavior: A multimethod study. *Journal of Personality and Social Psychology, 57*(1), 55–66. doi:10.1037/0022-3514.57.1.55

Eisenberg, N., Fabes, R. A., Schaller, M., Miller, P., Carlo, G., Poulin, R., . . . Shell, R. (1991). Personality and socialization correlates of vicarious emotional responding. *Journal of Personality and Social Psychology, 61*(3), 459–470. doi:10.1037/0022-3514.61.3.459

Harrison, N. A., Singer, T., Rotshtein, P., Dolan, R. J., & Critchley, H. D. (2006). Pupillary contagion: Central mechanisms engaged in sadness processing. *Social Cognitive and Affective Neuroscience, 1*(1), 5–17. doi:10.1093/scan/nsl006

Hofelich, A. J., & Preston, S. D. (2011). The meaning in empathy: Distinguishing conceptual encoding from facial mimicry, trait empathy, and attention to emotion. *Cognition and Emotion, 26*(1), 119–128. doi:10.1080/02699931.2011.559192

Hume, D. (1990). *A treatise of human nature* (7th impression of 2nd ed.). Oxford, UK: Clarendon Press. (Originally published in 1739-1740).

Insel, T. R., & Young, L. J. (2001). The neurobiology of attachment. *Nature Reviews Neuroscience, 2*, 129–135.

Kirschbaum, C., Pirke, K-M., & Hellhammer, D. H. (1993). The "Trier Social Stress Test"- A tool for investigating psychobiological stress responses in a laboratory setting. *Neuropsychobiology, 28*, 76–81.

Kosfeld, M., Heinrichs, M., Zak, P. J., Fischbacher, U., & Fehr, E. (2005). Oxytocin increases trust in humans. *Nature, 435*, 673–676.

Krebs, D. (1975). Empathy and altruism. *Journal of Personality and Social Psychology, 32*(6), 1134–1146. doi:10.1037/0022-3514.32.6.1134

Latané, B. (1969). A lady in distress: Inhibiting effects of friends and strangers on bystander intervention. *Journal of Experimental Social Psychology, 5*(2), 189–202.

Lipps, T. (1903). Einfühlung, innere Nachahmung und Organempfindung. *Archiv für die gesamte Psychologie, 1*, 465–519.

Lonstein, J. S., & Morrell, J. I. (2007). Neuroendocrinology and neurochemistry of maternal motivation and behavior. In A. Lajtha & J. D. Blaustein (Eds.), *Handbook of neurochemistry and molecular neurobiology* (3rd ed., pp. 195–245). Berlin, Germany: Springer-Verlag.

Lovallo, W. R., Wilson, M. F., Pincomb, G. A., Edwards, G. L., Tompkins, P., & Brackett, D. (1985). Activation patterns to aversive stimulation in man: Passive exposure versus effort to control. *Psychophysiology, 22*, 283–291.

Lundberg, U., & Frankenhaeuser, M. (1980). Pituitary-adrenal and sympathetic-adrenal correlates of distress and effort. *Journal of Psychosomatic Research, 24*(3–4), 125–130.

Mason, J. W. (1968). A review of psychoendocrine research on the sympathetic-adrenal medullary system. *Psychosomatic Medicine, 30*(5, Suppl.), 631–653.

McDougall, W. (1908/1923). *An introduction to social psychology* (18th ed.). London, UK: Methuen & Co.

Merleau-Ponty, M. (1962/1970). *Phenomenology of perception* (5th ed.). London, UK/ New York, NY: Routledge & Kegan Paul/The Humanities Press.

Miczek, K. A., de Almeida, R. M., Kravitz, E. A., Rissman, E. F., de Boer, S. F., & Raine, A. (2007). Neurobiology of escalated aggression and violence. *Journal of Neuroscience, 27*, 11806–11809.

Numan, M., & Insel, T. R. (2003). *The neurobiology of parental behavior.* New York, NY: Springer-Verlag.

Pierrehumbert, B., Torrisi, R., Ansermet, F., Borghini, A., & Halfon, O. (2012). Adult attachment representations predict cortisol and oxytocin responses to stress. *Attachment and Human Development, 14*(5), 453–476.

Pierrehumbert, B., Torrisi, R., Laufer, D., Halfon, O., Ansermet, F., & Beck Popovic, M. (2010). Oxytocin response to an experimental psychosocial challenge in adults exposed to traumatic experiences during childhood or adolescence. *Neuroscience, 166*(1), 168–177.

Post, S. G. (2003). *Unlimited love: Altruism, compassion, and service.* Philadelphia, PA: Templeton Foundation Press.

Preston, S. D. (2013). Examining the origins of altruism in offspring care. *Psychological Bulletin, 139*(6), 1305–1341.

Preston, S. D., Bechara, A., Damasio, H., Grabowski, T. J., Stansfield, R. B., Mehta, S., & Demasio, A. R. (2007). The neural substrates of cognitive empathy. *Society for Neuroscience, 2*(3–4), 254–275. doi:10.1080/17470910701376902

Preston, S. D., & de Waal, F. B. M. (2002). Empathy: Its ultimate and proximate bases. *Behavioral and Brain Sciences, 25*(1), 1–71. doi:10.1017/S0140525X02000018

Preston, S. D., & Hofelich, A. J. (2012). The many faces of empathy: Parsing empathic phenomena through a proximate, dynamic-systems view of representing the other in the self. *Emotion Review, 4*(1), 24–33. doi:10.1177/1754073911421378

Prinz, W. (1997). Perception and action planning. *European Journal of Cognitive Psychology, 9*(2), 129–154.

Rand, D. G., Greene, J. D., & Nowak, M. A. (2012). Spontaneous giving and calculated greed. *Nature, 489*(7416), 427–430.

Rapson, R. L., Hatfield, E., & Cacioppo, J. T. (1993). *Emotional contagion.* New York, NY: Cambridge University Press.

Sapolsky, R. M. (1994). *Why zebras don't get ulcers: A guide to stress, stress-related diseases, and coping.* New York, NY: W. H. Freeman.

Sapolsky, R. M. (2009). Stress, glucocorticoids, and damage to the nervous system: The current state of confusion. *Stress, 1*(1), 1–19. doi:10.3109/10253899609001092

Sapolsky, R. M., Romero, L. M., & Munck, A. U. (2000). How do glucocorticoids influence stress responses? Integrating permissive, suppressive, stimulatory, and preparative Actions. *Endocrine Reviews, 21*(1), 55–89. doi:10.1210/er.21.1.55

Schulkin, J. (2000). *Roots of social sensibility and neural function.* Cambridge, MA: The MIT Press.

Singer, T. (2006). The neuronal basis and ontogeny of empathy and mind reading: Review of literature and implications for future research. *Neuroscience and Biobehavioral Review, 30*(6), 855–863. doi:10.1016/j.neubiorev.2006.06.011

Singer, T., Seymour, B., O'Doherty, J., Kaube, H., Dolan, R. J., & Frith, C. D. (2004). Empathy for pain involves the affective but not sensory components of pain. *Science, 303*(5661), 1157–1162. doi: 10.1126/science.1093535

Taylor, S. F., Klein, L. C., Lewis, B. P., Gruenewald, T. L., Gurung, R. A. R., & Updegraff, J. A. (2000). Biobehavioral responses to stress in females: Tend-and-befriend, not fight-or-flight. *Psychological Review, 107*(3), 411–429. doi:10.1037//0033-295X.107.3.411

Toi, M., & Batson, C. D. (1982). More evidence that empathy is a source of altruistic motivation. *Journal of Personality and Social Psychology, 43*(2), 281–292.

von Dawans, B., Fischbacher, U., Kirschbaum, C., Fehr, E., & Heinrichs, M. (2012). The social dimension of stress reactivity: Acute stress increases prosocial behavior in humans. *Psychological Science, 23*, 651–660.

Wispe, L. (1986). The distinction between sympathy and empathy: To call forth a concept, a word is needed. *Journal of Personality and Social Psychology, 50*(2), 314–321.

Zahn-Waxler, C., & Radke-Yarrow, M. (1990). The origins of empathic concern. *Motivation and Emotion, 14*(2), 107–130.

7

Amygdala Tuning Toward
Self and Other

VINCENT MAN, DANIEL L. AMES, ALEXANDER TODOROV,
AND WILLIAM A. CUNNINGHAM ■

Human action is often proposed to be immoral at worst, amoral at best. According to such a worldview, people are inherently selfish and will act primarily to maximize their self-interested goals. Yet people have a surprising ability to forego their own self-interested desires to help others. For example, in economic games, people give far more than what would be expected from self-interest alone, and news reports provide many accounts of people putting themselves into risky situations for the benefit of others. What this suggests is that although people may be selfish, this selfishness is clearly bounded. In this chapter and project we examine how selfless goals can tune neural systems previously linked to self-preservation behavior. We highlight how the amygdala—once thought to be the seat of unconscious fear, threat, and negativity—may also be at the heart of compassion and other-focused motivation.

PROSOCIAL FEELINGS

Traditional Western thought has long conceptualized human nature to be selfish at its core. Philosophers and psychologists have contrasted reason against passion, or cognition against emotion, characterizing the former as an active, deliberate mode of behavior driven by rational considerations that inhibit animal drives and allow for appropriate social conduct, and the latter as an impulsive, reactionary mode that is driven by the world we encounter (Zelazo &

Cunningham, 2007). For example, in Plato's *Phaedrus*, the character Socrates describes the tripartite model of the soul, which separated reason or intellect from the "dark" appetitive passions (Plato, 1997). The Stoic philosophers extended this division by describing reason as a virtue, which one follows to become free from passion. Importantly, the Stoic philosophers characterized the passions as automatic and passive, and reason as an active, deliberative process that exerts control over the passions (Graver, 2009). To the extent that reason and the accompanying conscious control of passion is a virtue, iniquity and vice arise out of being overwhelmed by the automatic impulses that make up passion. Such impulses are described as drives and were originally directed toward objects relevant for self-preservation (White, 1979). Reflecting philosophical thought, early psychological theories similarly divided the human psyche and described interactions among its components (e.g., Freud, 1990).

Yet subsequent thought illustrated the importance of processes, once thought to be immoral, for moral behaviors. The philosopher David Hume argued that reason provided information about the means to an end whereas passion provided the drives to engage in deliberated actions (Hume, 2000). The psychological literature too followed this shift in conceptualizing the interaction between the two putatively separate systems. For example, contemporary perspectives on moral judgments have shifted the emphasis away from rationalist approaches where morality was regarded as a consequence of reasoning operations, and emphasized the role of moral emotions as direct inputs for such evaluations (Haidt, 2001). Moral emotions are distinct in that they inherently involve interpersonal features, and contrary to deliberative deductive processes, such emotions contribute to decision making through rapid and automatic appraisals of moral situations (Haidt, 2001). The neurologist Antonio Damsio posited the *Somatic Marker Hypothesis*, which describes the way in which associations between emotional physiological states and encountered stimuli are processed in the ventral medial prefrontal cortex and, in conjunction with the amygdala, serve directing roles in decision making, particularly for complex or ambiguous situations (Damasio et al., 1996). In other words, emotions, or "passions," are useful in marking aspects of a situation and contribute to information used in reasoning to navigate through situations (Damasio, 1994).

This emerging perspective was echoed in subsequent work in the behavioral sciences. For example, many studies in the field of experimental economics have employed a "dictator game" paradigm as a way of examining the degree to which an individual benefits oneself over others. In this paradigm, a fund is given to a participant which can be split and shared with another individual. However, the participant is also free to keep all of the endowment. Contrary to the decision that would maximize self-interest, the literature has extensively documented that most people do not keep all the money, instead sharing some portion of it with the other individual (Hoffman, McCabe, & Smith, 1996). Demonstrations of fair behavior have held across manipulations of this experimental paradigm. For example, variants of the dictator game have been employed to demonstrate altruistic reciprocal behavior (Diekmann, 2004), where despite a decrease in fair behavior when the transparency of a participant's actions is reduced, people continue to share some portion of their fund rather than keep all of it for themselves (Dana, Weber, & Kuang, 2007). Other psychological research has demonstrated how situational changes influence selfish and selfless behavior. For example, recent work has shown that when people are placed under increased cognitive load, they demonstrate an increase in cooperative behavior (Rand, Greene, & Nowak, 2012). Using a variety of economic games, the authors demonstrated that individuals who make faster decisions contribute more money toward others, and experimental demands that force faster decisions promote similarly cooperative behavior. Not only does such a finding challenge the view that automatic processes are directed toward only self-focused interests, but it also shows that rather than working completely in self-interest, people are able to demonstrate sensitivity toward others.

RETHINKING THE AMYGDALA

Although there are many systems involved in self- and other-focused processing, we restrict our focus to the amygdala for several reasons. Theory regarding amygdala function has mirrored the assumed division of the human psyche. Whereas the frontal cortices have been thought to be involved in reason and human virtue, the amygdala was thought to be related to our more "reptilian" brain—providing emotional signals that cloud human thought and are at the heart of anxiety, depression, and prejudice. Indeed, much of the early social neuroscience literature focused on how one could inhibit the amygdala during tasks for better emotional or self-regulatory outcomes. Furthermore, the amygdala has been traditionally thought to be at the heart of negative emotion specifically. In this project and chapter, we highlight that the amygdala does not simply function in the service of negative emotions, but it may also support positive emotions, reward processing, and prosocial behavior.

Though the amygdala is often referred to as a unitary structure with designated functions, the view we put forward here instead aligns with research situating the distinct yet interconnected nuclei that comprise the structure within unique neural circuits that underlie different functional systems (LeDoux, 2004). The extended amygdala is comprised of several nuclei, each with its own cellular (cytoarchitectonic) properties and connections to surrounding areas of the brain (e.g., Sah, Faber, De Armentia, & Power, 2003). These include the lateral, basal, and accessory basal nuclei, which make up the "basolateral amygdala," as well as the surrounding central, medial, and cortical nuclei (Davis & Whalen, 2001). From this perspective, the extended amygdala can support multiple specialized functions such as attention, reward reinforcement, and fear representation, depending on the amygdala subsystem (i.e., the particular pattern of neural populations within and across the subnuclei, and the larger networks to which they project). One approach to understanding how these nuclei interact and give rise to the multitude of functions associated with the extended amygdala is through the connection pathways between the structure and various subcortical and cortical regions of the brain. Output projections from subcortical regions, particularly the thalamus and hippocampus, carry sensory and stimulus-driven information to the basolateral amygdala, whereas pathways from cortical regions such as the prefrontal cortex modulate the amygdala via top-down processes. The amygdala serves as an informational, affect-driven hub between inferior temporal cortex regions involved in the perception and identification of salient stimuli and prefrontal regions involved in decision-making and executive functions.

From the basolateral amygdala, output pathways to various cortical and subcortical regions are associated with particular functions depending on the region to which they project. For example, the connectivity between the basolateral nucleus of the amygdala and the prefrontal cortex guides behavior based on valuation processes. The output of information to the orbitofrontal cortex (OFC) is important for decision-making processes and guiding goal-directed behavior (Anderson, Bechara, Damasio, Tranel, & Damasio, 1999; Schoenbaum, Chiba, & Gallagher, 1998). Research has strongly supported the role of the OFC in decision-making and goal-directed behavior (Bechara, Damasio, Tranel, & Damasio, 1997), and lesions to this region especially impair social and moral behavior (Anderson et al., 1999). Cells in the OFC activate to information relayed from the basolateral amygdala in order to make choices and guide behavior (Schoenbaum et al., 1998). Along similar principles, outputs from the basolateral amygdala to the hippocampus influence other functions such as memory for emotional events and spatial learning (see Davis & Shi, 2000, for an overview). Indeed, which target area the amygdala activates is dependent upon the reinforcement signal of the information received by the basolateral amygdala, such as the nature of the sensory information from the thalamus (Davis & Whalen, 2001).

The importance of connectivity in supporting various functions is apparent in the contributions of the amygdala to reward circuits and appetitive behavior. Connections between the basolateral amygdala and striatal structures, particularly the dopaminergic systems of the nucleus accumbens (NAcc) (McDonald, 1991), are relevant to reward learning in the context of conditioned reinforcement (Cador, Robbins, & Everitt, 1989; Davis & Whalen, 2001; Hatfield, Han, Conley, Gallagher, & Holland, 1996). Projections from the basolateral amygdala to the NAcc in the ventral striatum, and dopamine terminals in the adjacent ventral tegmental area (VTA), underlie two functional processes that give rise to approach (i.e., appetitive or reward-seeking) behavior (McDonald, 1991). Information from the amygdala about reward contingencies (e.g., associations between conditioned and unconditioned stimuli in a reward paradigm) is sent to the NAacc, where the dopaminergic system amplifies and outputs the signal (Davis & Whalen, 2001). Moreover, lesions of the basolateral amygdala have been found to reduce approach behavior (Cador et al., 1989). More broadly, the basolateral amygdala is critically involved in stimulus valuation, such as the representation of unconditioned stimuli via connectivity to the perirhinal cortex (Gewirtz & Davis, 1998). Studies supporting this role of the basolateral amygdala have employed unconditioned stimulus (US) devaluation paradigms, where a neutral stimulus is paired with an intrinsically rewarding unconditioned stimulus, and the unconditioned stimulus is subsequently paired with an intrinsically aversive stimulus (Davis & Whalen, 2001). Typical animals show reduced conditioned response to the neutral stimulus, but animals with lesions to the basolateral, but not the central, amygdala, block US devaluation (Hatfield et al., 1996). This pattern of lesions also blocks second-order conditioning in animals, which similarly relies on value representation (Everitt, Cador, & Robbins, 1989; Everitt, Morris, O'Brien, & Robbins, 1991).

Despite the documented place of the amygdala along neuronal circuits of reward and appetitive behavior, the amygdala has been regarded under prevailing theories as a structure involved in fear apprehension and aversion response (see LeDoux, 2000) through the provision of arousal cues that direct attention to the immediate environment. Earlier research restricted the amygdala's functional profile to negative affective states. For example, the amygdala, particularly the central nucleus (Davis & Whalen, 2001), has been heavily conceptualized as a crucial structure in an automatic system that detects threatening information in one's environment and directs subsequent behavior (Freese & Amaral, 2009). Research using functional magnetic resonance imaging (fMRI) in humans has shown that the amygdala is involved in the detection of threat and representation of negative affective states across multiple stimulus modalities, including the perception (Adolphs et al., 1999; Calder, Keane, Manes, Antoun, & Young, 2000; Morris et al., 1996) and evaluation (Adolphs & Tranel, 2004; Anderson, Spencer, Fullbright, & Phelps, 2000) of negative facial expressions, threat-related words (Isenberg et al., 1999), and aversive odors (Zald & Pardo, 1997). This region is also known to play a critical role in the representation of fear, including the acquisition of fear responses through operant conditioning and the behavioral expression of the fear experiences (LaBar, Gatenby, Gore, LeDoux, & Phelps, 1998; LeDoux 1998, 2000; Phelps et al., 2001). Given that this increased amygdala activation to fearful faces is not accompanied by subjective reports of fear (Morris et al., 1998), the functional role of the amygdala is specified to the processing of affective information rather than the entirety of emotional experience. The amygdala has been implicated in such functions by directing attention toward relevant information via projections from the central nucleus to the cholinergic systems of the basal forebrain (Everitt & Robbins, 1997; Holland & Gallagher, 1999).

The manner in which the amygdala utilizes such arousal cues to direct attention toward negative affective information has been further shown to be automatic, particularly in the context of perceptual attention (Anderson & Phelps, 2001). For example, when individuals were presented with fearful and happy faces for a perceptually subthreshold period, followed by longer presentations of neutral faces, such that the individuals only had explicit experiences of apprehending the neutral faces and consequently did not show noticeable changes in their emotional arousal state, the amygdala demonstrated relatively greater signal intensity to masked fearful faces than to masked happy faces (Whalen, Shin, McInerney, & Rauch, 1998). Neurons in the central nucleus of the amygdala have been shown to change their firing rate as a function of tones that predict shock in a fear conditioning paradigm (Kapp, Silvestri, & Guarrci, 1996; Kapp, Silvestri, Guarraci, Moynihan, & Cain, 1997). It has been suggested that the automaticity of amygdala activation toward negative information could reflect habitual vigilance for negative stimuli through individual experience, or that it could reflect evolutionary and genetic forces that bias the automatic capture of attention (Cunningham, Raye, & Johnson, 2005).

Extending beyond the apprehension of negative stimuli alone, developments in attentional theories of the amygdala have further supported its role in processing various forms of meaningful information. Early neuroimaging studies examining the role of the amygdala in threat and fear processing documented greater activation of the region toward ambiguous stimuli, which requires further information before the engagement of approach or avoidance behavior (Whalen, 1998). For example, it was found that stimuli classified as being of high interest, which participants reported to be more difficult to interpret, elicited greater focal activation in the left amygdala (Hamann, Ely, Hoffman, & Kilts, 2002). The notion that the amygdala is sensitive to the uncertainty of stimulus contingencies may also account for the relative bias toward the amygdala representing negative information in the literature. It has been argued that fearful faces may have been found to be more effective in activating the amygdala (Whalen et al., 1998) due to the ambiguity inherent in the lack of information about the source of a threat, rather than the specific emotional content itself (Davis & Whalen, 2001). The mechanism underlying this vigilant role of the amygdala was purported to be the amygdala-mediated lowering of neuronal thresholds in structures that comprise sensory systems such as the basal forebrain, via the modulation of acetylcholine. Similarly, the amygdala influences the activation of neurons with receptors particular to other neurotransmitters such as dopamine and serotonin, which then affects thalamic sensory processes (Whalen, 1998). The lowering of neuronal thresholds results in greater sensitivity to ambiguous stimuli and increases neural vigilance toward potentially important information.

More recent studies have shown that the amygdala is not only sensitive to fearful or negative stimuli but also to positive information. Again, this has been shown across various stimulus modalities, such as visual (Garavan, Pendergrass, Ross, Stein, & Risinger, 2001; Hamann et al., 2002; Liberzon, Phan, Decker, & Taylor, 2003) and verbal stimuli (Hamann & Mao, 2002). Thus, recent reviews demonstrate that amygdala activation is better characterized by a quadratic or U-shaped function, where the BOLD response is greater to both highly positive and highly negative stimuli, compared to neutrally valenced stimuli (Cunningham & Brosch, 2012; Cunningham & Kirkland, 2013; Cunningham et al., 2005; Mende-Siedlecki, Said, & Todorov, 2013). In fact, when the overall emotional intensity of the stimuli is controlled, there remains no relationship between positivity or negativity and amygdala activation (Anderson et al., 2003; Anderson & Sobel, 2003; Cunningham, Raye, & Johnson, 2004; Small et al., 2003; though see Anders, Eippert, Weiskopf, & Veit, 2008). This demonstrates that rather than sensitivity to specific valence, the amygdala is involved in processing stimuli of great affective intensity, that is, highly salient information.

This perspective of the amygdala as a brain region involved in processes that direct attention toward salient information, rather than soley tracking negative stimuli, is enforced by views that emphasize its role in integrating information from multiple sources. Though the implication of the amygdala in bottom-up processes has been described both here and extensively in the literature, there is also support for a role of the structure in top-down pathways: Amygdala response can be controlled through prefrontal processes (Ochsner & Gross, 2005). A recent magnetoencephalography study compared the fit of two models of amygdala function: a "dual" model that included both cortical and subcortical pathways to the amygdala, and a "cortical" model that excluded the subcortical pathways (Garrido, Barnes, Sahani, & Dolan, 2012). Data supported the dual model over the cortical model, demonstrating the importance of the subcortical pathway, particularly for early stimulus processing and automatic appraisals of salient information. In fact, the position that the amygdala is specific only to negativity may be a consequence of regarding the amygdala only as a functional unit, rather than accounting for the numerous connections between its component nuclei and other regions of the brain. Our emphasis on distinguishing between the related functions of the amygdala based on its subsystems allows for the conceptualization of a flexible amygdala that tunes toward multiple types of relevant information and supports appropriate consequent processes.

As much as the amygdala demonstrates a general flexibility toward various forms of input information, there are still patterns of individual differences in the activity profile of the structure. For example, individuals with greater promotion focus, a motivational orientation characterized by relatively greater sensitivity to gains (Higgins, 1997), showed greater amygdala activation to positive stimuli, whereas individuals with greater prevention focus, a motivational orientation characterized by relatively greater sensitivity to preventing loss, showed greater amygdala activation to negative stimuli (Cunningham et al., 2005). Furthermore, the personality factors of extraversion and neuroticism are associated with increased amygdala responding to positive and negative information, respectively (Canli et al., 2001; Canli, Sivers, Whitfield, Gotlib, & Gabrieli, 2002; Cunningham et al., 2010). There are thus both general patterns of amygdala response as well as variations due to trait factors.

One way to account for both these features of amygdala activity is by conceptualizing the amygdala as a structure involved in the processing of motivationally relevant stimuli (e.g., Sander, Grafman, & Zalla, 2003). Following this initial relevance evaluation, additional resources are recruited to facilitate situation-appropriate responses (Brosch, Sander, Pourtois, & Scherer, 2008). This suggestion is based on appraisal theories of emotion (see Ellsworth & Scherer, 2003), which stand in contrast to the inflexible pattern-matching mechanism put forward by basic theories of emotion, and emphasize instead the importance of the subjective evaluation of a stimulus according to its importance for the individual. Thus, the amygdala functions as part of a larger affect system that informs us about what is important in the environment, and then facilitates the modulation of appropriate perceptual, attentional, autonomic, or conceptual processes in order to respond to present challenges or opportunities. On this view, differences in amygdala response between individuals and to various situations are not undefined noise, but rather the critical variation to be understood. Specifically, we expect that amygdala activation should vary as a function of the needs, goals, and values of the organism.

What is considered relevant can be defined by the usefulness of a stimulus for any momentary motivational structure of an individual. Because multiple goals can be important, the salience and priority of specific needs, goals, and values shape responses. Therefore, motivational contingencies, and consequently the relevance of a given stimulus, may change continuously. For example, when one is hungry, food will be more relevant, whereas when one is in a dangerous neighborhood, potential criminals will be more relevant. Consistent with this idea, one study investigated neural mechanisms underlying attention toward food in participants both when hungry and satiated, thus varying the motivational relevance of the food stimuli within participants (Mohanty, Gitelman, Small, & Mesulam, 2008). When hungry, participants not only showed increased amygdala activation to pictures of food but also faster attentional orienting toward food cues and increased connectivity between limbic areas and parietal attention regions, compared to when participants were satiated. This point is also illustrated by the way in which more abstract social goals influence the apprehension of, and response to, encountered stimuli. A study that manipulated the processing goals of participants to evaluate only negative, only positive, or both positive and negative aspects of presented names found that amygdala activity was more strongly associated with the particular aspects of each name that signaled goal relevance (Cunningham, Van Bavel, & Johnsen, 2008), providing further support that the amygdala is engaged in processing aspects of stimuli that fit the current situational demands.

This pattern of results also suggests that previous research on social perception and prejudice may need to be updated. Specifically, studies using fMRI to study racial attitudes have suggested a role for the amygdala in the processing of threat associated with automatic prejudice (Cunningham et al., 2004; Lieberman, Hariri, Jarcho, Eisenberger, & Bookheimer, 2005; Phelps et al., 2000). Yet, if the amygdala responds to motivationally relevant stimuli rather than threat per se, it may be possible to reverse these effects and find greater amygdala activity to in-group members, to the extent that these people are deemed motivationally relevant. Situations like this should not be unexpected: People who accurately identify, value, and cooperate with in-group members enjoy numerous functional benefits, including the fulfillment of their basic psychological needs (Allport, 1954). To test for this, in an fMRI study participants were randomly assigned to a mixed-race team, and brain regions involved in the processing of novel in-group and out-group members were examined (Van Bavel, Packer, & Cunningham, 2008). Though previous research on intergroup perception found amygdala activity, typically interpreted to reflect negative processing, in response to social out-groups, greater activity in the amygdala was found when participants viewed novel in-group faces compared to novel out-group faces.

This shift in our understanding of the role of the amygdala in social perception allows for important reinterpretations of previous amygdala findings. For example, Wheeler and Fiske (2005) found that amygdala response to faces from Black and White social groups differed as a function of social goals. Under a social categorization goal, the amygdala was significantly more responsive to racial out-groups than in-groups. However, this pattern disappeared when participants had a goal to individuate each target or to visually inspect the targets' faces. Whereas out-group faces may have been deemed more relevant when social categories were being judged, in-group faces may have been deemed more important when a need to individuate was present. Thus, although these data were originally proposed to suggest that people could control their prejudiced responses, they may rather suggest that the relevance of the faces in the two conditions changed.

THE AMYGDALA AND PROSOCIAL BEHAVIOR

Given that humans are a highly social species, other people are highly relevant to most aspects of life. As such, it is important to process information about other individuals within and outside of one's group, as well as engage in the appropriate social behaviors. The *Social Brain Hypothesis* posits that larger brain size and expanded volume in particular brain regions reflect the increased computational demands inherent to social organization in higher primates, including humans (Dunbar, 1998). Recently, evidence has been found for a link between amygdala volume and social network size and complexity in humans (Bickart et al., 2011). This relationship suggests that the amygdala may be part of a system that allows for the development of social relationships, community, and perhaps appropriate social behavior.

The amygdala is important for processing many forms of information that contribute toward more complex social judgments. Human faces are of particular significance for social evaluations, given the amount and relevance of information conveyed in facial expressions. Though the evaluation of human faces can rely on different dimensions (Todorov, Said, Engell, & Oosterhof, 2008), the trustworthiness of a face is one dimension important for most social outcomes (Oosterhof &Todorov, 2008). The critical role of the amygdala in supporting such evaluations of perceived trustworthiness in faces has been documented well, for both the untrustworthy (Engell, Haxby, & Todorov, 2007; Winston, Strange, O'Doherty, & Dolan, 2002) and trustworthy (Said, Baron, & Todorov, 2009; Todorov et al., 2008) poles of the dimension. Complimentary neuropsychology research has supported this role of the amygdala; for example, patients with bilateral amygdala lesions were found to have deficits in evaluations of trustworthiness based on facial features (Adolphs, Tranel, & Damasio, 1998). Together, the convergent evidence demonstrates the importance of facial expressions for navigating complex social environments.

To maneuver within such complex environments moreover necessitates judging the intentions, decisions, and actions of other individuals, all of which are implicated in moral evaluations. Research has demonstrated that the formulation of moral judgments is an abstract social process also supported by multiple neural systems. Earlier fMRI studies have delineated the structures that support emotional processes broadly, including the extended amygdala and other subcortical nuclei, as well as those particularly necessary for moral emotions and evaluations, such as the superior temporal sulcus, medial frontal gyrus, and right medial orbitofrontal cortex (Moll, de Oliveira-Souza, Bramati, & Grafman, 2002; Moll, Oliveira-Souza, Eslinger, et al., 2002). Given the increase in functional connectivity between these regions for morally relevant stimuli, it is plausible that each of these structures supports different components, which together comprise the apprehension and evaluation of morally relevant information.

Although the evidence thus far implicates the amygdala in the processing of apprehended social and moral information, its contributory role in the expression of social behaviors has also been elucidated. Social behaviors vary in the degree to which the enacting agent, or other individuals, acquires gains, where prosocial behaviors consist of acts that confer benefits upon other individuals. One exceptional manifestation of prosocial behavior is altruism, which describes behaviors that extend assistance or confer advantages to others without anticipation of reward or at some cost to oneself (Piliavin & Charng, 1990). Altruism could be understood as a construct built upon component processes such as empathy and theory of mind; that is, to be altruistic requires empathetic ability. To the extent that empathy is involved in prosocial behavior then, the importance of the amygdala has also been shown (Decety & Jackson, 2004). Specifically, this role of the amygdala in empathetic and other prosocial behaviors is modulated by the neuropeptide oxytocin (Hurlemann et al., 2010). Oxytocin attenuates amygdala response to fear, resulting in a decrease in functional coupling between the amygdala and upper brainstem regions involved in autonomic responses to threat (Kirsch et al., 2005) by disrupting projections from the central nucleus (see Huber, Veinante, & Stoop, 2005). Decreases in fear processing and response may contribute to decreased distrust of others and, consequently, greater prosocial behavior (Labuschagne et al., 2010). Furthermore, given that empathetic behaviors necessitate adopting the perspective of another person and sharing their affective state (Decety & Jackson, 2006), there should be much overlap in the mechanisms supporting theory of mind and empathy. Indeed, greater amygdala activation has been found during performance on tasks that require theory of mind processes (Baron-Cohen et al., 1999), and convergent neuropsychological evidence demonstrated impairment in performance on such tasks after amygdala damage (Adolphs, Baron-Cohen, & Tranel, 2002).

THE AMYGDALA AND THE GOALS OF SELF AND OTHER

Because goals shape amygdala activation (see Cunningham & Brosch, 2012, for a review), with the appropriate goal, the amygdala can become vigilant to the needs of others. To the extent that the amygdala is tuned to detect the needs of others, people will be able to more quickly detect those in need in a complex social environment and, as a result, be able to direct resources to these people. On this view, our "impulses" do not distract us from moral behavior, but rather can help guide us unconsciously to moral behavior.

To explore this hypothesis, we conducted a behavioral and fMRI experiment designed to systematically explore how positive self-focused and other-focused goals (i.e., helping oneself and helping others, respectively) shape amygdala function. In our study, participants were asked to identify people who would either (a) be most useful to help them with a goal (self-focused condition) or (b) be most in need of help from them given a particular context (other-focused condition). Given the adaptability of amygdala function in accordance with contextual demands, we predicted that with the appropriate goal, the amygdala would be sensitive to the needs of others. Consequently, we hypothesized that people should be able to more quickly detect individuals in need within a complex social environment and, as a result, be able to direct resources to these people.

Preliminary results from our study support this hypothesis. Specifically, although we found that the amygdala responded to the most trustworthy and untrustworthy faces regardless of whether participants were attending to themselves or others, we found that trait levels of empathy moderated the magnitude of this U-shaped function. Specifically, for participants lower in trait empathy, we found an altered U-shaped function with relatively greater activation for the self-focus than the other-focus condition. This effect is consistent with the idea that people are more sensitive to trustworthiness when they are seeking information that can be used to further their own goals. Importantly, this effect was reversed for participants who were higher in trait empathy. For these participants, activation was relatively greater when making other-focused judgments. In other words, high empathy appears to not only modulate amygdala response towards others, but more empathetic people may also be more sensitive to information about trustworthiness when making decisions to help others.

Perhaps paradoxically, shifting focus away from the self and helping others may be among the most reliable paths to personal well-being and flourishing. For instance, a broad and representative longitudinal survey found that engagement in volunteer work enhances happiness, life satisfaction, self-esteem, sense of control over one's life, and physical and mental health (Thoits & Hewitt, 2001). Studies comparing elderly volunteers to nonvolunteers reveal that those who engage in volunteer work report greater life satisfaction, a stronger will to live, increased self-respect, and fewer psychological symptoms of depression and anxiety (Hunter & Linn, 1981), while experiencing lower mortality rates compared to nonvolunteers (Oman, Thoresen, & McMahon, 1999). More generally, a sizable corpus of research on altruism suggests a robust relationship between helping others and personal well-being (for reviews, see Post, 2005; Thoits & Hewitt, 2001). Thus, selfless acts undertaken at a cost to the self confer tremendous benefits upon the actor. In additional analyses of this data set, we will examine the extent to which these effects, the ability to shift to the needs of others, may be associated with compassionate behavior and well-being.

CONCLUSION

This research project builds on the idea that our evolutionarily older brain systems are not solely a source of immorality and selfishness, but when tuned by our goals, can contribute to moral and just behavior. Thus, human flourishing does not come from the suppression of aspects of the self, but rather through the integration of all relevant processes together into a unified response. Specifically, theories of amygdala function suggest that it provides arousal cues to direct attention and facilitate effective responses to the environment. Previous conceptions of amygdala function restricted these responses to the self-focused objective of "avoiding personal harm." However, under our framework, the attentional benefits that the amygdala confers upon social perceivers can be leveraged to promote better prosocial decisions and, by extension, more effective prosocial actions. The amygdala is of critical importance to many of the social processes that make up the core of positive psychology, including empathy (Carr et al., 2003), attachment (Lemche et al., 2005), trust (Said et al., 2009), prosocial behavior (Cushing et al., 2008), and morality (Raine & Yang, 2006). In short, a detailed understanding of the amygdala's involvement in human social behavior holds great promise for elucidating the fundamental nature of positive psychology.

REFERENCES

Adolphs, R., Baron-Cohen, S., & Tranel, D. (2002). Impaired recognition of social emotions following amygdala damage. *Journal of Cognitive Neuroscience, 14*(8), 1264–1274.

Adolphs, R., & Tranel, D. (2004). Impaired judgments of sadness but not happiness following bilateral amygdala damage. *Journal of Cognitive Neuroscience, 16*(3), 453–462.

Adolphs, R., Tranel, D., & Damasio, A. R. (1998). The human amygdala in social judgment. *Nature, 393*(6684), 470–474.

Adolphs, R., Tranel, D., Hamann, S., Young, A. W., Calder, A. J., Phelps, E. A., . . . Damasio, A. R. (1999). Recognition of facial emotion in nine individuals with bilateral amygdala damage. *Neuropsychologia, 37*(10), 1111–1117.

Allport, G. W. (1954). *The nature of prejudice.* Reading, MA: Addison-Wesley.

Anders, S., Eippert, F., Weiskopf, N., & Veit, R. (2008). The human amygdala is sensitive to the valence of pictures and sounds irrespective of arousal: An fMRI study. *Social Cognitive and Affective Neuroscience, 3*(3), 233–243.

Anderson, A. K., Christoff, K., Stappen, I., Panitz, D., Ghahremani, D. G., Glover, G., . . . Sobel, N. (2003). Dissociated neural representations of intensity and valence in human olfaction. *Nature Neuroscience, 6*(2), 196–202.

Anderson, A. K., & Phelps, E. A. (2001). Lesions of the human amygdala impair enhanced perception of emotionally salient events. *Nature, 411*(6835), 305–309.

Anderson, A. K., & Sobel, N. (2003). Dissociating intensity from valence as sensory inputs to emotion. *Neuron, 39*(4), 581–583.

Anderson, A. K., Spencer, D. D., Fullbright, R. K., & Phelps, E. A. (2000). Contribution of the anteromedial temporal lobes to the evaluation of facial emotion. *Neuropsychology, 14*(4), 526–536.

Anderson, S. W., Bechara, A., Damasio, H., Tranel, D., & Damasio, A. R. (1999). Impairment of social and moral behavior related to early damage in human prefrontal cortex. *Nature Neuroscience, 2*(11), 1032–1037.

Baron-Cohen, S., Ring, H. A., Wheelwright, S., Bullmore, E. T., Brammer, M. J., Simmons, A., & Williams, S. C. (1999). Social intelligence in the normal and autistic brain: An fMRI study. *European Journal of Neuroscience, 11*(6), 1891–1898.

Bechara, A., Damasio, H., Tranel, D., & Damasio, A. R. (1997). Deciding advantageously before knowing the advantageous strategy. *Science, 275*(5304), 1293–1295.

Bickart, K. C., Wright, C. I., Dautoff, R. J., Dickerson, B. C., & Barrett, L. F. (2011). Amygdala volume and social network size in humans. *Nature Neuroscience, 14*(2), 163–164.

Brosch, T., Sander, D., Pourtois, G., & Scherer, K. R. (2008). Beyond fear rapid spatial orienting toward positive emotional stimuli. *Psychological Science, 19*(4), 362–370.

Cador, M., Robbins, T. W., & Everitt, B. J. (1989). Involvement of the amygdala in stimulus-reward associations: Interaction with the ventral striatum. *Neuroscience, 30*(1), 77–86.

Calder, A., Keane, J., Manes, F., Antoun, N., & Young, A. W. (2000). Impaired recognition and experience of disgust following brain injury. *Nature Neuroscience, 3*(11), 1077–1078.

Canli, T., Sivers, H., Whitfield, S. L., Gotlib, I. H., & Gabrieli, J. D. (2002). Amygdala response to happy faces as a function of extraversion. *Science, 296*(5576), 2191–2191.

Canli, T., Zhao, Z., Desmond, J. E., Kang, E., Gross, J., & Gabrieli, J. D. (2001). An fMRI study of personality influences on brain reactivity to emotional stimuli. *Behavioral Neuroscience, 115*(1), 33–42.

Carr, L., Iacoboni, M., Dubeau, M., Mazziotta, J. C., & Lenzi, G. L. (2003). Neural mechanisms of empathy in humans: A relay from neural systems for imitation to limbic areas. *Proceedings of the National Academy of Sciences USA, 100*(9), 5497–5502.

Cunningham, W. A., Arbuckle, N. L., Jahn, A., Mowrer, S. M., & Abduljalil, A. M. (2010). Aspects of neuroticism and the amygdala: Chronic tuning from motivational styles. *Neuropsychologia, 48*(12), 3399–3404.

Cunningham, W. A., & Brosch, T. (2012). Motivational salience amygdala tuning from traits, needs, values, and goals. *Current Directions in Psychological Science, 21*(1), 54–59.

Cunningham, W. A., & Kirkland, T. (2013). The joyful, yet balanced, amygdala: Moderated responses to positive but not negative stimuli in trait happiness. *Social Cognitive and Affective Neuroscience, 9*(6), 760–766. doi:10.1093/scan/nst045

Cunningham, W. A., Raye, C. L., & Johnson, M. K. (2004). Implicit and explicit evaluation: fMRI correlates of valence, emotional intensity, and control in the processing of attitudes. *Journal of Cognitive Neuroscience, 16*(10), 1717–1729.

Cunningham, W. A., Raye, C. L., & Johnson, M. K. (2005). Neural correlates of evaluation associated with promotion and prevention regulatory focus. *Cognitive, Affective, and Behavioral Neuroscience, 5*(2), 202–211.

Cunningham, W. A., Van Bavel, J. J., & Johnsen, I. R. (2008). Affective flexibility evaluative processing goals shape amygdala activity. *Psychological Science, 19*(2), 152–160.

Cushing, B. S., Perry, A., Musatov, S., Ogawa, S., & Papademetriou, E. (2008). Estrogen receptors in the medial amygdala inhibit the expression of male prosocial behavior. *Journal of Neuroscience, 28*(41), 10399–10403.

Damasio, A. (1994). *Descartes' error: Emotion, reason, and the human brain.* New York, NY: Penguin Putnam.

Damasio, A. R., Everitt, B. J., & Bishop, D. (1996). The somatic marker hypothesis and the possible functions of the prefrontal cortex. *Philosophical Transactions of the Royal Society of London B, Biological Sciences, 351*(1346), 1413–1420.

Dana, J., Weber, R. A., & Kuang, J. X. (2007). Exploiting moral wiggle room: Experiments demonstrating an illusory preference for fairness. *Economic Theory, 33*(1), 67–80.

Davis, M., & Whalen, P. J. (2001). The amygdala: Vigilance and emotion. *Molecular Psychiatry, 6*(1), 13–34.

Davis, M., & Shi, C.-J. (2000). The amygdala. *Current Biology, 10*, R131.

Decety, J., & Jackson, P. L. (2004). The functional architecture of human empathy. *Behavioral and Cognitive Neuroscience Reviews, 3*(2), 71–100.

Decety, J., & Jackson, P. (2006). A social-neuroscience perspective on empathy. *Current Directions in Psychological Science, 15*(2), 54–58.

De Martino, B., Kumaran, D., Seymour, B., & Dolan, R. J. (2006). Frames, biases, and rational decision-making in the human brain. *Science, 313*(5787), 684–687.

Diekmann, A. (2004). The power of reciprocity fairness, reciprocity, and stakes in variants of the dictator game. *Journal of Conflict Resolution*, 48(4), 487–505.

Dunbar, R. (1998). The social brain hypothesis. *Evolutionary Anthropology*, 6(5), 178–190.

Ellsworth, P. C., & Scherer, K. R. (2003). Appraisal processes in emotion. *Handbook of Affective Sciences*, 572, V595.

Engell, A. D., Haxby, J. V., & Todorov, A. (2007). Implicit trustworthiness decisions: Automatic coding of face properties in the human amygdala. *Journal of Cognitive Neuroscience*, 19(9), 1508–1519.

Everitt, B. J., Cador, M., & Robbins, T. W. (1989). Interactions between the amygdala and ventral striatum in stimulus-reward associations: Studies using a second-order schedule of sexual reinforcement. *Neuroscience*, 30(1), 63–75.

Everitt, B. J., Morris, K. A., O'Brien, A., & Robbins, T. W. (1991). The basolateral amygdala-ventral striatal system and conditioned place preference: Further evidence of limbic-striatal interactions underlying reward-related processes. *Neuroscience*, 42(1), 1–18.

Everitt, B. J., & Robbins, T. W. (1997). Central cholinergic systems and cognition. *Annual Review of Psychology*, 48(1), 649–684.

Freese, J. L., & Amaral, D. G. (2009). Neuroanatomy of the primate amygdala. In P. J. Whalen & E. A. Phelps (Eds.), *The human amygdala* (pp. 3–42). New York, NY: Guilford Press.

Freud, S. (1990). *Beyond the pleasure principle*. (J. Strachey, Trans.). New York, NY: Norton.

Garavan, H., Pendergrass, J. C., Ross, T. J., Stein, E. A., & Risinger, R. C. (2001). Amygdala response to both positively and negatively valenced stimuli. *Neuroreport*, 12(12), 2779–2783.

Garrido, M. I., Barnes, G. R., Sahani, M., & Dolan, R. J. (2012). Functional evidence for a dual route to amygdala. *Current Biology*, 22(2), 129–134.

Gewirtz, J. C., & Davis, M. (1998). Application of Pavlovian higher-order conditioning to the analysis of the neural substrates of fear conditioning. *Neuropharmacology*, 37, 453–459.

Graver, M. R. (2009). *Stoicism and emotion* (2nd ed.). Chicago, IL: University of Chicago Press.

Haidt, J. (2001). The emotional dog and its rational tail: A social intuitionist approach to moral judgment. *Psychological Review*, 108(4), 814–834.

Hamann, S. B., Ely, T. D., Hoffman, J. M., & Kilts, C. D. (2002). Ecstasy and agony: Activation of the human amygdala in positive and negative emotion. *Psychological Science*, 13(2), 135–141.

Hamann, S., & Mao, H. (2002). Positive and negative emotional verbal stimuli elicit activity in the left amygdala. *Neuroreport*, 13(1), 15–19.

Hatfield, T., Han, J. S., Conley, M., Gallagher, M., & Holland, P. (1996). Neurotoxic lesions of basolateral, but not central, amygdala interfere with Pavlovian second-order conditioning and reinforcer devaluation effects. *Journal of Neuroscience*, 16(16), 5256–5265.

Higgins, E. T. (1997). Beyond pleasure and pain. *American Psychologist*, 52(12)8, 1280–1300.

Hoffman, E., McCabe, K., & Smith, V. L. (1996). Social distance and other-regarding behavior in dictator games. *American Economic Review, 86*(3), 653–660.

Holland, P., & Gallagher, M. (1999). Amygdala circuitry in attentional and representational processes. *Trends in Cognitive Sciences, 3*(2), 65–73.

Huber, D., Veinante, P., & Stoop, R. (2005). Vasopressin and oxytocin excite distinct neuronal populations in the central amygdala. *Science, 308*(5719), 245.

Hume, D. (2000). *Treatise of human nature.* (D. F. Norton & M. J. Norton, Eds.). New York, NY: Oxford University Press.

Hunter, K. I., & Linn, M. W. (1981). Psychosocial differences between elderly volunteers and non-volunteers. *International Journal of Aging and Human Development, 12*(3), 205–213.

Hurlemann, R., Patin, A., Onur, O. A., Cohen, M. X., Baumgartner, T., Metzler, S., . . . Kendrick, K. M. (2010). Oxytocin enhances amygdala-dependent, socially reinforced learning and emotional empathy in humans. *Journal of Neuroscience, 30*(14), 4999–5007.

Isenberg, N., Silbersweig, D., Engelien, A., Emmerich, S., Malavade, K., Beattie, B. A., . . . Stern, E. (1999). Linguistic threat activates the human amygdala. *Proceedings of the National Academy of Sciences USA, 96*(18), 10456–10459.

Kapp, B. S., Silvestri, A. J., & Guarraci, F. A. (1996). Amygdaloid central nucleus neuronal activity: Correlations with EEG arousal. *Neuroscience Abstracts, 22*, 2049.

Kapp, B. S., Silvestri, A. J., Guarraci, F. A., Moynihan, J. E., & Cain, M. E. (1997). Associative and EEG arousal-related characteristics of amygdaloid central nucleus neurons in the rabbit. *Neuroscience Abstracts, 23*, 787.

Kirsch, P., Esslinger, C., Chen, Q., Mier, D., Lis, S., Siddhanti, S., . . . Meyer-Lindenberg, A. (2005). Oxytocin modulates neural circuitry for social cognition and fear in humans. *Journal of Neuroscience, 25*(49), 11489–11493.

LaBar, K. S., Gatenby, J. C., Gore, J. C., LeDoux, J. E., & Phelps, E. A. (1998). Human amygdala activation during conditioned fear acquisition and extinction: A mixed-trial fMRI study. *Neuron, 20*(5), 937–945.

Labuschagne, I., Phan, K. L., Wood, A., Angstadt, M., Chua, P., Heinrichs, M., . . . Nathan, P. J. (2010). Oxytocin attenuates amygdala reactivity to fear in generalized social anxiety disorder. *Neuropsychopharmacology, 35*(12), 2403–2413.

LeDoux, J. (1998). *The emotional brain: The mysterious underpinnings of emotional life.* New York, NY: Simon & Schuster.

LeDoux, J. E. (2000). Emotion circuits in the brain. *Annual Review of Neuroscience, 23*, 155–184.

LeDoux, J. E. (2004). The amygdala. *Current Biology, 17*(20), 868–874.

Lemche, E., Giampietro, V. P., Surguladze, S. A., Amaro, E. J., Andrew, C. M., Williams, S. C. R., . . . Philips, M. L. (2006). Human attachment security is mediated by the amygdala: Evidence from combined fMRI and psychophysiological measures. *Human Brain Mapping, 27*(8), 623–635.

Liberzon, I., Phan, K. L., Decker, L. R., & Taylor, S. F. (2003). Extended amygdala and emotional salience: A PET activation study of positive and negative affect. *Neuropsychopharmacology, 28*(4), 726–733.

Lieberman, M. D., Hariri, A., Jarcho, J. M., Eisenberger, N. I., & Bookheimer, S. Y. (2005). An fMRI investigation of race-related amygdala activity in African-American and Caucasian-American individuals. *Nature Neuroscience, 8*(6), 720–722.

McDonald, A. J. (1991). Organization of amygdaloid projections to the prefrontal cortex and associated striatum in the rat. *Neuroscience, 44*(1), 1–14.

Mende-Siedlecki, P., Said, C. P., & Todorov, A. (2013). The social evaluation of faces: A meta-analysis of functional neuroimaging studies. *Social Cognitive and Affective Neuroscience, 8*(3), 285–299.

Mohanty, A., Gitelman, D. R., Small, D. M., & Mesulam, M. M. (2008). The spatial attention network interacts with limbic and monoaminergic systems to modulate motivation-induced attention shifts. *Cerebral Cortex, 18*(11), 2604–2613.

Moll, J., de Oliveira-Souza, R., Bramati, I. E., & Grafman, J. (2002). Functional networks in emotional moral and nonmoral social judgments. *Neuroimage, 16*(3), 696–703.

Moll, J., de Oliveira-Souza, R., Eslinger, P. J., Bramati, I. E., Mourão-Miranda, J., Andreiuolo, P. A., & Pessoa, L. (2002). The neural correlates of moral sensitivity: A functional magnetic resonance imaging investigation of basic and moral emotions. *Journal of Neuroscience, 22*(7), 2730–2736.

Morris, J. S., Frith, C. D., Perrett, D. I., Rowland, D., Young, A. W., Calder, A. J., & Dolan, R. J. (1996). A differential neural response in the human amygdala to fearful and happy facial expressions. *Nature, 383*(6603), 812.

Ochsner, K. N., & Gross, J. J. (2005). The cognitive control of emotion. *Trends in Cognitive Sciences, 9*(5), 242–249.

Oman, D., Thoresen, C. E., & McMahon, K. (1999). Volunteerism and mortality among the community-dwelling elderly. *Journal of Health Psychology, 4*(3), 301–316.

Oosterhof, N. N., & Todorov, A. (2008). The functional basis of face evaluation. *Proceedings of the National Academy of Sciences USA, 105*(32), 11087–11092.

Phelps, E. A., O'Connor, K. J., Cunningham, W. A., Funayama, E. S., Gatenby, J. C., Gore, J. C., & Banaji, M. R. (2000). Performance on indirect measures of race evaluation predicts amygdala activation. *Journal of Cognitive Neuroscience, 12*(5), 729–738.

Phelps, E. A., O'Connor, K. J., Gatenby, J. C., Gore, J. C., Grillon, C., & Davis, M. (2001). Activation of the left amygdala to a cognitive representation of fear. *Nature Neuroscience, 4*(4), 437–441.

Piliavin, J., & Charng, H. (1990). Altruism: A review of recent theory and research. *Annual Review of Sociology, 16*, 27–65.

Plato. (1997). *Phaedrus*. (A. Nehamas & P. Woodruff, Trans.). In J. M. Cooper & D. S. Hutchinson (Eds.), *Complete works* (pp. 506–556). Indianapolis, IN: Hackett.

Post, S. G. (2005). Altruism, happiness, and health: It's good to be good. *International Journal of Behavioral Medicine, 12*(2), 66–77.

Raine, A., & Yang, Y. (2006). Neural foundations to moral reasoning and antisocial behavior. *Social Cognitive and Affective Neuroscience, 1*(3), 203–213.

Rand, D. G., Greene, J. D., & Nowak, M. A. (2012). Spontaneous giving and calculated greed. *Nature, 489*(7416), 427–430.

Sah, P., Faber, E. S. L., De Armentia, M. L., & Power, J. (2003). The amygdaloid complex: Anatomy and physiology. *Physiological Reviews, 83*(3), 803–834.

Said, C. P., Baron, S. G., & Todorov, A. (2009). Nonlinear amygdala response to face trustworthiness: Contributions of high and low spatial frequency information. *Journal of Cognitive Neuroscience, 21*(3), 519–528.

Sander, D., Grafman, J., & Zalla, T. (2003). The human amygdala: An evolved system for relevance detection. *Reviews in the Neurosciences, 14*(4), 303–316.

Schoenbaum, G., Chiba, A. A., & Gallagher, M. (1998). Orbitofrontal cortex and basolateral amygdala encode expected outcomes during learning. *Nature Neuroscience, 1*(2), 155–159.

Small, D. M., Gregory, M. D., Mak, Y. E., Gitelman, D., Mesulam, M. M., & Parrish, T. (2003). Dissociation of neural representation of intensity and affective valuation in human gustation. *Neuron, 39*(4), 701.

Thoits, P. A., & Hewitt, L. N. (2001). Volunteer work and well-being. *Journal of Health and Social Behavior, 42*(2), 115–131.

Todorov, A., Said, C. P., Engell, A. D., & Oosterhof, N. N. (2008). Understanding evaluation of faces on social dimensions. *Trends in Cognitive Sciences, 12*(12), 455–460.

Van Bavel, J. J., Packer, D. J., & Cunningham, W. A. (2008). The neural substrates of ingroup bias: A functional magnetic resonance imaging investigation. *Psychological Science, 19*(11), 1131–1139.

Whalen, P. J. (1998). Fear, vigilance, and ambiguity: Initial neuroimaging studies of the human amygdala. *Current Directions in Psychological Science, 7*(6), 177–188.

Whalen, P. J., Shin, L. M., McInerney, S. C., & Rauch, S. L. (1998). Greater fMRI activation to fearful vs angry facial expression in the amygdaloid region. *Neuroscience Abstracts, 24*, 692.

Wheeler, M. E., & Fiske, S. T. (2005). Controlling racial prejudice social-cognitive goals affect amygdala and stereotype activation. *Psychological Science, 16*(1), 56–63.

White, N. P. (1979). The basis of Stoic ethics. *Harvard Studies in Classical Philology, 83*, 143–178.

Winston, J. S., Strange, B. A., O'Doherty, J., & Dolan, R. J. (2002). Automatic and intentional brain responses during evaluation of trustworthiness of faces. *Nature Neuroscience, 5*(3), 277–283.

Zald, D. H., & Pardo, J. V. (1997). Emotion, olfaction, and the human amygdala: Aamygdala activation during aversive olfactory stimulation. *Proceedings of the National Academy of Sciences USA, 94*(8), 4119–4124.

Zelazo, P. D., & Cunningham, W. (2007). Executive function: Mechanisms underlying emotion regulation. In J. Gross (Ed.), *Handbook of emotion regulation* (pp. 135–158). New York, NY: Guilford Press.

8

Toward a Neuroscience
of Compassion

A Brain Systems–Based Model
and Research Agenda

YONI K. ASHAR, JESSICA R. ANDREWS-HANNA,
SONA DIMIDJIAN, AND TOR D. WAGER ■

Love and compassion are necessities, not luxuries. Without them,
humanity cannot survive.

—THE DALAI LAMA

Compassion is regarded as a central virtue by many cultures and value systems. It is an essential ingredient of healthy interactions with others at every
scale, from the everyday interactions within a local community to the interactions among nations that shape human well-being and suffering in profound
ways. Though compassion is interpersonal, it has also been empirically linked
with personal benefits, including increased positive emotions (Dunn, Aknin,
& Norton, 2014; Fredrickson, Cohn, Coffey, Pek, & Finkel, 2008), improved
physical health (Carson et al., 2005; Kok et al., 2013), and a reduced immu-
nological stress response (Pace et al., 2009, 2010). Unfortunately, despite the
personal and interpersonal advantages of a compassionate stance, people
often respond to others' suffering with indifference, aversion, or even gloating. A scientific understanding of *how* and *when* compassion arises could help
promote a more compassionate society.

To illustrate the complexity of responding to others' suffering, imagine encountering a disheveled elderly women begging for money on the street corner. Perhaps she seems desperately needy and frantic, or perhaps she seems jaded and worn from years of begging. Basic affective feelings—the desire to approach or avoid, elementary forms of distress, tenderness, and aversion—arise immediately, often unbidden. Simultaneously, an assortment of thoughts may present themselves, such as "It's her fault she's homeless," "She probably has nowhere to sleep," "My $2 won't do her much good anyways," "She seems like a sweet person," "I can't trust her to spend the money wisely," and so forth. In some cases, this information is integrated to construct a schematized, gestalt "emotional meaning" (Roy, Shohamy, & Wager, 2012) regarding the situation, such as compassionately perceiving the woman as deserving of help or angrily blaming her for her suffering. All of these feelings, judgments, and emotional meanings interact, and each can constrain the evolution of the others, in a process potentially resulting in behavioral decisions such as helping or distancing. Understanding these interactions, particularly the factors that lead to the evolution of compassion versus disgust or schadenfreude, could support the development of targeted interventions to increase compassion and compassionate behavior.

There are many obstacles to studying compassion, not least among them that scholars define compassion in different ways (see Batson, 2011; Goetz, Keltner, & Simon-Thomas, 2010; Singer & Lamm, 2009 for discussions), and the boundaries between affective feelings, judgments, and emotions are conceptually permeable. The concept of "compassion" can potentially include feelings, thoughts, emotions, and behaviors (helping). Here, we operationally define compassion as a mental state arising in response to another's suffering that motivates behavior intended to relieve their suffering. The conceptual ambiguity inherent in defining psychological processes such as "compassion" and "emotion" is a major reason to anchor concepts and definitions in the study of brain systems. Mapping compassion and its psychological ingredients to brain systems can provide a stable framework for identifying processes independent of semantic definitions, and a basis for their objective measurement.

In the first section of this chapter, we emphasize that compassion and compassionate behavior comprise multiple processes, including affective feelings, social inferences, and emotional meanings, each supported by distinct brain networks. In the second section, we describe the relationships between these component processes, illustrating how the attractor-like properties of their underlying brain networks facilitate a dynamic interplay of patterns of neural activity. In the third section, we identify several future directions for the field of compassion research, focusing especially on compassion-training interventions.

NEURAL UNDERPINNINGS OF COMPASSION

A growing body of research suggests that at least two distinct neural networks underlie empathy, the sharing and understanding of another's experience (de Waal, 2008; Decety & Jackson, 2004; Fan, Duncan, de Greck, & Northoff, 2011; Shamay-Tsoory, Aharon-Peretz, & Perry, 2009; Van Overwalle & Baetens, 2009; Zaki & Ochsner, 2012). One network comprising the dorsal medial prefrontal cortex (dmPFC), temporoparietal junction (TPJ), and posterior cingulate cortex (PCC) supports *social-inferential* properties of empathy, as when inferring the perspectives, beliefs, and feelings of other people. A second, distinct network centered on the anterior insula (aI) and the dorsal anterior cingulate cortex (dACC) engages when individuals experience *affective* responses to others' suffering.

While these brain systems support sharing in and understanding another's suffering, a distinct brain system underlies the valuing of others and prosocial motivation to help them (Harbaugh, Mayr, & Burghart, 2007; Hare, Camerer, Knoepfle, & Rangel, 2010; Moll et al., 2006; Zaki & Ochsner, 2012). We posit that the valuing of others' welfare and consequent prosocial motivation is supported by a medial prefrontal-striatal network constructing (potentially compassionate) emotional meanings (Roy et al., 2012).

Social Inference

Compassion and compassionate behavior depend first and foremost on the inference of another person's unmet needs (Batson, 2011). Additionally, compassion and compassionate behavior have been empirically shown to depend on a number of other social inferences (Goetz et al., 2010; Yarkoni, Ashar, & Wager, 2015), including attributions of responsibility (Rudolph, Roesch, Greitemeyer, & Weiner, 2004), trustworthiness (Sargeant & Lee, 2004; van't Wout & Sanfey, 2008), and in some cases self-similarity (Batson, Lishner, Cook, & Sawyer, 2005; Vollhardt & Staub, 2011). Social inferences depend on the ability to understand and make attributions regarding others' mental states, a process often referred to as "mentalizing" or "theory of mind." A system of cortical structures including the dorsal medial prefrontal cortex (dmPFC), posterior cingulate cortex (PCC), and temporoparietal junction (TPJ) (Figure 8.1a), is widely thought to support these processes (Zaki & Ochsner, 2012). This network is recruited when rating the intensity of others' emotional suffering (Bruneau, Dufour, & Saxe, 2012; Bruneau, Pluta, & Saxe, 2012), passing moral judgment on others (Koster-Hale, Saxe, Dungan, &

Young, 2013), and accurately inferring others' emotions (Zaki, Weber, Bolger, & Ochsner, 2009).

Affective Feeling

A second system, including the ventral mid-anterior insular cortex (aI), dorsal anterior cingulate (dACC), and their connections with the amygdala, supports affective responses to others' suffering (Figure. 81a) (Decety, Norman, Berntson, & Cacioppo, 2012; Lamm, Decety, & Singer, 2011; Singer & Lamm, 2009; Zaki & Ochsner, 2012). Affective feelings here refer to basic, rudimentary feelings, with motivational properties, but without elaborated conceptual schemas (Russell & Barrett, 1999).

Two types of affective responses, related but conceptually distinct, may arise in response to others' suffering: (a) distress responses, and (b) "tender" responses (Decety & Lamm, 2011; Eisenberg & Eggum, 2011; Singer & Klimecki, 2014). Distress is characterized by negative arousal, and can be associated with escape behavior (Batson, 2011), or, with increased helping (Ashar et al., in press). Tenderness is characterized by warm, positive feelings toward the other and helping behavior (Ashar et al., in press). Tender responding may be additionally supported by the neural systems underlying parental care-giving (P. Kim, Strathearn, & Swain, 2015; Lonstein, Lévy, & Fleming, 2015).

The relationship between affective feeling and compassionate behavior is complex. The interpersonal implications of an emotion, rather than its basic affective properties, seem to be most predictive of compassion. For example, we found that both positively valenced emotions (tenderness) and distress were positively associated with increased charitable donation (Ashar et al., in press), suggesting that valence alone is not linearly related to helping. Relatedly and somewhat paradoxically, Condon and Barrett found that compassion is conceptualized as a positively valenced emotion, but the experience of compassion leads to heightened negative affect (Condon & Feldman Barrett, 2013).

Emotional Meaning

Compassion can be characterized by an emotional appraisal of one's relationship to a suffering other, informed by the suffering other's personal significance to the self and by contextual features of the situation. For example, compassionate responses are critically determined by how much ones cares about helping veterans specifically, or by the personal significance of a particular disease afflicting another (i.e., if a loved one also has the same disease). We propose that a ventromedial prefrontal-subcortical network (Figure 8.1a) subserves these processes, which we describe as the construction of "emotional meaning" (Roy et al., 2012). The ventromedial prefrontal cortex (vmPFC) connects systems involved in episodic memory, representation of the affective qualities of sensory events, social cognition, and interoceptive signals, and it plays a unique role in representing conceptual information and in transducing concepts into affective behavioral and physiological responses (Haber & Knutson, 2010). Additionally, the vmPFC has the requisite connections to the social inference and associative affect networks outlined earlier, as well as to the striatum, hypothalamus, and brainstem, allowing it to coordinate system-wide affective physiological and behavioral responses (Roy et al., 2012). This network shows increased activity when participants are asked to adopt a compassionate stance toward others' suffering (Engen & Singer, 2015; J.-W. Kim et al., 2009; Klimecki, Leiberg, Lamm, & Singer, 2012), and connectivity within this network correlates with sadness when viewing a film about another's suffering (Raz et al., 2012).

The emotional meaning constructed around another's suffering includes how much a person "cares" about the suffering other. Caring about another person's welfare is a fundamental antecedent of compassion (Batson, 2011) and is closely related to evaluating the other's relevance for the self (Goetz et al., 2010). Neuroimaging studies confirm that activity in vmPFC-subcortical circuits tracks the closeness of another person (Harris & Fiske, 2007; Krienen, Tu, & Buckner, 2010), even when closeness is crossed with valence: For Arabs and Jewish Israelis, considering the suffering of in-group or out-group members activated the vmPFC equally, while this region showed relatively less activity when considering South Americans (a distant group) (Bruneau, Dufour, et al., 2012).

Numerous studies have found that activity in the vmPFC and ventral striatum is associated with prosocial behavior, such as increased charitable donations (Genevsky, Västfjäll, Slovic, & Knutson, 2013; Harbaugh et al., 2007; Hare et al., 2010; Moll et al., 2006), decisions to give more equitably (Zaki & Mitchell, 2011), and kind behavior toward a socially excluded person (Masten, Morelli, & Eisenberger, 2011). This neural activity has often been interpreted as reflecting a common neural currency of valuing: since vmPFC/mOFC activity tracks value across a range of domains, including food, money, social rewards, and more (Levy & Glimcher, 2012), it may also represent how much we value other people's welfare. This valuation would be closely related to the emotional meaning we ascribe to the other's suffering, and their significance to the self.

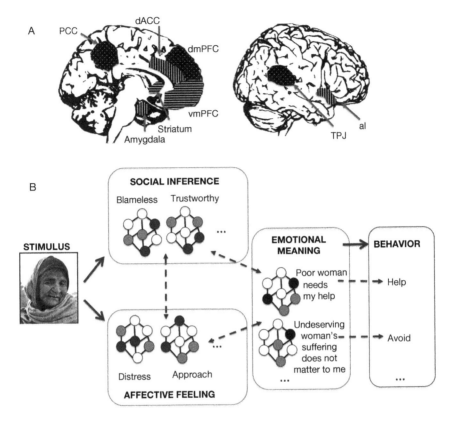

Figure 8.1 (A) Key brain systems hypothesized to support compassion. An insular-cingulate network supports *affective feelings* such as aversion or approach motivation, resulting either from sharing the affective state of the other or reacting directly to the stimulus. A distinct cortical network supports *social inferences* and attributions regarding the other's internal state, such as "She is poor" or "It's her fault she is poor." A third prefrontal-subcortical network synthesizes conceptual and affective information to evaluate the gestalt, situated *emotional meaning* of the stimulus (Roy et al., 2012). aI, anterior insula; dACC, dorsal anterior cingulate cortex; dmPFC, dorsomedial prefrontal cortex; PCC, posterior cingulate cortex; TPJ, temporoparietal junction; vmPFC, ventromedial prefrontal cortex. Regional boundaries are approximate. (B) The suffering of another person is initially represented as social inferences and affective feelings. Information in these two networks contributes to the formation of an emotional meaning, which may guide the observer's behavior. These systems can be conceptualized as attractor networks, such that dynamic, interacting patterns of activity both within and between networks characterize the possible responses to others' suffering. With training, these networks can learn to adopt prosocial patterns more readily.

Additional Brain Systems

Though not the focus of the present review, a number of additional brain systems may also play an important role in generating a compassionate response to a suffering individual. If the individual is a familiar other, neural circuits subserving memory retrieval, including the medial temporal lobe, retrosplenial cortex, and posterior inferior parietal lobule, may facilitate the retrieval of prior information relevant to the individual. Frontoparietal control systems, including those involved in emotion regulation, may additionally help the observer inhibit his prepotent emotional or behavioral response, or resolve his internal conflict regarding the possible courses of action. Additionally, the "mirror neuron" system, including the intraparietal sulcus, posterior superior temporal sulcus (pSTS), and premotor cortex, plays an important role in understanding others' motor goals and actions (Van Overwalle & Baetens, 2009). Finally, neural systems supporting parental care-giving behavior may also be recruited during the experience of compassion (P. Kim et al., 2015; Lonstein et al., 2015).

A DYNAMIC PROCESS-CONTENT MODEL OF COMPASSION

Thus far, we have described three distinct brain networks, each implicated by prior research as supporting a category of processes critical for compassion to arise. We now describe the interrelationship of these processes, focusing especially on the *content* of these processes, i.e., the specific social inference, affective feeling, or gestalt appraisal arising.

In our model, a potential recipient of compassionate behavior (i.e., a suffering woman) can be processed both in a feed-forward fashion, in which information flow through the brain is primarily unidirectional (Figure 8.1b, left-to-right directionality), and in an iterative, recurrent fashion, like an attractor network (Figure 8.1b, within- and between-network arrows), where information flows multidirectionally within and between networks.

After early visual processing of the stimulus (i.e., a suffering person), one or many affective feelings may arise. The precise nature of these feelings (their *content*) may be represented as unique *patterns* of neural activity within an insular-cingulate network. Simultaneously, the observer may form social inferences about the mental state and condition of the suffering individual, represented by distinct patterns of neural activity within the network comprising the dmPFC, TPJ, and PCC (Kragel & LaBar, 2015; Peelen, Atkinson, & Vuilleumier, 2010; Saarimaki et al., 2015). The patterns of activity in these two networks are next integrated in the medial prefrontal-striatal network, along with additional information, to form an emotional meaning of the suffering individual, integrating contextual features. The strength and nature of the emotional meaning will ultimately guide behavior toward the suffering other.

The networks supporting social inference and affective feelings act as "rate-limiting processes" such that diminished function in either will greatly reduce the likelihood of a compassionate emotional meaning arising. Likewise, helping behavior toward the other is unlikely unless a critical intensity of emotional meaning is reached. Thus, the presence of these three processes—feelings, social inference, and meaning—is necessary for compassion and compassionate behavior. The absence of these processes would be indicative of apathy.

Each network functions as an attractor network: The activity of any one population of neurons impacts other populations of neurons, causing changes to iteratively reverberate throughout the network, such that the network will progress through different states. At a system-wide level, the three networks also function as an attractor network: Activity in one network will impact the other two, which will then impact the first network, and so on, evolving until a stable system-wide pattern potentially emerges. Thus, quicker responses (such as a startle response or fast aversion) and their concordant neural activations may yield to slower, potentially trained responses, including compassion.

To illustrate the proposed model, we return to our opening example. Upon first sight of the homeless woman, feelings of aversion and/or a desire to engage are represented as fast, competing patterns in an amygdala/insula/ACC network. In tandem, social inferences—such as she is suffering, she wants me to give her money, she is hungry, and so on—arise as different patterns in the dmPFC/PCC/TPJ network. Within each network, populations of neurons progress through different states, representing these competing or coexisting social inferences and affective feelings. An emotional meaning emerges as the individual constructs a situated, gestalt representation of the situation congruent with the woman's personal significance to the individual, such as "this poor woman needs my help" or "this woman is disgusting to me and deserves her suffering." The content in different networks may mutually influence each other. For example, feelings of disgust may strengthen social inferences of blame, while a simultaneous prosocial emotional meaning will strengthen competing social inferences of blamelessness, and activity in all three networks will adapt accordingly. Compassion and other distinctive responses such as gloating are characterized by the formation of a stable, coherent, system-wide representation of the feelings, thoughts, and narrative surrounding the encounter, leading to coordinated behaviors, including helping. Conversely, an individual may continue to feel torn, characterized by continuous oscillations between various network configurations, and coordinated behavior may not emerge.

Implications for Compassion Deficits

Our model of compassion is consistent with established findings regarding the dissociable neural bases of compassion deficits in specific clinical populations. Psychopathy, schizophrenia, and narcissism are characterized by deficits in affective feeling but not necessarily social inference, while autism, bipolar disorder, and borderline traits are associated with impairment in social inference but not affective feeling (Cox et al., 2012).

Similar mechanisms may underlie the dehumanization of devalued others. In dehumanization, compassion may fail to arise because of difficulty inferring others' internal states (Harris & Fiske, 2007; Haslam, 2006), because affective responses are suppressed (Xu, Zuo, Wang, & Han, 2009), or because the content of social inferences and/or affective responses supports gloating, cruelty, dismissal, or other non-compassionate responses (Hein, Silani, Preuschoff, Batson, & Singer, 2010). Dehumanization can be supported by distorted emotional meanings as well, such as narratives depicting others as sexual objects (Bernard, Gervais, Allen, Campomizzi, & Klein, 2012) or depicting them as "parasites," a dehumanizing image used in genocidal campaigns.

COMPASSION TRAINING AND OTHER FUTURE DIRECTIONS

Many open, important questions remain in compassion research. Here we highlight a few prominent future directions, with an eye toward compassion training due to its potential for large-scale use and its clear societal implications.

Linking Cognitive Neuroscience With Compassion Training

Recent evidence suggests that people can be trained both to feel and act more compassionately toward others (Galante, Galante, Bekkers, & Gallacher, 2014). Compassion training programs have typically been based on compassion meditation and/or loving-kindness meditation, contemplative practices cultivating feelings of care, connection, and love for others, and/or asking practioners to reflects on others' suffering and on human interdependence (Hofmann, Grossman, & Hinton, 2011). Relative to a variety of control conditions, compassion training programs have been shown to increase prosocial behavior in a video game (Leiberg, Klimecki, & Singer, 2011), accuracy in discerning others' emotions (Mascaro, Rilling, Tenzin Negi, & Raison, 2013), affective responses to suffering others (Ashar et al., in press.; Hutcherson, Seppala, & Gross, 2008; Klimecki et al., 2012), altruistic redistribution of funds to benefit others treated unfairly (Weng et al., 2013), charitable donation amounts (Ashar et al., in press), and real-world helping behavior to strangers in need (Condon, Desbordes, Miller, & DeSteno, 2013). Compassion training has also been found to decrease stress-related neuroendocrine responding (Pace et al., 2009, 2010, 2013).

Evidence is accumulating that such programs leads to changes in neural function as well. Relative to control groups, compassion training programs have lead to increased enhanced neural activity in the right amygdala (Desbordes et al., 2012), inferior parietal lobule and dorsolateral PFC (Weng et al., 2013), and striatum and right medial orbitofrontal cortex (Klimecki et al., 2012) when witnessing human suffering. Compassion training has also been shown to increase neural activity in the inferior frontal gyrus and dorsomedial PFC when attempting to infer others' emotions (Mascaro & Rilling, 2012). Relatedly, expert compassion meditators showed enhanced neural processing in the TPJ, posterior superior temporal sulcus, amygdalae, and insula in response to sounds of human distress (Lutz, Greischar, Perlman, & Davidson, 2009) and in the ventral striatum and medial OFC when viewing suffering others (Engen & Singer, 2015; Klimecki et al., 2012). The diversity of brain regions represented likely reflects the underlying diversity of compassion training and measurement paradigms employed.

Advances in the basic science of compassion will pave the way for interventions to more precisely target and assess specific processes and neural networks, enabling robust, replicable interventions. Using our dynamic model of compassion as a platform, we propose that compassion training may increase prosocial behavior by targeting the component processes highlighted earlier, in addition to the underlying nature of their content. An intervention might aim to enhance prosocial inferences, positive affective feelings and/or empathetic suffering, and more compassionate emotional meanings. For example, we recently developed a quantitative psychological model of six specific feelings and attributions strongly predictive of charitable donation. We then targetted these specific process in a compassion training program. We found that a composite measure of these feelings and attributions mediated the effects of the training program on charitable donation (Ashar et al., in press). This suggests that precisely characterizing the psychological and neural processes supporting compassion can enhance efforts to train compassion.

Our model also has implications for how compassion-related brain activity can be detected and measured using functional magnetic resonance imaging (fMRI) and other technologies. While overall regional activity may distinguish between compassion and apathy (i.e., Harbaugh et al., 2007; Hare et al., 2010; Klimecki et al., 2012), distinguishing between different responses of similar intensities (such as compassion and schadenfreude) will require examining within-network patterns of activity, rather than overall regional activity. For example, evidence is accumulating that both compassion (Harbaugh et al., 2007; Klimecki et al., 2012) and schadenfreude (Dvash, Gilam, Ben-Ze'ev, Hendler, & Shamay-Tsoory, 2010; Hein et al., 2010) activate the striatum, a component of the emotional meaning network. Likewise, Arabs and Jewish Israelis report feeling less compassion for the suffering of an out-group member, but they showed no differences in overall regional neural activity in the vmPFC, PCC, or rTPJ compared to the in-group member (Bruneau, Dufour, et al., 2012). Similarly, patterns of activity—rather than overall regional activity—in the rTPJ were associated with inferences about others' blameworthiness (Koster-Hale et al., 2013). Thus, within-region *patterns* of neural activity may be more informative than overall activity levels in some cases. Consequently, multivoxel pattern analysis (MVPA), a multivariate technique allowing detection of spatially distributed patterns of activation, may be a useful tool in differentiating between different, but equally intense, responses to others' suffering.

Additionally, our model posits a theoretical mechanism by which training occurs: As the networks practice stabilizing in compassionate states, these prosocial patterns will become more readily accessible and adopted more quickly. This prediction could be explored by measuring the time delay for a participant to reach a "compassionate" neural state, quantifiable with spatial patterns of activation previously linked to compassion-related psychological processes.

Improved Measurement of Compassion and Compassionate Behavior

Investigations of compassion and compassionate behavior are limited by the tools we use to measure these phenomena. A common approach is collecting self-reported compassion. This approach is vulnerable to demand characteristics both from the specific experimental context and from the general social desirability of adopting a compassionate stance (DellaVigna, List, & Malmendier, 2012; Izuma, Saito, & Sadato, 2010). Facial expression may be valuable for measuring compassion (Eisenberg et al., 1989), particularly with the recent advent of automated facial expression recognition software. Neuroimaging results can be difficult to interpret in psychological terms; relating neural activity to in-scanner behavior, such as in-scanner charitable donation (Harbaugh et al., 2007; Hare et al., 2010) or empathic accuracy tasks (Mascaro & Rilling, 2012) helps guide interpretation. Lastly, real-world measures of compassionate behavior in which the participant is unaware of being observed will serve an important role in improving the ecological validity of compassion assessment. Some examples of ecologically valid paradigms include whether a person gives up his or her seat to another person on crutches (Condon et al., 2013) and audio sampling of daily life to assess compassionate speech and behavior.

We observed a partial disassociation between charitable donation and self-report of compassion (Ashar et al., in press). About one quarter of participants did not donate money at all in an online real-money donation task, despite reporting similar levels of compassion relative to donating participants. We speculate that this is because charitable donation is influenced by many factors not related to compassion (i.e., financial distress, negative beliefs about charities), highlighting the difficulty of developing robust measures of compassionate behavior.

Translating Compassion Into Compassionate Behavior

Compassion will benefit others to the extent that it leads to compassionate behavior. Individuals feeling compassion will choose not to help if the costs associated with helping outweigh the anticipated benefits (Batson, 2011). Because the material costs of helping are small in many situations (i.e., $2, 5 minutes of one's time, etc.), it is likely that other social, cognitive, or emotional costs likely deter helping behavior. For example, the presence of other individuals ("bystander effect") has been robustly demonstrated to hinder helping behavior (Fischer et al., 2011). Conversely, social pressure and perceived social norms can increase helping (DellaVigna et al., 2012; Izuma et al., 2010). Additionally, the discomfort or distress often experienced in approaching a suffering person can inhibit helping. Further research examining factors facilitating and inhibiting the behavioral expression of compassion, and the responsiveness of those factors to training, will be of great value to intervention research.

Sustaining Compassion

The "burning out" of individuals in caregiving positions is a well-documented, costly phenomenon (Zenasni, Boujut, Woerner, & Sultan, 2012). It is possible that particular ways of empathizing will lead to burnout, while others will not (Klimecki & Singer, 2012). Specifcally, high levels of distress may exhaust a care-giver's emotional resources, while feelings of tenderness and care might offer a more sustainable way of empathizing (see also Batson et al., 1987; Eisenberg et al., 1989). Compassion training programs may counteract or prevent these effects by increasing tender, caring, positive emotions in the face of suffer-ing (Ashar et al., in press; Klimecki et al., 2012; Singer & Klimecki, 2014). In our investigation, participants who were repeatedly exposed to suffering sub-stantially decreased in reported compassion and helping behavior—perhaps reflecting a sort of "burnout" or desenstization to other's suffering—but a compassion training program protected against these decreases (Ashar et al., in press). Studies are needed directly testing whether training caregivers to empathize in particular ways can prevent professional burnout.

CONCLUSION

We have proposed here a dynamic, process-content model of compassion, whereby social inference and affective feelings support the construction of potentially compassionate emotional meanings regarding a suffering other. This model also functions as a dynamic system, like an attractor state net-work, where patterns of neural activity both within and across networks engage in a dynamic, interactive process, potentially leading to behavioral decisions. Importantly, advancing the basic science of compassion, as we have tried to do here, can empower intervention research. Although accumulating evidence suggests that compassionate feeling, behavior, and neural function do respond to training, the neuropsychological mechanisms supporting these changes are unclear. By carefully targeting and measuring specific neural and psychological processes, we will ultimately be able to design more powerful, robust, and generalizable compassion training programs, building toward a kinder world.

REFERENCES

Ashar, Y. K., Andrews-Hanna, J. R., Yarkoni, T., Sills, J., Halifax, J., Dimidjian, S., & Wager, T. D. (n.d.). Effects of Compassion Meditation on a psychological model of charitable donation. *Emotion*.

Batson, C. D. (2011). *Altruism in humans*. Oxford University Press.

Batson, C. D., Lishner, D. a, Cook, J., & Sawyer, S. (2005). Similarity and Nurturance: Two Possible Sources of Empathy for Strangers. *Basic and Applied Social Psychology*, 27(1), 37–41. doi:10.1207/s15324834basp2701

Bernard, P., Gervais, S. J., Allen, J., Campomizzi, S., & Klein, O. (2012). Integrating sexual objectification with object versus person recognition: the sexualized-body-inversion hypothesis. *Psychological Science*, *23*(5), 469–71. doi:10.1177/0956797611434748

Bruneau, E. G., Dufour, N., & Saxe, R. (2012). Social cognition in members of conflict groups: behavioural and neural responses in Arabs, Israelis and South Americans to each other's misfortunes. *Philosophical Transactions of the Royal Society of London. ; Series B, Biological Sciences*, *367*(1589), 717–30. doi:10.1098/rstb.2011.0293

Bruneau, E. G., Pluta, A., & Saxe, R. (2012). Distinct roles of the "Shared Pain" and "Theory of Mind" networks in processing others' emotional suffering. *Neuropsychologia*, *50*(2), 219–231. doi:10.1016/j.neuropsychologia.2011.11.008

Carson, J. W., Keefe, F. J., Lynch, T. R., Carson, K. M., Goli, V., Fras, A. M., & Thorp, S. R. (2005). Loving-kindness meditation for chronic low back pain: results from a pilot trial. *Journal of Holistic Nursing : Official Journal of the American Holistic Nurses' Association*, *23*(3), 287–304. doi:10.1177/0898010105277651

Condon, P., Desbordes, G., Miller, W. B., & DeSteno, D. (2013). Meditation increases compassionate responses to suffering. *Psychological Science*, *24*(10), 2125–7. doi:10.1177/0956797613485603

Condon, P., & Feldman Barrett, L. (2013). Conceptualizing and experiencing compassion. *Emotion*, *13*, 817–21. doi:10.1037/a0033747

Cox, C. L., Uddin, L. Q., Di martino, A., Castellanos, F. X., Milham, M. P., & Kelly, C. (2012). The balance between feeling and knowing: Affective and cognitive empathy are reflected in the brain's intrinsic functional dynamics. *Social Cognitive and Affective Neuroscience*, *7*(6), 727–737. doi:10.1093/scan/nsr051

de Waal, F. B. M. (2008). Putting the altruism back into altruism: the evolution of empathy. *Annual Review of Psychology*, *59*, 279–300. doi:10.1146/annurev.psych.59.103006.093625

Decety, J., & Jackson, P. L. (2004). The functional architecture of human empathy. *Behavioral and Cognitive Neuroscience Reviews*, *3*(2), 71–100. doi:10.1177/1534582304267187

Decety, J., & Lamm, C. (2011). Empathy versus Personal Distress: Recent Evidence from Social Neuroscience. In J. Decety & W. Ickes (Eds.), *The Social Neuroscience of Empathy* (1st ed., pp. 199–214). Cambridge, Massachusetts: MIT Press.

Decety, J., Norman, G. J., Berntson, G. G., & Cacioppo, J. T. (2012). A neurobehavioral evolutionary perspective on the mechanisms underlying empathy. *Progress in Neurobiology*, *98*(1), 38–48. doi:10.1016/j.pneurobio.2012.05.001

DellaVigna, S., List, J. A., & Malmendier, U. (2012). Testing for Altruism and Social Pressure in Charitable Giving. *The Quarterly Journal of Economics*, *127*(1), 1–56. doi:10.1093/qje/qjr050

Desbordes, G., Negi, L. T., Pace, T. W. W., Wallace, B. A., Raison, C. L., & Schwartz, E. L. (2012). Effects of mindful-attention and compassion meditation training on amygdala response to emotional stimuli in an ordinary, non-meditative state. *Frontiers in Human Neuroscience*, *6*(November), 1–15. doi:10.3389/fnhum.2012.00292

Dunn, E. W., Aknin, L. B., & Norton, M. I. (2014). Prosocial Spending and Happiness: Using Money to Benefit Others Pays Off. *Current Directions in Psychological Science*, *23*(1), 41–47. doi:10.1177/0963721413512503

Dvash, J., Gilam, G., Ben-Ze'ev, A., Hendler, T., & Shamay-Tsoory, S. G. (2010). The envious brain: the neural basis of social comparison. *Human Brain Mapping*, *31*(11), 1741–50. doi:10.1002/hbm.20972

Eisenberg, N., & Eggum, N. D. (2011). Empathic Responding: Sympathy and Personal Distress. In J. Decety & W. Ickes (Eds.), *The Social Neuroscience of Empathy* (1st ed., pp. 71–85). Cambridge, Massachusetts: MIT Press.

Eisenberg, N., Fabes, R. a, Miller, P. a, Fultz, J., Shell, R., Mathy, R. M., & Reno, R. R. (1989). Relation of sympathy and personal distress to prosocial behavior: a multi-method study. *Journal of Personality and Social Psychology*, *57*(1), 55–66. doi:10.1037/0022-3514.57.1.55

Engen, H. G., & Singer, T. (2015). Compassion-based emotion regulation up-regulates experienced positive affect and associated neural networks. *Social Cognitive and Affective Neuroscience*, *10*(9), 1291–1301. doi:10.1093/scan/nsv008

Fan, Y., Duncan, N. W., de Greck, M., & Northoff, G. (2011). Is there a core neural network in empathy? An fMRI based quantitative meta-analysis. *Neuroscience and Biobehavioral Reviews*, *35*(3), 903–911. doi:10.1016/j.neubiorev.2010.10.009

Fischer, P., Krueger, J. I., Greitemeyer, T., Vogrincic, C., Kastenmüller, A., Frey, D., . . . Kainbacher, M. (2011). The bystander-effect: a meta-analytic review on bystander intervention in dangerous and non-dangerous emergencies. *Psychological Bulletin*, *137*(4), 517–537.

Fredrickson, B. L., Cohn, M. a, Coffey, K. a, Pek, J., & Finkel, S. M. (2008). Open hearts build lives: positive emotions, induced through loving-kindness meditation, build consequential personal resources. *Journal of Personality and Social Psychology*, *95*(5), 1045–1062. doi:10.1037/a0013262

Galante, J., Galante, I., Bekkers, M.-J., & Gallacher, J. (2014). Effect of Kindness-Based Meditation on Health and Well-Being: A Systematic Review and Meta-Analysis. *Journal of Consulting and Clinical Psychology*, No–Specified. doi:10.1037/a0037249

Genevsky, A., Västfjäll, D., Slovic, P., & Knutson, B. (2013). Neural underpinnings of the identifiable victim effect: affect shifts preferences for giving. *The Journal of Neuroscience : The Official Journal of the Society for Neuroscience*, *33*(43), 17188–96. doi:10.1523/JNEUROSCI.2348-13.2013

Goetz, J. L., Keltner, D., & Simon-Thomas, E. (2010). Compassion: an evolutionary analysis and empirical review. *Psychological Bulletin*, *136*(3), 351–374. doi:10.1037/a0018807

Haber, S. N., & Knutson, B. (2010). The Reward Circuit: Linking Primate Anatomy and Human Imaging. *Neuropsychopharmacology*, *35*(1), 4–26. doi:10.1038/npp.2009.129

Harbaugh, W. T., Mayr, U., & Burghart, D. R. (2007). Neural responses to taxation and voluntary giving reveal motives for charitable donations. *Science (New York, N.Y.)*, *316*(5831), 1622–5. doi:10.1126/science.1140738

Hare, T. A., Camerer, C. F., Knoepfle, D. T., & Rangel, A. (2010). Value computations in ventral medial prefrontal cortex during charitable decision making incorporate input from regions involved in social cognition. *The Journal of Neuroscience : The Official Journal of the Society for Neuroscience*, *30*(2), 583–90. doi:10.1523/JNEUROSCI.4089-09.2010

Harris, L. T., & Fiske, S. T. (2007). Social groups that elicit disgust are differentially processed in mPFC. *Social Cognitive and Affective Neuroscience*, *2*(1), 45–51. doi:10.1093/scan/nsl037

Haslam, N. (2006). Dehumanization: An Integrative Review. *Personal and Social Psychology Review, 10*, 214–234. doi:10.1207/s15327957pspr1003

Hein, G., Silani, G., Preuschoff, K., Batson, C. D., & Singer, T. (2010). Neural responses to ingroup and outgroup members' suffering predict individual differences in costly helping. *Neuron, 68*(1), 149–60. doi:10.1016/j.neuron.2010.09.003

Hofmann, S. G., Grossman, P., & Hinton, D. E. (2011). Loving-kindness and compassion meditation: Potential for psychological interventions. *Clinical Psychology Review, 31*(7), 1126–1132. doi:10.1016/j.cpr.2011.07.003

Hutcherson, C. a, Seppala, E. M., & Gross, J. J. (2008). Loving-kindness meditation increases social connectedness. *Emotion (Washington, D.C.), 8*(5), 720–724. doi:10.1037/a0013237

Izuma, K., Saito, D. N., & Sadato, N. (2010). Processing of the incentive for social approval in the ventral striatum during charitable donation. *Journal of Cognitive Neuroscience, 22*(4), 621–31. doi:10.1162/jocn.2009.21228

Kim, J.-W., Kim, S.-E., Kim, J.-J., Jeong, B., Park, C.-H., Son, A. R., . . . Ki, S. W. (2009). Compassionate attitude towards others' suffering activates the mesolimbic neural system. *Neuropsychologia, 47*(10), 2073–81. doi:10.1016/j.neuropsychologia.2009.03.017

Kim, P., Strathearn, L., & Swain, J. E. (2015). The maternal brain and its plasticity in humans. *Hormones and Behavior*, 1–11. doi:10.1016/j.yhbeh.2015.08.001

Klimecki, O. M., Leiberg, S., Lamm, C., & Singer, T. (2012). Functional Neural Plasticity and Associated Changes in Positive Affect After Compassion Training. *Cerebral Cortex (New York, N.Y. : 1991), 23*, 1–10. doi:10.1093/cercor/bhs142

Klimecki, O. M., & Singer, T. (2012). Empathic Distress Fatigue Rather Than Compassion Fatigue? Integrating Findings from Empathy Research in Psychology and Social Neuroscience. In B. Oakley, A. Knafo, G. Madhavan, & D. S. Wilson (Eds.), *Pathological altruism* (pp. 368–383). New York: Oxford University Press.

Kok, B. E., Coffey, K. a, Cohn, M. a, Catalino, L. I., Vacharkulksemsuk, T., Algoe, S. B., . . . Fredrickson, B. L. (2013). How positive emotions build physical health: perceived positive social connections account for the upward spiral between positive emotions and vagal tone. *Psychological Science, 24*, 1123–32. doi:10.1177/0956797612470827

Koster-Hale, J., Saxe, R., Dungan, J., & Young, L. L. (2013). Decoding moral judgments from neural representations of intentions. *Proceedings of the National Academy of Sciences of the United States of America, 110*(14), 5648–53. doi:10.1073/pnas.1207992110

Kragel, P. A., & LaBar, K. S. (2015). Multivariate neural biomarkers of emotional states are categorically distinct. *Social Cognitive and Affective Neuroscience*, nsv032–. doi:10.1093/scan/nsv032

Krienen, F. M., Tu, P.-C., & Buckner, R. L. (2010). Clan Mentality: Evidence That the Medial Prefrontal Cortex Responds to Close Others. *Journal of Neuroscience, 30*(41), 13906–13915. doi:10.1523/JNEUROSCI.2180-10.2010

Lamm, C., Decety, J., & Singer, T. (2011). Meta-analytic evidence for common and distinct neural networks associated with directly experienced pain and empathy for pain. *NeuroImage, 54*(3), 2492–2502. doi:10.1016/j.neuroimage.2010.10.014

Leiberg, S., Klimecki, O. M., & Singer, T. (2011). Short-term compassion training increases prosocial behavior in a newly developed prosocial game. *PLoS ONE, 6*(3), e17798. doi:10.1371/journal.pone.0017798

Levy, D. J., & Glimcher, P. W. (2012). The root of all value: a neural common currency for choice. *Current Opinion in Neurobiology, 22*(6), 1027–38. doi:10.1016/j.conb.2012.06.001

Lonstein, J. S., Lévy, F., & Fleming, A. S. (2015). Common and divergent psychobiological mechanisms underlying maternal behaviors in non-human and human mammals. *Hormones and Behavior, 73*, 156–185. doi:10.1016/j.yhbeh.2015.06.011

Lutz, A., Greischar, L. L., Perlman, D. M., & Davidson, R. J. (2009). BOLD signal in insula is differentially related to cardiac function during compassion meditation in experts vs. novices. *NeuroImage, 47*(3), 1038–1046. doi:10.1016/j.neuroimage.2009.04.081

Mascaro, J. S., Rilling, J. K., Tenzin Negi, L., & Raison, C. L. (2013). Compassion meditation enhances empathic accuracy and related neural activity. *Social Cognitive and Affective Neuroscience, 8*(1), 48–55. doi:10.1093/scan/nss095

Masten, C. L., Morelli, S. a., & Eisenberger, N. I. (2011). An fMRI investigation of empathy for "social pain" and subsequent prosocial behavior. *NeuroImage, 55*(1), 381–388. doi:10.1016/j.neuroimage.2010.11.060

Moll, J., Krueger, F., Zahn, R., Pardini, M., de Oliveira-Souza, R., & Grafman, J. (2006). Human fronto-mesolimbic networks guide decisions about charitable donation. *Proceedings of the National Academy of Sciences of the United States of America, 103*(42), 15623–15628. doi:10.1073/pnas.0604475103

Pace, T. W. W., Negi, L. T., Adame, D. D., Cole, S. P., Sivilli, T. I., Brown, T. D., . . . Raison, C. L. (2009). Effect of compassion meditation on neuroendocrine, innate immune and behavioral responses to psychosocial stress. *Psychoneuroendocrinology, 34*(1), 87–98. doi:10.1016/j.psyneuen.2008.08.011

Pace, T. W. W., Negi, L. T., Dodson-Lavelle, B., Ozawa-de Silva, B., Reddy, S. D., Cole, S. P., . . . Raison, C. L. (2013). Engagement with Cognitively-Based Compassion Training is associated with reduced salivary C-reactive protein from before to after training in foster care program adolescents. *Psychoneuroendocrinology, 38*, 294–299. doi:10.1016/j.psyneuen.2012.05.019

Pace, T. W. W., Negi, L. T., Sivilli, T. I., Issa, M. J., Cole, S. P., Adame, D. D., & Raison, C. L. (2010). Innate immune, neuroendocrine and behavioral responses to psychosocial stress do not predict subsequent compassion meditation practice time. *Psychoneuroendocrinology, 35*(2), 310–315. doi:10.1016/j.psyneuen.2009.06.008

Peelen, M. V, Atkinson, A. P., & Vuilleumier, P. (2010). Supramodal representations of perceived emotions in the human brain. *The Journal of Neuroscience : The Official Journal of the Society for Neuroscience, 30*(30), 10127–10134. doi:10.1523/jneurosci.2161-10.2010

Raz, G., Winetraub, Y., Jacob, Y., Kinreich, S., Maron-Katz, A., Shaham, G., . . . Hendler, T. (2012). Portraying emotions at their unfolding: A multilayered approach for probing dynamics of neural networks. *NeuroImage, 60*(2), 1448–1461. doi:10.1016/j.neuroimage.2011.12.084

Roy, M., Shohamy, D., & Wager, T. D. (2012). Ventromedial prefrontal-subcortical systems and the generation of affective meaning. *Trends in Cognitive Sciences, 16*(3), 147–156. doi:10.1016/j.tics.2012.01.005

Rudolph, U., Roesch, S. C., Greitemeyer, T., & Weiner, B. (2004). A meta-analytic review of help giving and aggression from an attributional perspective: Contributions to a general theory of motivation. *Cognition & Emotion, 18*(6), 815–848. doi:10.1080/02699930341000248

Russell, J. A., & Barrett, L. F. (1999). Core affect, prototypical emotional episodes, and other things called emotion: dissecting the elephant. *Journal of Personality and Social Psychology, 76*(5), 805–19.

Saarimaki, H., Gotsopoulos, A., Jaaskelainen, I. P., Lampinen, J., Vuilleumier, P., Hari, R., . . . Nummenmaa, L. (2015). Discrete Neural Signatures of Basic Emotions. *Cerebral Cortex*, 1–11. doi:10.1093/cercor/bhv086

Sargeant, A., & Lee, S. (2004). Donor trust and relationship commitment in the U.K. charity sector: the impact on behavior. *Nonprofit And Voluntary Sector Quarterly, 33*(2), 185–202.

Shamay-Tsoory, S. G., Aharon-Peretz, J., & Perry, D. (2009). Two systems for empathy: A double dissociation between emotional and cognitive empathy in inferior frontal gyrus versus ventromedial prefrontal lesions. *Brain, 132*(Pt 3), 617–627. doi:10.1093/brain/awn279

Singer, T., & Klimecki, O. M. (2014). Empathy and compassion. *Current Biology : CB, 24*(18), R875–8. doi:10.1016/j.cub.2014.06.054

Singer, T., & Lamm, C. (2009). The social neuroscience of empathy. *Annals of the New York Academy of Sciences, 1156*, 81–96. doi:10.1111/j.1749-6632.2009.04418.x

Van Overwalle, F., & Baetens, K. (2009). Understanding others' actions and goals by mirror and mentalizing systems: A meta-analysis. *NeuroImage, 48*(3), 564–584. doi:10.1016/j.neuroimage.2009.06.009

van't Wout, M., & Sanfey, A. G. (2008). Friend or foe: the effect of implicit trustworthiness judgments in social decision-making. *Cognition, 108*(3), 796–803. doi:10.1016/j.cognition.2008.07.002

Vollhardt, J. R., & Staub, E. (2011). Inclusive altruism born of suffering: The relationship between adversity and prosocial attitudes and behavior toward disadvantaged outgroups. *American Journal of Orthopsychiatry, 81*(3), 307–315. doi:10.1111/j.1939-0025.2011.01099.x

Weng, H. Y., Fox, A. S., Shackman, A. J., Stodola, D. E., Caldwell, J. Z. K., Olson, M. C., . . . Davidson, R. J. (2013). Compassion training alters altruism and neural responses to suffering. *Psychological Science, 24*, 1171–1180. doi:10.1177/0956797612469537

Xu, X., Zuo, X., Wang, X., & Han, S. (2009). Do you feel my pain? Racial group membership modulates empathic neural responses. *The Journal of Neuroscience : The Official Journal of the Society for Neuroscience, 29*(26), 8525–8529. doi:10.1523/JNEUROSCI.2418-09.2009

Yarkoni, T., Ashar, Y. K., & Wager, T. D. (2015). Interactions between donor Agreeableness and recipient characteristics in predicting charitable donation and positive social evaluation. *PeerJ*.

Zaki, J., & Mitchell, J. P. (2011). Equitable decision making is associated with neural markers of intrinsic value. *Proceedings of the National Academy of Sciences of the United States of America, 108*(49), 19761–19766. doi:10.1073/pnas.1112324108

Zaki, J., & Ochsner, K. (2012). The neuroscience of empathy: progress, pitfalls and promise. *Nature Neuroscience, 15*(5), 675–680. doi:10.1038/nn.3085

Zaki, J., Weber, J., Bolger, N., & Ochsner, K. (2009). The neural bases of empathic accuracy. *Proceedings of the National Academy of Sciences, 106*(27), 11382–11387. doi:10.1073/pnas.0902666106

Zenasni, F., Boujut, E., Woerner, A., & Sultan, S. (2012). Burnout and empathy in primary care. *British Journal of General Practice, 62*(602), 462. doi:10.3399/bjgp12X654515

9

Extraordinary Altruism

A Cognitive Neuroscience Perspective

ABIGAIL A. MARSH ■

The thing he wanted to do seemed like a natural choice to him—almost inevitable, "Like dominoes falling," he said. And yet it could not have seemed more unnatural to everyone else. "Lunatic" they called people like him (Henderson et al., 2003). His wife intimated they might be right. It would certainly be painful. It might make him sick. There was a slim chance it could kill him—although, fortunately, it did not. Today, years later, he still thinks about the day it finally happened when he wakes up every morning. It brought him, as he sees it, only positive outcomes. But the practice was only permitted in the United States beginning in 1999, and it is still forbidden in many countries. This is despite the fact that it is proven to save lives. What is this natural but unnatural, painful but positive, beneficent but banned act? It is the nondirected, or altruistic, donation of a kidney to a stranger. And this man is one of roughly 1,400 people in the United States who have ever chosen to undertake it.

Nondirected altruistic kidney donors request that one of their own working kidneys be surgically removed and implanted into a stranger. Whether that stranger is male or female, young or old, compassionate or callous they may never know. Some donors meet their recipient before the surgery, but more often they do not. They may never meet, either because the recipient prefers to remain anonymous, or, in some cases, because the recipient dies. Recovery from donation can be painful—sometimes excruciatingly so—and results in weeks of lost work. Debates continue about its long-term effects on health and longevity (Leichtman et al., 2011; Massey et al., 2010). In rare cases, donors have lost their health insurance when their insurer declared the removal of a kidney to be a preexisting condition (Rabin, 2012; Yang, Thiessen-Philbrook,

Klarenbach, Vlaicu, & Garg, 2007). If there is such a thing as altruism, altruistic kidney donation surely qualifies.

Altruism—behavior intended to benefit another person instead of the self—is among the most mysterious and controversial behaviors in the human repertoire. Longstanding questions persist about what qualifies as altruism, what drives it, and what neurocognitive processes support it. This chapter will explore these questions and consider how a better understanding of extraordinary altruists like altruistic kidney donors may help to answer them. Answering these questions may provide us with not only a deeper understanding of extraordinary altruism, but of ordinary altruism as well, and the basic social and affective capacities of the human brain that support it.

WHAT IS ALTRUISM?

A dominant belief among many contemporary scientists, philosophers, and policymakers is that human altruism does not exist (Miller, 1999). For most of Western history, the prevailing view has been that every human action is ultimately motivated by self-serving goals—and that this is as it should be. It is both a descriptive and a prescriptive belief (Batson, 1991). Arguments in favor of the existence of genuine altruism are generally based on some form of the *empathy-altruism hypothesis*, which holds that an other-oriented motivational state, termed empathy, can drive us to act on behalf of others even at cost (or at least at no benefit) to ourselves (Batson & Shaw, 1991). Understanding altruism, according to this hypothesis, requires understanding empathy.

Efforts to understand empathy and altruism are often hampered by the use of these two terms to describe a variety of distinct processes (de Waal, 2008). To begin with, it is essential to distinguish among three distinct phenomena to which the term empathy may refer: emotional empathy, cognitive empathy, and empathic concern. Emotional empathy usually refers to a low-level emotional response to another person's distress. This form of empathy is sometimes termed "emotional contagion," in reference to the idea that emotional information may be transmitted from sender to receiver via low-level or unconscious processes (de Waal, 2008). This form of empathy can be identified using any method that can detect an emotional response, including measurements of brain activation, peripheral physiology, facial movements, or self-reported emotion. Correctly identifying another person's emotional state is also considered an index of emotional empathy (Nichols, 2001). So if, for example, witnessing another person's distress causes the viewer to show increased physiological arousal (e.g., increased heart rate or sweating), to exhibit facial behavior similar to the distressed person's (e.g., knitting the brows together), or to correctly identify the distressed person's distress, we can infer that emotional empathy has occurred.

At the neural level, accumulating evidence supports the idea that emotional empathy represents the activation of shared representations for personal and vicarious experiences of emotion (Bernhardt & Singer, 2012). For example, a large body of research demonstrates that viewing or inferring another person to be experiencing pain results in the activation of cortical and subcortical structures, such as the anterior insula and dorsal anterior cingulate cortex, that also respond during personally experienced pain, a phenomenon that may enable the viewer to generate a representation of the social and affective components of another person's pain by mapping it onto his or her own experiences (Lamm, Decety, & Singer, 2011). Parallel processes may also underlie emotional empathy for fear, disgust, and perhaps anger (Goldman & Sripada, 2005; Marsh, 2011). Critically, theories of shared neural representations require that empathizing with distinct emotional states relies upon distinct neural processes, such that a person can be skilled in empathizing with some emotions but not others. Emotional empathy can be contrasted with cognitive empathy, which refers to the understanding of others' cognitive states, such as beliefs and intentions (Baron-Cohen, 1997). The brain regions that subserve cognitive empathy overlap minimally, if at all, with those that subserve emotional empathy, underscoring the importance of resisting the tendency to conflate the two phenomena (Blair, 2008; Gallagher & Frith, 2003).

Cognitive and emotional empathy index how well the empathizer interprets the internal state of another person. The third form of empathy, empathic concern, departs from this emphasis. This form of empathy entails *caring* about the other person's internal state. Beyond simply understanding another person's internal state, empathic concern entails feeling *for* them—wishing, in the case of another's distressed emotional state, that it were better and desiring to make it so (Eisenberg, 2007). Whereas both cognitive and emotional empathy apply to a variety of internal states, empathic concern generally occurs in response to distress (Nichols, 2001). There have been suggestions that empathic concern constitutes a distinct emotional state with distinct physiological signatures (Eisenberg et al., 1989), but the primary means of assessing this form of empathy is via self-report. Empathic concern appears not to be closely tied to cognitive empathy (Blair, 1999a). By contrast, emotional empathy, at least some forms of it, appears to be critical for experiencing empathic concern (Nichols, 2001). Empathic concern—an other-oriented motivational state associated with wanting to improve another's welfare—is the form of empathy thought to drive altruism (Batson, 1991, 2010), at least, when altruism is defined psychologically, in terms of its motivation.

THE IMPORTANCE OF INDIVIDUAL DIFFERENCES

Some of the best evidence for the existence of empathic concern-driven altruism derives, paradoxically, from psychopaths. Psychopathy is a condition characterized by persistent antisocial behaviors like aggression, theft, and deceit, and by personality traits like a lack of remorse, guilt, or empathic concern, which are termed *callous-unemotional traits* (Blair, Peschardt, Budhani, Mitchell, & Pine, 2006; Hare & Neumann, 2008). Psychopathic traits vary continuously in the population, such that a given person can be minimally, moderately, or highly psychopathic, and these are differences of degree, not kind (Edens, Marcus, Lilienfeld, & Poythress, 2006; Guay, Ruscio, Knight, & Hare, 2007). Highly psychopathic individuals consider the needs and rights of others minimally or not at all and fill the ranks of the world's notorious serial murders, con artists, and repeat offenders (Hare, 2006). How can such a population support the possibility of altruism? Because, very simply, they are unlike everybody else. That psychopaths exist requires that other people exist who are not psychopaths—who have *some* capacity for empathic concern.

These facts also support the possibility of extraordinary altruists. If psychopaths occupy the low end of an empathic concern spectrum, it stands to reason others would exist who are the mirror image of psychopaths: "antipsychopaths", who experience more empathic concern than average. Altruistic kidney donors seem, potentially, like excellent representatives of this population. Rather than being set apart by their antisocial behavior, they are set apart by their prosocial behavior, often engaging in a variety of other prosocial acts, such as donating blood or registering as marrow donors (Henderson et al., 2003). Their behavior is clearly altruistic in the biological sense. Donors are forbidden from benefitting materially (e.g., being paid), and it is debatable whether donation results in more abstract gains like increased social esteem (Massey et al., 2010). And when queried about their motivations for donating, most altruistic donors cite the desire to help another person as their foremost consideration (Lennerling, Forsberg, Meyer, & Nyberg, 2004; Massey et al., 2010). Even stronger evidence that donors are driven by empathic concern would be evidence that donors possess qualities that experimental research paradigms have previously linked to psychological altruism.

LABORATORY STUDIES OF ALTRUISM

Studies of human altruism in the laboratory show that it is primarily elicited by the distress of a victim, and the more sensitive to distress participants are, the more likely they are to behave altruistically (Eisenberg & Miller,

1987; Nichols, 2001). Extensive research conducted by Batson and colleagues shows that sensitivity to distress can be experimentally manipulated (Batson & Shaw, 1991), prompting altruism in even the unlikeliest of circumstances. In one study, Batson and Ahmad (2001) stacked the deck solidly in favor of selfish behavior: University student participants played a one-trial prisoner's dilemma against an anonymous partner they would never meet. Payoffs were made concrete and real in the form of raffle tickets for a $30 gift certificate at a store of the winner's choice. Ostensibly by chance, the partner was always selected to play first, and she always defected. Participants could either defect in return, earning 5 tickets (the partner would also earn 5 tickets), or cooperate, whereby the participant would win 0 tickets and the partner 25. Why would any player cooperate in response to defection from an anonymous stranger? Most theoretical frameworks predict defection, which maximizes personal gain and satisfies norms of reciprocity, fairness, and distributive justice (Batson, 2010). Defection was in fact universal (20/20 participants) when participants received no communication from their partner. But responses changed dramatically when participants read a short note from the partner describing her distress about recent events in her life. This prompt induced an altruistic response in nearly half (9/20) of the participants who read it following instructions to imagine how the partner was feeling.

The results of this and similar studies demonstrate the effectiveness with which distress-induced empathy produces altruism. It also shows than any given distress cue will be more effective in eliciting altruism from some people than others, since even in the empathy condition of this experiment more than half the participants still defected. This, together with a long tradition of research on bystander intervention showing that the clarity or interpretability of a target's distress predicts helping in bystanders (Clark & Word, 1974; Shotland & Huston, 1979), suggests that individual differences in the ability to correctly interpret others' distress cues will predict individual differences in altruism.

Studies conducted by my colleagues and I have confirmed this to be the case. We have measured altruistic behavior in the laboratory and found that the ability to recognize emotional expressions that convey distress, particularly fear, predicts altruism in the laboratory (Marsh, Kozak, & Ambady, 2007). Individual differences in fear recognition predicted altruism more accurately than gender, mood, and self-reported empathic concern. These findings support the contention that the ability to simply recognize when others are experiencing distress (a low-level form of emotional empathy) is the most important requirement for experiencing empathic concern (Nichols, 2001). Together with abundant evidence that psychopathy impairs the recognition of fearful expressions (Dawel, O'Kearney, McKone, & Palermo, 2012; Marsh & Blair, 2008), these findings suggest that the ability to recognize others' fear is a strong indicator of where an individual falls on the empathic concern spectrum.

Predicting Extraordinary Altruism

In light of this prior evidence, we developed a paradigm aimed at assessing neural and behavioral responses to others' distress in altruistic kidney donors to test the hypothesis that their altruistic behavior may result from increased sensitivity to others' distress (Marsh et al., 2014). We recruited 19 altruistic kidney donors and 20 matched controls who all underwent brain scanning while viewing fearful, neutral, and angry facial expressions. Later, participants were asked to identify these expressions in a separate task conducted outside the scanner and then completed a large number of self-report scales and measures such as self-reported empathy and psychopathy. Our first hypothesis was that altruists would exhibit enhanced amygdala activation in response to fearful facial expressions during brain scanning. This hypothesis was based on abundant evidence that, in healthy adults, activity in the amygdala, a subcortical structure in the temporal lobes, is greater when participants view fearful facial expressions relative to any other type of emotional expression (Fusar-Poli et al., 2009; Murphy, Nimmo-Smith, & Lawrence, 2003), and that this response is attenuated in individuals with psychopathic traits (Blair, 1999b; Dolan & Fullam, 2009; Jones, Laurens, Herba, Barker, & Viding, 2009; Marsh et al., 2008; White et al., 2012). Because the amygdala is a structure that is critical to generating the experience of fear (Davis, 1992; Feinstein, Adolphs, Damasio, & Tranel, 2011; LaBar, LeDoux, Spencer, & Phelps, 1995), heightened amygdala responses to others' fearful expressions may represent manifestations of the emotional empathy upon which empathic concern depends (Goldman & Sripada, 2005; Marsh, 2011). We also hypothesized that altruists' heightened amygdala activation would correspond to heightened accuracy for recognizing these expressions. Finally, we hypothesized that altruistic kidney donors would be less psychopathic than healthy controls.

All three hypotheses were confirmed: the amygdalae of altruistic kidney donors were more active in response to fearful expressions, a pattern that corresponded to improved recognition of these expressions, and they reported reduced psychopathic traits. These findings support the idea of altruists exhibiting enhanced empathic responses to others' distress, and therefore their donations reflect genuinely heightened concern for others' well-being, a conclusion of considerable importance to the transplantation community (Levey, Danovitch, & Hou, 2011). Even today, some transplantation centers will not perform transplants using non-directed donors (Woodle et al., 2010), in part due to concerns that these decisions reflect psychological disorders or irrational expectations of self-benefit rather than genuine altruism (Henderson et al., 2003). The finding that, neurocognitively, altruistic donors fit the profile of individuals who experience unusually high levels of empathic concern and psychological altruism may mitigate these concerns. This is of particular importance given the critical and growing need for donor kidneys in the United States (Coresh et al., 2007).

More generally, an exploration of what sets extraordinary altruists apart from other individuals may also help to answer basic psychological and neuroscientific questions about the nature of altruism. That altruistic kidney donors exhibit hallmarks of altruism as determined by laboratory work provides support for the possibility that empathic processes do in fact underlie acts of extraordinary altruism, and this may help to illuminate the fundamental neurocognitive processes that support these behaviors.

UNANSWERED QUESTIONS

A number of questions about altruism remain, however, that are unlikely to be addressed from a study of extraordinary altruists without further development of the theoretical understanding of altruism and its origins. Among the central remaining questions about altruism is the question of what drives the leap from emotional empathy to empathic concern. A historically favored explanation (MacDougall, 1908) that has seen a recent resurgence (e.g., Batson, 2010; Bell, 2001; de Waal, 2008; Marsh, Adams, & Kleck, 2005; Preston, 2014) is that empathic concern is a more generalized form of the parental nurturing response. Parental nurturing requires an organism to place the needs of another organism before its own, sometimes at great expense and for protracted periods, and its emergence marked an extraordinary development in the evolution of vertebrate behavior (Eibl-Eibesfeldt, 1996). Parental nurturing is primarily a mammalian behavior—indeed, the word "mammal" is a reminder of the resources mammals expend nurturing and raising their young relative to their evolutionary progenitors. This development was facilitated by the emergence of the oxytocin system. Oxytocin is a mammalian hormone produced in the hypothalamus that, via dedicated receptors in the brain and body, promotes a variety of essential parental behaviors (Carter & Altemus, 1997).

The oxytocin system may be especially critical to the emergence of a mammalian behavior closely linked to altruism, which is *alloparenting* (Keebaugh & Young, 2011; Ross et al., 2009). Alloparenting is the provision of care and protection to unrelated young within the social group, and it has been observed in over 100 mammalian species, including elephants, dolphins, wolves, and many species of primate, including humans (Riedman, 1982). Characteristics of species in which alloparenting occurs include organization into small, close-knit, and cooperative groups and infants being born relatively helpless and dependent on care from adults. Among alloparenting species, adults provide parental care not only for their own offspring but for offspring in general, and they possess strong mechanisms to prevent aggression in response to infantile cues.

It is hypothesized that because alloparenting mammals respond to generalized offspring cues with parental nurturing and the inhibition of aggression, fear and submission cues in these species evolved to mimic infantile cues, exploiting the parental nurturing response to inhibit aggression toward vulnerable adults (Lorenz, 1966). For example, wolves' stereotyped fear and submission behaviors include rolling on the back, pinning back the ears, and tucking in the tail, all of which mimic appearance cues of pups and are thought to serve an appeasement function (Schenkel, 1967). Similar processes may occur in humans. Like other alloparenting species, humans respond to a variety of infant-like cues with parental nurturance. Abundant evidence demonstrates that nurturing responses are elicited by many stimuli that resemble infants, including adults with babyish facial features (Zebrowitz, 1997). Human fear and submission behaviors may also exploit this tendency by mimicking infantile cues. Fearful expressions are perceived to be morphologically similar to infantile faces, sharing with them features like wide eyes, high brows, a flat brow ridge, and a generally rounded appearance, and eliciting attributions of dependence, weakness, submissiveness, and babyishness (Marsh et al., 2005). This may explain why fearful expressions are perceived as highly affiliative (Hess, Blairy, & Kleck, 2000), elicit behavioral approach (Marsh, Ambady, & Kleck, 2005; Hammer & Marsh, 2014), and promote empathic concern (Marsh & Ambady, 2007). These findings support the idea that humans' tendency to care for distressed infants is the progenitor of their tendency to experience empathic concern toward adults who display distress cues like fearful expressions that mimic the appearance of infants.

Considering how parenting and alloparenting responses relate to psychological altruism may help guide the development of future questions about the neurocognitive basis of human altruism. The role of primitive subcortical structures like the hypothalamus and periaqueductal gray should be investigated, given the important role these structures play in parental nurturance (Bartels & Zeki, 2004; Champagne, Diorio, Sharma, & Meaney, 2001; Francis, Young, Meaney, & Insel, 2002; Sheehan, Paul, Amaral, Numan, & Numan, 2001). Recent findings support the possibility that these structures' role in human altruism and empathic concern can be assessed using current technologies (Moll et al., 2012; Simon-Thomas et al., 2012). Whether responses in these regions mediate altruistic responses to distress cues like fearful expressions merits investigation. Another potentially fruitful avenue of investigation may be oxytocinergic function in altruists, given the importance of the oxytocin system for alloparenting. Differences in the oxytocin receptor gene have been shown to influence responses to novel human infant faces, especially following the inhalation of intranasal oxytocin (Marsh et al., 2012).

CONCLUSION

Whether humans possess the capacity to genuinely care about others' welfare affects not only our beliefs about ourselves and others, but how we construct our societies. A normative belief that humans can only ever be driven by self-interest leads to the creation of social institutions that reflect that belief (Miller, 1999). The existence of transplant centers that refuse organs from altruistic donors due to doubts that these donations reflect genuine altruism is only one such example. Undoubtedly, many patients in need of a donor kidney have died as a result. An improved understanding of extraordinary altruism has the potential, then, to change the lives of those whose health depends on the altruism of others, and perhaps in the process to transform humans' understanding of ourselves and the evolutionary forces and neural processes that undergird our most profound and mysterious social behaviors.

REFERENCES

Baron-Cohen, S. (1997). *Mindblindness*. Cambridge, MA: MIT Press.

Bartels, A., & Zeki, S. (2004). The neural correlates of maternal and romantic love. *Neuroimage, 21*, 1155–1166.

Batson, C. D. (1991). *The altruism question*. Hillsdale, NJ: Erlbaum.

Batson, C. D. (2010). The naked emperor: Seeking a more plausible genetic basis for psychological altruism. *Economics and Philosophy, 26*, 149–164.

Batson, C. D., & Ahmad, N. (2001). Empathy-induced altruism in a prisoner's dilemma II: What if the target of empathy has defected? *European Journal of Social Psychology, 31*, 25–36.

Batson, C. D., & Shaw, L. L. (1991). Evidence for altruism: Toward a pluralism of prosocial motives. *Psychological Inquiry, 2*, 107–122.

Bell, D. C. (2001). Evolution of parental caregiving. *Personality and Social Psychology Review, 5*, 216–229.

Bernhardt, B. C., & Singer, T. (2012). The neural basis of empathy. *Annual Review of Neuroscience, 35*, 1–23.

Blair, R. J. (2008). Fine cuts of empathy and the amygdala: Dissociable deficits in psychopathy and autism. *Quarterly Journal of Experimental Psychology, 61*, 157–170.

Blair, R. J., Peschardt, K. S., Budhani, S., Mitchell, D. G., & Pine, D. S. (2006). The development of psychopathy. *Journal of Child Psychology and Psychiatry, 47*, 262–276.

Blair, R. J. R. (1999a). Psychophysiological responsiveness to the distress of others in children with autism. *Personality and Individual Differences, 26*, 477–485.

Blair, R. J. R. (1999b). Responsiveness to distress cues in the child with psychopathic tendencies. *Personality and Individual Differences, 27*, 135–145.

Carter, C. S., & Altemus, M. (1997). Integrative functions of lactational hormones in social behavior and stress management. *Annals of the New York Academy of Sciences, 807*, 164–174.

Champagne, F., Diorio, J., Sharma, S., & Meaney, M. J. (2001). Naturally occurring variations in maternal behavior in the rat are associated with differences in estrogen-inducible central oxytocin receptors. *Proceedings of the National Academy of Sciences USA, 98*, 12736–12741.

Clark, R. D., & Word, L. E. (1974). Where is the apathetic bystander? Situational characteristics of the emergency. *Journal of Personality and Social Psychology, 29*, 279–287.

Coresh, J., Selvin, E., Stevens, L. A., Manzi, J., Kusek, J. W., Eggers, P., . . . Levey, A. S. (2007). Prevalence of chronic kidney disease in the United States. *Journal of the American Medical Association, 298*, 2038–2047.

Davis, M. (1992). The role of the amygdala in fear and anxiety. *Annual Review of Neuroscience, 15*, 353–375.

Dawel, A., O'Kearney, R., McKone, E., & Palermo, R. (2012). Not just fear and sadness: Meta-analytic evidence of pervasive emotion recognition deficits for facial and vocal expressions in psychopathy. *Neuroscience and Biobehavioral Reviews, 36*, 2288–2304.

de Waal, F. B. (2008). Putting the altruism back into altruism: The evolution of empathy. *Annual Review of Psychology, 59*, 279–300.

Dolan, M. C., & Fullam, R. S. (2009). Psychopathy and functional magnetic resonance imaging blood oxygenation level-dependent responses to emotional faces in violent patients with schizophrenia. *Biological Psychiatry, 66*, 570–577.

Edens, J. F., Marcus, D. K., Lilienfeld, S. O., & Poythress, N. G. J. (2006). Psychopathic, not psychopath: Taxometric evidence for the dimensional structure of psychopathy. *Journal of Abnormal Psychology, 115*, 131–144.

Eibl-Eibesfeldt, I. (1996). *Love and Hate: The Natural History of Behavior Patterns.* Chicago: Aldine.

Eisenberg, N. (2007). Empathy-related responding and prosocial behavior. *Novartis Foundation Symposium, 278*, 71–80.

Eisenberg, N., Fabes, R. A., Miller, P. A., Fultz, J., Shell, R., Mathy, R. M., & Reno, R. R. (1989). Relation of sympathy and personal distress to prosocial behavior: A multimethod study. *Journal of Personality and Social Psychology, 57*, 55–66.

Eisenberg, N., & Miller, P. A. (1987). The relation of empathy to prosocial and related behaviors. *Psychological Bulletin, 101*, 91–119.

Feinstein, J. S., Adolphs, R., Damasio, A., & Tranel, D. (2011). The human amygdala and the induction and experience of fear. *Current Biology, 21*, 34–38.

Francis, D. D., Young, L. J., Meaney, M. J., & Insel, T. R. (2002). Naturally occurring differences in maternal care are associated with the expression of oxytocin and vasopressin (V1a) receptors: Gender differences. *Journal of Neuroendocrinology, 14*, 349–353.

Fusar-Poli, P., Placentino, A., Carletti, F., Landi, P., Allen, P., Surguladze, S., . . . Politi, P. (2009). Functional atlas of emotional faces processing: A voxel-based meta-analysis of 105 functional magnetic resonance imaging studies. *Journal of Psychiatry and Neuroscience, 34*, 418–432.

Gallagher, H. I., & Frith, C. D. (2003). Functional imaging of "theory of mind." *Trends in Cognitive Sciences, 7*, 77–83.

Goldman, A. I., & Sripada, C. S. (2005). Simulationist models of face-based emotion recognition. *Cognition, 94*, 193–213.

Guay, J. P., Ruscio, J., Knight, R. A., & Hare, R. D. (2007). A taxometric analysis of the latent structure of psychopathy: Evidence for dimensionality. *Journal of Abnormal Psychology, 116*, 701–716.

Hammer, J. L., & Marsh, A. A. (2015). Why do fearful facial expressions elicit behavioral approach? Evidence from a combined approach-avoidance implicit association test. *Emotion, 15*, 223–231.

Hare, R. D. (2006). Psychopathy: A clinical and forensic overview. *Psychiatry Clinics of North America, 29*, 709–724.

Hare, R. D., & Neumann, C. S. (2008). Psychopathy as a clinical and empirical construct. *Annual Review of Clinical Psychology, 4*, 217–246.

Henderson, A. J., Landolt, M. A., McDonald, M. F., Barrable, W. M., Soos, J. G., Gourlay, W., . . . Landsberg, D. N. (2003). The living anonymous kidney donor: Lunatic or saint? *American Journal of Transplantation, 3*, 203–213.

Hess, U., Blairy, S., & Kleck, R. E. (2000). The influence of facial emotion displays, gender, and ethnicity on judgments of dominance and affiliation. *Journal of Nonverbal Behavior, 24*, 265–283.

Jones, A. P., Laurens, K. R., Herba, C. M., Barker, G. J., & Viding, E. (2009). Amygdala hypoactivity to fearful faces in boys with conduct problems and callous-unemotional traits. *American Journal of Psychiatry, 166*, 95–102.

Keebaugh, A. C., & Young, L. J. (2011). Increasing oxytocin receptor expression in the nucleus accumbens of pre-pubertal female prairie voles enhances alloparental responsiveness and partner preference formation as adults. *Hormones and Behavior, 60*, 498–504.

LaBar, K. S., LeDoux, J. E., Spencer, D. D., & Phelps, E. A. (1995). Impaired fear conditioning following unilateral temporal lobectomy in humans. *Journal of Neuroscience, 15*, 6846–6855.

Lamm, C., Decety, J., & Singer, T. (2011). Meta-analytic evidence for common and distinct neural networks associated with directly experienced pain and empathy for pain. *NeuroImage, 54*, 2492–2502.

Leichtman, A., Abecassis, M., Barr, M., Charlton, M., Cohen, D., Confer, D., . . . Matas, A. J. (2011). Living kidney donor follow-up: State-of-the-art and future directions, conference summary and recommendations. *American Journal of Transplantation, 11*, 2561–2568.

Lennerling, A., Forsberg, A., Meyer, K., & Nyberg, G. (2004). Motives for becoming a living kidney donor. *Nephrology Dialysis Transplantation, 19*, 1600–1605.

Levey, A. M., Danovitch, G., & Hou, S. (2011). Living donor kidney transplantation in the United States—Looking back, looking forward. *American Journal of Kidney Disease, 58*, 343–348.

Lorenz, K. (1966). *On aggression.* London, UK: Methuen.

MacDougall, W. (1908). *An introduction to social psychology.* London, UK: Methuen.

Marsh, A. A. (2011). Empathy and compassion: A cognitive neuroscience perspective. In J. Decety (Ed.), *Empathy: From bench to bedside* (pp. 191–206). Cambridge, MA: MIT Press.

Marsh, A. A., Adams, R. B., Jr., & Kleck, R. E. (2005). Why do fear and anger look the way they do? Form and social function in facial expressions. *Personality and Social Psychology Bulletin, 31*, 73–86.

Marsh, A. A., & Ambady, N. (2007). The influence of the fear facial expression on prosocial responding. *Cognition and Emotion, 21*, 225–247.

Marsh, A. A., Ambady, N., & Kleck, R. E. (2005). The effects of fear and anger facial expressions on approach- and avoidance-related behaviors. *Emotion, 5*, 119–124.

Marsh, A. A., & Blair, R. J. (2008). Deficits in facial affect recognition among antisocial populations: A meta-analysis. *Neuroscience and Biobehavioral Reviews, 32*, 454–465.

Marsh, A. A., Finger, E., Mitchell, D. G. V., Reid, M. E., Sims, C., Kosson, D. S., . . . Blair, R. J. R. (2008). Reduced amygdala response to fearful expressions in children and adolescents with callous-unemotional traits and disruptive behavior disorders. *American Journal of Psychiatry, 165*, 712–720.

Marsh, A. A., Kozak, M. N., & Ambady, N. (2007). Accurate identification of fear facial expressions predicts prosocial behavior. *Emotion, 7*, 239–251.

Marsh, A. A., Stoycos, S. A., Brethel-Haurwitz, K. M., Robinson, P., & Cardinale, E. M. (2014). Neural and cognitive characteristics of extraordinary altruists. *Proceedings of the National Academy of Sciences, 111*, 15036–15041.

Marsh, A. A., Yu, H. H., Pine, D. S., Gorodetsky, E. K., Goldman, D., & Blair, R. J. (2012). The influence of oxytocin administration on responses to infant faces and potential moderation by OXTR genotype. *Psychopharmacology, 224*, 469–476.

Massey, E. K., Kranenburg, L. W., Zuidema, W. C., Hak, G., Erdman, R. A., Hilhorst, M., . . . Weimar, W (2010). Encouraging psychological outcomes after altruistic donation to a stranger. *American Journal of Transplantation, 10*, 1445–1452.

Miller, D. T. (1999). The norm of self-interest. *American Psychologist, 54*, 1053–1060.

Moll, J., Bado, P., de Oliveira-Souza, R., Bramati, I. E., Lima, D. O., Paiva, F. F., . . . Zahn, R. (2012). A neural signature of affiliative emotion in the human septohypothalamic area. *Journal of Neuroscience, 32*, 12499–12505.

Murphy, F. C., Nimmo-Smith, I., & Lawrence, A. D. (2003). Functional neuroanatomy of emotions: A meta-analysis. *Cognitive Affective and Behavioral Neuroscience, 3*, 207–233.

Nichols, S. (2001). Mindreading and the cognitive architecture underlying altruistic motivation. *Mind and Language, 16*, 425–455.

Preston, S. D. (2013). The origins of altruism in offspring care. *Psychological Bulletin, 139*, 1305–1341.

Rabin, R. C. (2012, June 11). The reward for donating a kidney: No insurance. *The New York Times*. Retrieved November 2015, from http://well.blogs.nytimes.com/2012/06/11/the-reward-for-donating-a-kidney-no-insurance/?_r=0

Riedman, M. L. (1982). The evolution of alloparental care and adoption in mammals and birds. *Quarterly Review of Biology, 57*, 405–435.

Ross, H. E., Freeman, S. M., Spiegel, L. L., Ren, X., Terwilliger, E. F., & Young, L. J. (2009). Variation in oxytocin receptor density in the nucleus accumbens has differential effects on affiliative behaviors in monogamous and polygamous voles. *Journal of Neuroscience, 29*, 1312–1318.

Schenkel, R. (1967). Submission: Its features in the wolf and dog. *American Zoologist, 7*, 319–329.

Sheehan, T., Paul, M., Amaral, E., Numan, M. J., & Numan, M. (2001). Evidence that the medial amygdala projects to the anterior/ventromedial hypothalamic nuclei to inhibit maternal behavior in rats. *Neuroscience, 106*, 341–356.

Shotland, R. L., & Huston, T. L. (1979). Emergencies: What are they and do they influence bystanders to intervene? *Journal of Personality and Social Psychology, 37*, 1822–1834.

Simon-Thomas, E. R., Godzik, J., Castle, E., Antonenko, O., Ponz, A., Kogan, A., & Keltner, D. J. (2012). An fMRI study of caring vs self-focus during induced compassion and pride. *Social Cognitive and Affective Neuroscience, 7*, 635–648.

White, S. F., Marsh, A. A., Fowler, K. A., Schechter, J. C., Adalio, C., Pope, K., & Blair, R. J. (2012). Reduced amygdala response in youths with disruptive behavior disorders and psychopathic traits: Decreased emotional response versus increased top-down attention to nonemotional features. *American Journal of Psychiatry, 169*, 750–78.

Woodle, E. S., Daller, J. A., Aeder, M., Shapiro, R., Sandholm, T., Casingal, V., ... Siegler, M. (2010). Ethical considerations for participation of nondirected living donors in kidney exchange programs. *American Journal of Transplantation, 10*, 1460–1467.

Yang, R. C., Thiessen-Philbrook, H., Klarenbach, S., Vlaicu, S., & Garg, A. X. (2007). Insurability of living organ donors: A systematic review. *American Journal of Transplantation, 7*, 1542–1551.

Zebrowitz, L. A. (1997). *Reading faces*. Boulder, CO: Westview Press.

PART III

Resilience and Creativity

10

Increasing Positive Emotion in Negative Contexts

Emotional Consequences, Neural Correlates, and Implications for Resilience

KATERI MCRAE AND IRIS B. MAUSS ■

Responses to stress, while unpleasant, can be useful in that they promote adaptive behavior (Frijda, 1986; Keltner & Gross, 1999; Tamir, 2009). However, when stress responses are overwhelming, inappropriate, or chronically activated, they can cause a wide range of long-term negative consequences (Lupien, McEwen, Gunnar, & Heim, 2009; McEwen, 2000). Stress responses can be triggered by a variety of different types of stressors, including daily hassles, traumatic events, chronic stress, and stressful life events. We focus here on one particularly pervasive type of stressor that can have pernicious effects on psychological health: stressful life events (SLEs; Kendler, Karkowski, & Prescott, 1999; Kessler, 1997; Tamir, 2009; Tennant, 2002). SLEs have been most commonly defined as unexpected, significant, and negative events, and include events such as the death of a loved one, divorce, or serious illness (Kendler et al., 1999; Kessler, 1997; Lin, Simeone, Ensel, & Kuo, 1979). SLEs have been implicated in the onset, maintenance, and escalation of a number of debilitating psychological and physical disorders as well as decreased well-being (Kendler et al., 1999; Kessler, 1997; Pagano et al., 2004; Tennant, 2002; Tosevski & Milovancevic, 2006). However, SLEs are not associated with negative long-term outcomes in *all* individuals.[1] Some individuals exhibit impressive resilience, achieving maintained or even improved mental health and well-being after SLEs (Bonanno, 2005; Freitas & Downey, 1998; Lucas, Clark, Georgellis, & Diener, 2003; Ryff, Singer, Love, & Essex, 1998).[2]

How can we explain the remarkable human ability to not merely subsist, but to thrive in the face of potential ruin? Two lines of inquiry point to two potent facilitators of resilience. The first is positive emotion, which has been shown to evoke powerful changes in emotional trajectory (Fredrickson & Levenson, 1998). The second is cognitive emotion regulation (the most prominent example of which is reappraisal), which refers to the utilization of cognitive strategies to modulate emotion intensity and duration (Davidson, 2000; Gross, 1998b; Thompson, 1994). In this chapter, we unite these two perspectives, arguing that using reappraisal to self-generate positive emotion ("positive reappraisal") is a particularly potent path to resilience.

POSITIVE REAPPRAISAL AND RESILIENCE: A CONCEPTUAL FRAMEWORK

Individuals can regulate their emotions in a number of different ways (Davidson, 2000; Gross, 1998b; Thompson, 1994). One type of emotion regulation appears to be particularly adaptive, namely, cognitive reappraisal. Reappraisal is an emotion regulation strategy in which the individual cognitively reevaluates an emotional situation to change its emotional impact (Gross, 1998b). Reappraisal has been shown experimentally to be useful even in powerfully negative situations (Gross, 1998a; Mauss, Cook, Cheng, & Gross, 2007; Ochsner, Bunge, Gross, & Gabrieli, 2002) and is strongly implicated in psychological health (Folkman, 1997; Garnefski & Kraaij, 2006; Gross & John, 2003), especially after SLEs (Bryant, Moulds, & Guthrie, 2001; Carrico, Antoni, Weaver, Lechner, & Schneiderman, 2005; Kraaij, Pruymboom, & Garnefski, 2002; Troy, Wilhelm, Shallcross, & Mauss, 2010; Wrosch, Heckhausen, & Lachman, 2000).

Together, these considerations motivate a conceptual framework that suggests reappraisal as a key factor in adjustment after SLEs. Importantly, as illustrated in Figure 10.1, reappraisal can target two different emotional states: One could either decrease negative emotion or increase positive emotion (Mauss & Tamir, in press). For example, if we have an argument with a good friend, we can reappraise the conflict as a natural part of friendship that will soon resolve (and thereby decrease our negative emotions), or we can remind ourselves how lucky we are to have our perspectives on the issue broadened by passionate, articulate company (and thereby increase our positive emotions). Because positive emotions are distinct from, and not the mere antithesis to, negative emotions (Watson, Wiese, Vaidya, & Tellegen, 1999), these two types of reappraisal might have different effects on emotions in the short term. Specifically,

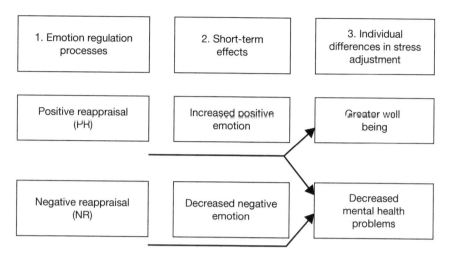

Figure 10.1 Short-term and long-term effects of positive and negative reappraisal.

using reappraisal to increase positive emotion (positive reappraisal, PR) might in the short term increase positive emotions without necessarily decreasing negative emotions.

Positive emotion has pervasive beneficial effects on psychological health and well-being (Fredrickson, 1998; Lyubomirsky, King, & Diener, 2005). For example, positive emotion can speed recovery from negative emotional events (Fredrickson & Levenson, 1998). Thus, the short-term effects of PR might over time translate into decreased mental health problems and greater well-being (resilience). Increasing positive emotion without removing negative emotion might present a particularly feasible and adaptive way to cope with stressors, because some negative emotion is important to experience in the context of SLEs. In the following sections, we examine the idea that PR has distinct short-term emotional consequences, discuss the neural correlates that might accompany it, and predict that it will lead to increased resilience. While negative reappraisal (NR) likely plays an important role in resilience, it is our hypothesis that PR has the potential to lead to even greater resilience, above and beyond NR.

SHORT-TERM EFFECTS: EMOTIONAL CONSEQUENCES AND NEURAL CORRELATES OF POSITIVE REAPPRAISAL

Our framework leads to the prediction that PR increases positive emotion, even in the context of negative stimuli. Although most studies of reappraisal focus on manipulating the negative emotion elicited by a negative stimulus (NR), these studies can give some insight into the potential consequences of PR (Gross, 1998a; Jackson, Malmstadt, Larson, & Davidson, 2000; Ochsner et al., 2002).

Short-Term Emotional Consequences of Positive Reappraisal

Studies on reappraisal often involve the presentation of negative images or films, paired with instructions to either respond naturally or to use reappraisal. Using this method, NR has been shown to successfully decrease several aspects of emotional responding, including self-reported negative emotion (Gross, 1998a), startle eyeblink magnitude (Dillon & LaBar, 2005; Jackson et al., 2000), and corrugator response (Jackson et al., 2000; Ray, McRae, Ochsner, & Gross, 2010). Neuroimaging studies have replicated and extended the effects of NR by demonstrating that NR decreases the event-related potentials associated with emotional arousal (Deveney & Pizzagalli, 2008; Foti & Hajcak, 2008; Hajcak & Nieuwenhuis, 2006) as well as amygdala activation (Kim & Hamann, 2007; Ochsner et al., 2002; Schaefer et al., 2002), which is thought to process emotionally salient information and organize peripheral physiological responding and behavioral emotional responses. Therefore, NR can be an effective way to curtail negative affective responding at many levels.

In addition, PR can be used to increase several aspects of emotional responding, including self-reported positive emotion, and sympathetic nervous system activation (Giuliani, McRae, & Gross, 2008), as well as activation in the amygdala and ventral striatum (a region associated with positive emotion and reward; Kim & Hamann, 2007). It is important to note that using PR in a positive context results in *greater* levels of amygdala activation (Kim & Hamann, 2007). Although amygdala activation is often associated with negative emotion, it also responds to positive emotion, novelty, and arousal (Anderson et al., 2003; Cunningham, Van Bavel, & Johnsen, 2008; Whalen, 1998). Together, these studies suggest that people can use reappraisal not just to manipulate negative emotional responses in negative contexts but also positive emotional responses in positive contexts.

Our central interest, however, is whether reappraisal can be used to increase positive emotion even in the context of negative emotional stimuli. And if so, how do the effects of PR compare to the effects of NR? A small number of studies have established that positive emotional experience is increased by PR in a negative context, to a greater extent than NR (McRae, Ciesielski, & Gross, 2012; Shiota & Levenson, 2012). One such study compared PR to a distancing NR tactic in the context of negative film clips. Relative to distancing, PR resulted in shortened cardiac interbeat interval paired with reduced blood pressure (Shiota & Levenson, 2012). This cardiovascular response profile has been previously associated with a "challenge" rather than a "threat" mindset (Tomaka, Blascovich, Kibler, & Ernst, 1997). A separate investigation measured skin conductance level (SCL) while using PR or NR in response to negative pictures. Based on the elevated amygdala activation observed when using PR in a positive context (Kim & Hamann, 2007), we predicted that PR would involve greater physiological activation than NR. In line with these predictions, this study reports smaller decreases in SCL when participants used PR compared to NR (McRae, Ciesielski, & Gross, 2012). Therefore, it is clear that PR and NR have different emotional and psychophysiological consequences.

To date, no neuroimaging studies we are aware of have directly compared NR and PR in a negative context. However, because typically participants are not restricted from increasing positive emotion while reappraising, some participants might make use of PR when asked to use NR. In fact, we have found that some individuals engage the ventral striatum, which is associated with positive emotion, to a greater extent than others while reappraising (McRae, Ochsner, Mauss, Gabrieli, & Gross, 2008). In addition, the relationship between control-related ventral PFC activation and reappraisal success is mediated by two separate neural pathways (Wager, Davidson, Hughes, Lindquist, & Ochsner, 2008). The first pathway involves decreases in amygdala activation, which may reflect NR, and the second involves increases in ventral striatum activation, which may reflect PR. If these two pathways represent NR and PR, respectively, it is reasonable to predict that PR engages the amygdala and the ventral striatum more strongly than does NR. Together with the self-report and psychophysiological findings, these studies support the conclusion that there are unique emotional effects of PR compared to NR. More specifically, they indicate that PR, compared with NR, might have an activating effect.

Control Regions Engaged by Positive Reappraisal

In addition to studying the emotional consequences of PR and NR, neuroimaging studies allow for the identification of the neural regions associated with implementing reappraisal, which implicate specific cognitive processes. Again, most research to date has examined NR. This research suggests that several prefrontal and parietal regions are recruited consistently during NR, which are thought to be implicated in cognitive control (Miller & Cohen, 2001; Ochsner, Silvers, & Buhle, 2012; Smith & Jonides, 1999; Wager et al., 2008). Importantly, some studies have identified the regions engaged to a greater degree during reappraisal used to down-regulate negative emotion compared with the regions engaged to up-regulate negative emotion. These studies demonstrate that down-regulation of negative emotion recruits right lateral prefrontal cortex and lateral orbitofrontal cortex regions to a greater extent than up-regulation. These regions are thought to be involved in inhibiting pre-potent responses and tracking changing emotional values (Eippert et al., 2007; Kim & Hamann, 2007; Mak, Hu, Zhang, Xiao, & Lee, 2009).

Although PR might have distinct emotional consequences from NR, it is unclear whether it engages similar control regions. Very few studies have examined this directly. Some insight, however, can be derived from studies examining PR in positive contexts. Compared with increasing negative emotion, increasing positive emotion in a positive context uniquely recruits left lateral prefrontal regions as well as dorsal medial prefrontal cortex (Kim & Hamann, 2007). Therefore, PR compared to NR might involve greater recruitment of the typical left-sided control regions associated with reappraisal and medial prefrontal regions thought to represent self-referential processing (Kelley et al., 2002). By and large, however, it is important to recognize that studies examining PR demonstrate that there seems to be far more overlap than distinction in the control-related regions engaged during PR compared with NR (Kim & Hamann, 2007).

In sum, although few studies have examined PR in negative contexts, the existing research allows us some understanding of its short-term effects on emotion and its neural correlates. First, PR appears to allow people to activate positive emotions even in intensely negative contexts. Second, PR appears to rely on control-related regions mostly similar to those engaged during NR. Therefore, one working hypothesis is that PR and NR use the same cognitive "fuel" but result in the production of different emotional responses. In other words, when people utilize these shared cognitive processes for the purpose of PR, they might reap many of the unique benefits associated with positive emotion. This activated positive emotion might then be garnered to engage with and improve negative situations, rather than merely "riding out the storm." We next turn to the implications these short-term emotional benefits might have for longer term resilience.

LONGER TERM EFFECTS: POSITIVE REAPPRAISAL AND RESILIENCE

Several lines of research provide initial support for the idea that PR plays a crucial role in psychological adjustment to SLEs. As the previous section shows, PR is associated with increased positive emotion. In turn, multiple lines of evidence support that increased frequency and intensity of positive emotion are positively associated with resilience (Fredrickson, 2001; Harker & Keltner, 2001; King, Hicks, Krull, & Del Gaiso, 2006) and a wide range of positive outcomes (Fredrickson, 1998, 2001; Lyubomirsky et al., 2005). For example, interventions that increase positive emotion increase well-being and decrease psychological health problems (Fredrickson, Cohn, Coffey, Pek, & Finkel, 2008; Lyubomirsky & Layous, 2013). Importantly, some evidence supports the notion that these beneficial effects of increased positive emotions are independent of the effects of reduced negative emotions (Diener, 1994; Folkman & Moskowitz, 2000; Lyubomirsky et al., 2005). For example, well-being is characterized by high levels of positive emotion, not merely the absence of negative emotion (Brown, Chorpita, & Barlow, 1998; Bylsma, Morris, & Rottenberg, 2008; Clark & Watson, 1991; McMakin, Santiago, & Shirk, 2009).

Given these positive effects of positive emotions in general, it stands to reason that positive emotions are also beneficial in the context of SLEs (c.f. Folkman & Moskowitz, 2000; Lechner, Tennen, Affleck, Lopez, & Snyder, 2009). In fact, given that times of stress are characterized by a dearth of positive emotions, positive emotions may be especially useful during such times. Indeed, increased positive emotions have been shown to predict better outcomes after SLEs (Bonanno & Keltner, 1997; Burns et al., 2008; Cohn, Fredrickson, Brown, Mikels, & Conway, 2009; Fredrickson, Tugade, Waugh, & Larkin, 2003; Keltner & Bonanno, 1997; Moskowitz, Folkman, & Acree, 2003). Importantly, there is evidence to suggest that positive emotions are not just a correlate of successful coping but also a cause of it. For instance, interventions that increase positive emotion improve recovery from depression (Dichter et al., 2009; Dimidjian et al., 2006; Seligman, Rashid, & Parks, 2006; Sin & Lyubomirsky, 2009) and appear to enhance successful coping with stress (Moskowitz et al., 2012). Some studies have further shown that the effects of positive emotions on coping are distinct from those of negative emotion (Fredrickson & Joiner, 2002; Moskowitz, Epel, & Acree, 2008; Moskowitz et al., 2003). For example, Fredrickson and Joiner (2002) found that positive but not negative emotion was associated with broad-minded coping (a form of adaptive coping). It may be that increasing positive emotions is adaptive precisely because it does not necessarily involve decreasing negative emotions. After all, negative emotions can serve important functions such as keeping us and others motivated to address issues (Frijda, 1986; Tamir, 2009). Increasing positive emotion without removing negative emotion might thus yield particularly adaptive ways to cope with stressors.

Given these emerging beneficial effects of positive emotions in the context of SLEs, individuals' ability to *self-generate* positive emotion via emotion regulation might be a particularly powerful resilience factor for at least two reasons. First, during times of stress there are relatively few situational cues to positive emotion, and thus self-generation of positive emotion is especially useful. Second, the good feelings that accompany positive emotions, as well as their downstream effects such as cognitive broadening and enhanced social connection, might be particularly useful in times of stress, because they are most needed then (Folkman & Moskowitz, 2000; Tugade & Fredrickson, 2007). Thus, someone who can self-generate positive emotion when faced with a negative situation might be at a distinct advantage.

What evidence supports the notion that self-generating positive emotions via PR supports resilience? While few studies have directly examined PR and coping with SLEs, several pieces of converging evidence support that PR may contribute to resilience. In a correlational study, for example, Shiota (2006) found that participants who self-reported using PR in response to daily stressful events experienced greater positive mood. Some research suggests that such effects can be observed under highly stressful conditions and that they are prospective. In their research on partners of men with AIDS before and after their partner died, Moskowitz, Folkman, Collette, and Vittinghoff (1996) found that use of PR was associated with greater experience of positive mood. Importantly, PR was the only one of eight assessed coping strategies that showed these positive effects before and after bereavement, as well as when controlling for the previous month's mood and for the seven other types of coping.

In summary, research makes a strong case in support of the notion that the positive emotions that are enhanced by PR play a crucial positive role in resilience, and that they do so above and beyond decreases in negative emotion associated with NR. Moreover, the emerging research on PR suggests that people naturally use PR, that they apply it to ordinary as well as stressful events, and that PR is associated with positive psychological health outcomes, even under extreme stress. Thus, PR may be an important resilience factor.

CURRENT AND FUTURE RESEARCH

We reviewed emerging evidence in support of the ideas that PR has unique effects on positive emotion and that it constitutes a crucial resilience factor beyond other factors, including NR. Important next steps are to advance our understanding of, first, the nature of PR and, second, its role in resilience. To address these directions, we are currently conducting a set of studies funded by the Positive Neuroscience Project.

In one study, we instruct participants to use PR or to use NR while viewing negative emotional pictures. By doing this in a neuroimaging context, we aim to confirm predictions made by our framework, including that PR compared to NR will have different effects on brain regions associated with emotion (e.g., amygdala and ventral striatum), but that they will largely engage overlapping regions involved in cognitive control (e.g., dorsal and ventral lateral prefrontal cortex).

In terms of PR's role in resilience, one important goal is to elucidate the causal contributions of PR on resilience. To this end, we have designed an intervention that enhances PR in samples exposed to recent SLEs. We compare this intervention to an active control group to help us rule out important confounds, such as expectation for change or positive social contact. One important corollary of our argument is that PR may be especially useful because it allows people to completely *self-generate* positive emotion rather than relying on positive experiences. Thus, it may be particularly useful to people experiencing high levels of adversity, while other types of positive emotion interventions (e.g., counting blessings, gratitude, savoring; Emmons & McCullough, 2003; Sheldon & Lyubomirsky, 2006) might be most useful at lower levels of adversity. We plan to test this hypothesis by comparing the effects of our PR intervention in participants exposed to varying degrees of stressor severity.

Once the causal effects of PR on resilience have been more firmly established, it will be important to examine potential mediators (e.g., the ability to utilize PR, levels of positive and negative emotion; Kok & Fredrickson, 2010; Lyubomirsky & Layous, 2013). For example, we argued that PR might be beneficial because it enhances positive emotion without necessarily diminishing the experience of justified—and potentially useful—negative emotions. Mediation analyses will examine this type of hypothesis. Research should also take into consideration potential moderators and boundary conditions of PR interventions, including initial levels of well-being and PR, to help us understand for whom PR might be most useful. Lastly, to test the hypothesis that PR has unique effects on resilience, it will be important in future research to compare the effects of PR interventions to those of other interventions (Gruber, 2011; Mauss, Tamir, Anderson, & Savino, 2011).

CONCLUSION

Everyone experiences stressful life events (SLEs) at some point of another in their lives. While the experience of SLEs is an unavoidable part of human life, human reactions to SLEs can range from severe incapacitation to growth. What explains this vast variation in stress adjustment? Much prior research has focused on people's ability to dampen negative emotions as a linchpin process in stress adjustment. We argued here that, in addition, people's ability to self-generate positive emotions such as happiness, gratitude, and love, and to do so even in adverse situations, should be considered. One particularly powerful way to generate positive emotion is to transform the very meaning of the stressful situation one finds oneself in (positive reappraisal, or PR). Emerging research supports the idea that PR makes an important contribution, and that it does so over that of negative reappraisal. This is evident in its short-term emotional consequences as well as its long-term effects on resilience. Thus, PR may be uniquely poised to not merely side-step negative emotion but to use emotional engagement as fuel for resilience and growth.

NOTES

1. We use the term *adjustment* to refer to the full range of possible psychological health outcomes (negative to positive) after a stressor and the term *resilience* to refer to maintained or enhanced psychological health outcomes after a stressor (i.e., greater well-being and decreased mental health problems).

2. Although stress and emotion regulation have implications for physical as well as psychological health (Kubzansky & Kawachi, 2000; Marsland, Bachen, & Cohen, 2012; Mauss & Gross, 2004), we focus here on psychological health in the interest of space and because mechanisms underlying effects on physical health may at times differ from those on psychological health.

REFERENCES

Anderson, A. K., Christoff, K., Stappen, I., Panitz, D., Ghahremani, D. G., Glover, G., . . . Sobel, N. (2003). Dissociated neural representations of intensity and valence in human olfaction. *Nature Neuroscience, 6*, 196–202. doi:10.1038/nn1001

Bonanno, G. A. (2005). Resilience in the face of potential trauma. *Current Directions in Psychological Science, 14*(3), 135–138. doi:10.1111/j.0963-7214.2005.00347.x

Bonanno, G. A., & Keltner, D. (1997). Facial expressions of emotion and the course of conjugal bereavement. *Journal of Abnormal Psychology, 106*(1), 126–137. doi:10.1037//0021-843X.106.1.126

Brown, T. A., Chorpita, B. F., & Barlow, D. H. (1998). Structural relationships among dimensions of the DSM-IV anxiety and mood disorders and dimensions of negative affect, positive affect, and autonomic arousal. *Journal of Abnormal Psychology, 107*(2), 179–192. doi:10.1037//0021-843X.107.2.179

Bryant, R. A., Moulds, M., & Guthrie, R. M. (2001). Cognitive strategies and the resolution of acute stress disorder. *Journal of Traumatic Stress, 14*(1), 213–219. doi:10.1023/A:1007856103389

Burns, A. B., Brown, J. S., Sachs-Ericsson, N., Plant, E. A., Curtis, J. T., Fredrickson, B. L., & Joiner, T. E. (2008). Upward spirals of positive emotion and coping: Replication, extension, and initial exploration of neurochemical substrates. *Personality and Individual Differences, 44*(2), 360–370. doi:10.1016/j.paid.2007.08.015

Bylsma, L. M., Morris, B. H., & Rottenberg, J. (2008). A meta-analysis of emotional reactivity in major depressive disorder. *Clinical Psychology Review, 28*(4), 676–691. doi:10.1016/j.cpr.2007.10.001

Carrico, A. W., Antoni, M. H., Weaver, K. E., Lechner, S. C., & Schneiderman, N. (2005). Cognitive-behavioural stress management with HIV-positive homosexual men: Mechanisms of sustained reductions in depressive symptoms. *Chronic Illness,* *1*(3), 207–215. doi:10.1179/174239505X55996

Clark, L. A., & Watson, D. (1991). Tripartite model of anxiety and depression: Psychometric evidence and taxonomic implications. *Journal of Abnormal Psychology, 100*(3), 316–336. doi:10.1037//0021-843X.100.3.316

Cohn, M. A., Fredrickson, B. L., Brown, S. L., Mikels, J. A., & Conway, A. M. (2009). Happiness unpacked: Positive emotions increase life satisfaction by building resilience. *Emotion, 9*(3), 361–368. doi:10.1037/a0015952

Cunningham, W. A., Van Bavel, J. J., & Johnsen, I. R. (2008). Affective flexibility: Evaluative processing goals shape amygdala activity. *Psychological Science, 19*(2), 152–160. doi:10.1111/j.1467-9280.2008.02061.x

Davidson, R. J. (2000). Affective style, psychopathology, and resilience: Brain mechanisms and plasticity. *American Psychologist, 55*(11), 1196–1214. doi:10.1037//0003-066X.55.11.1196

Deveney, C. M., & Pizzagalli, D. A. (2008). The cognitive consequences of emotion regulation: An ERP investigation. *Psychophysiology, 45*(3), 435–444. doi:10.1111/j.1469-8986.2007.00641.x

Dichter, G. S., Felder, J. N., Petty, C., Bizzell, J., Ernst, M., & Smoski, M. J. (2009). The effects of psychotherapy on neural responses to rewards in major depression. *Biological Psychiatry, 66*(9), 886–897. doi:10.1016/j.biopsych.2009.06.021

Diener, E. (1994). Assessing subjective well-being: Progress and opportunities. *Social Indicators Research, 31*(2), 103–157.

Dillon, D. G., & LaBar, K. S. (2005). Startle-modulation during conscious emotion regulation is arousal-dependent. *Behavioral Neuroscience, 119*(4), 1118–1124. doi:10.1037/0735-7044.119.4.1118

Dimidjian, S., Hollon, S. D., Dobson, K. S., Schmaling, K. B., Kohlenberg, R. J., Addis, M. E., . . . Jacobson, N. S. (2006). Randomized trial of behavioral activation, cognitive therapy, and antidepressant medication in the acute treatment of adults with major depression. *Journal of Consulting and Clinical Psychology, 74*(4), 658–670. doi:10.1037/0022-006X.74.4.658

Eippert, F., Veit, R., Weiskopf, N., Erb, M., Birbaumer, N., & Anders, S. (2007). Regulation of emotional responses elicited by threat-related stimuli. *Human Brain Mapping, 28*(5), 409–423. doi:10.1002/hbm.20291

Emmons, R. A., & McCullough, M. E. (2003). Counting blessings versus burdens: An experimental investigation of gratitude and subjective well-being in daily life. *Journal of Personality and Social Psychology, 84*(2), 377.

Folkman, S. (1997). Positive psychological states and coping with severe stress. *Social Science and Medicine, 45*(8), 1207–1221. doi:10.1016/S0277-9536(97)00040-3

Folkman, S., & Moskowitz, J. T. (2000). Positive affect and the other side of coping. *American Psychologist, 55*(6), 647–654.

Foti, D., & Hajcak, G. (2008). Deconstructing reappraisal: Descriptions preceding arousing pictures modulate the subsequent neural response. *Journal of Cognitive Neuroscience, 20*(6), 977–988. doi:10.1162/jocn.2008.20066

Fredrickson, B. L. (1998). What good are positive emotions? *Review of General Psychology, 2,* 300–319. doi:10.1037/1089-2680.2.3.300

Fredrickson, B. L. (2001). The role of positive emotions in positive psychology: The broaden-and-build theory of positive emotions. *American Psychologist, 56*(3), 218–226. doi:10.1037//0003-066X.56.3.218

Fredrickson, B. L., Cohn, M. A., Coffey, K. A., Pek, J., & Finkel, S. M. (2008). Open hearts build lives: Positive emotions, induced through loving-kindness meditation, build consequential personal resources. *Journal of Personality and Social Psychology, 95*(5), 1045–1062. doi:10.1037/A0013262

Fredrickson, B. L., & Joiner, T. (2002). Positive emotions trigger upward spirals toward emotional well-being. *Psychological Science, 13*(2), 172–175. doi:10.1111/1467-9280.00431

Fredrickson, B. L., & Levenson, R. W. (1998). Positive emotions speed recovery from the cardiovascular sequelae of negative emotions. *Cognition and Emotion, 12*(2), 191–220. doi:10.1080/026999398379718

Fredrickson, B. L., Tugade, M. M., Waugh, C. E., & Larkin, G. R. (2003). What good are positive emotions in crisis? A prospective study of resilience and emotions following the terrorist attacks on the United States on September 11th, 2001. *Journal of Personality and Social Psychology, 84*, 365–376. doi:10.1037//0022-3514.84.2.365

Freitas, A. L., & Downey, G. (1998). Resilience: A dynamic perspective. *International Journal of Behavioral Development, 22*(2), 263–285. doi:10.1080/016502598384379

Frijda, N. H. (1986). *The emotions.* New York, NY: Cambridge University Press.

Garnefski, N., & Kraaij, V. (2006). Relationships between cognitive emotion regulation strategies and depressive symptoms: A comparative study of five specific samples. *Personality and Individual Differences, 40*(8), 1659–1669. doi:10.1016/J.Paid.2005.12.009

Giuliani, N. R., McRae, K., & Gross, J. J. (2008). The up- and down-regulation of amusement: Experiential, behavioral, and autonomic consequences. *Emotion, 8*(5), 714–719. doi:10.1037/a0013236

Gross, J. J. (1998a). Antecedent- and response-focused emotion regulation: Divergent consequences for experience, expression, and physiology. *Journal of Personality and Social Psychology, 74*(1), 224–237. doi:10.1037//0022-3514.74.1.224

Gross, J. J. (1998b). The emerging field of emotion regulation: An integrative review. *Review of General Psychology, 2*(3), 271–299. doi:10.1037//1089-2680.2.3.271

Gross, J. J., & John, O. P. (2003). Individual differences in two emotion regulation processes: implications for affect, relationships, and well-being. *Journal of Personality and Social Psychology, 85*(2), 348–362. doi:10.1037/0022-3514.85.2.348

Gruber, J. (2011). Can feeling too good be bad? Positive emotion persistence (PEP) in bipolar disorder. *Current Directions in Psychological Science, 20*(4), 217–221.

Hajcak, G., & Nieuwenhuis, S. (2006). Reappraisal modulates the electrocortical response to unpleasant pictures. *Cognitive, Affective, and Behavioral Neuroscience, 6*(4), 291–297. doi:10.3758/cabn.6.4.291

Harker, L., & Keltner, D. (2001). Expressions of positive emotion in women's college yearbook pictures and their relationship to personality and life outcomes across adulthood. *Journal of Personality and Social Psychology, 80*(1), 112–124. doi:10.1037//0022-3514.80.1.112

Jackson, D. C., Malmstadt, J. R., Larson, C. L., & Davidson, R. J. (2000). Suppression and enhancement of emotional responses to unpleasant pictures. *Psychophysiology, 37*(4), 515–522. doi:10.1111/1469-8986.3740515

Kelley, W. M., Macrae, C. N., Wyland, C. L., Caglar, S., Inati, S., & Heatherton, T. F. (2002). Finding the self? An event-related fMRI study. *Journal of Cognitive Neuroscience, 14*(5), 785–794. doi:10.1162/08989290260138672

Keltner, D., & Bonanno, G. A. (1997). A study of laughter and dissociation: Distinct correlates of laughter and smiling during bereavement. *Journal of Personality and Social Psychology, 73*(4), 687–702.

Keltner, D., & Gross, J. J. (1999). Functional accounts of emotions. *Cognition and Emotion, 13*(5), 467–480. doi:10.1080/026999399379140

Kendler, K. S., Karkowski, L. M., & Prescott, C. A. (1999). Causal relationship between stressful life events and the onset of major depression. *American Journal of Psychiatry, 156*(6), 837–848.

Kessler, R. C. (1997). The effects of stressful life events on depression. *Annual Review of Psychology, 48*, 191–214. doi:10.1146/annurev.psych.48.1.191

Kim, S. H., & Hamann, S. (2007). Neural correlates of positive and negative emotion regulation. *Journal of Cognitive Neuroscience, 19*(5), 776–798. doi:10.1162/jocn.2007.19.5.776

King, L. A., Hicks, J. A., Krull, J. L., & Del Gaiso, A. K. (2006). Positive affect and the experience of meaning in life. *Journal of Personality and Social Psychology, 90*(1), 179–196. doi:10.1037/0022-3514.90.1.179

Kok, B. E., & Fredrickson, B. L. (2010). Upward spirals of the heart: Autonomic flexibility, as indexed by vagal tone, reciprocally and prospectively predicts positive emotions and social connectedness. *Biological Psychology, 85*(3), 432–436.

Kraaij, V., Pruymboom, E., & Garnefski, N. (2002). Cognitive coping and depressive symptoms in the elderly: A longitudinal study. *Aging and Mental Health, 6*(3), 275–281. doi:10.1080/13607860220142387

Kubzansky, L. D., & Kawachi, I. (2000). Going to the heart of the matter: Do negative emotions cause coronary heart disease? *Journal of Psychosomatic Research, 48*, 323–337.

Lechner, S. C., Tennen, H., Affleck, G., Lopez, S. J., & Snyder, C. R. (2009). Benefit-finding and growth. In *Oxford handbook of positive psychology* (2nd ed., pp. 633–640). New York, NY: Oxford University Press.

Lin, N., Simeone, R. S., Ensel, W. M., & Kuo, W. (1979). Social support, stressful life events, and illness: A model and an empirical test. *Journal of Health and Social Behavior, 20*(2), 108–119. doi:10.2307/2136433

Lucas, R. E., Clark, A. E., Georgellis, Y., & Diener, E. (2003). Reexamining adaptation and the set point model of happiness: Reactions to changes in marital status. *Journal of Personality and Social Psychology, 84*(3), 527–539. doi:10.1111/j.1467-8721.2007.00479.x

Lupien, S. J., McEwen, B. S., Gunnar, M. R., & Heim, C. (2009). Effects of stress throughout the lifespan on the brain, behaviour and cognition. *Nature Reviews Neuroscience, 10*(6), 434–445. doi:10.1038/nrn2639

Lyubomirsky, S., King, L., & Diener, E. (2005). The benefits of frequent positive affect: Does happiness lead to success? *Psychological Bulletin, 131*(6), 803–855. doi:10.1037/0033-2909.131.6.803

Lyubomirsky, S., & Layous, K. (2013). How do simple positive activities increase well-being? *Current Directions in Psychological Science, 22*, 57–62. doi:10.1177/0963721412469809

Mak, A. K. Y., Hu, Z.-G., Zhang, J. X., Xiao, Z-W., & Lee, T. M. C. (2009). Neural correlates of regulation of positive and negative emotions: An fMRI study. *Neuroscience Letters, 457*(2), 101–106. doi:10.1016/j.neulet.2009.03.094

Marsland, A. L., Bachen, E. A., & Cohen, S. (2012). Stress, immunity, and susceptibility to upper respiratory infectious disease. In A. L. Marsland, E. A. Bachen & S. Cohen (Eds.), *Handbook of health psychology* (2nd ed., pp. 717–738). New York, NY: Psychology Press.

Mauss, I. B., Cook, C. L., Cheng, J. Y. J., & Gross, J. J. (2007). Individual differences in cognitive reappraisal: Experiential and physiological responses to an anger provocation. *International Journal of Psychophysiology, 66*(2), 116–124. doi:10.1016/j.ijpsycho.2007.03.017

Mauss, I. B., & Gross, J. J. (2004). Emotion suppression and cardiovascular disease: Is hiding your feelings bad for your heart? In L. R. Temoshok, A. Vingerhoets, & I. Nyklicek (Eds.), *The expression of emotion and health* (pp. 62–81). London, UK: Brunner-Routledge.

Mauss, I. B., & Tamir, M. (2013). Emotion goals: How their content, structure, and operation shape emotion regulation. In J. J. Gross (Ed.), *Handbook of emotion regulation* (2nd ed., pp. 361–375). New York, NY: Guilford Press.

Mauss, I. B., Tamir, M., Anderson, C. L., & Savino, N. S. (2011). Can seeking happiness make people unhappy? Paradoxical effects of valuing happiness. *Emotion, 11*(4), 807–815. doi:10.1037/a0022010

McEwen, B. S. (2000). The neurobiology of stress: From serendipity to clinical relevance. *Brain Research, 886*(1–2), 172–189. doi:10.1176/appi.ajp.163.12.2164

McMakin, D. L., Santiago, C. D., & Shirk, S. R. (2009). The time course of positive and negative emotion in dysphoria. *Journal of Positive Psychology, 4*(2), 182–192. doi:10.1080/17439760802650600

McRae, K., Ciesielski, B., & Gross, J. J. (2012). Unpacking cognitive reappraisal: Goals, tactics, and outcomes. *Emotion, 12*(2), 250–255. doi:10.1037/A0026351

McRae, K., Ochsner, K. N., Mauss, I. B., Gabrieli, J. J. D., & Gross, J. J. (2008). Gender differences in emotion regulation: An fMRI study of cognitive reappraisal. *Group Processes and Intergroup Relations, 11*(2), 143–162. doi:10.1177/1368430207088035

Miller, E. K., & Cohen, J. D. (2001). An integrative theory of prefrontal cortex function. *Annual Review of Neuroscience, 24*(1), 167–202. doi:10.1146/annurev.neuro.24.1.167

Moskowitz, J. T., Epel, E. S., & Acree, M. (2008). Positive affect uniquely predicts lower risk of mortality in people with diabetes. *Health Psychology, 27*(1 Suppl.), S73–82. doi:10.1037/0278-6133.27.1.S73

Moskowitz, J. T., Folkman, S., & Acree, M. (2003). Do positive psychological states shed light on recovery from bereavement? Findings from a 3-year longitudinal study. *Death Studies, 27*, 471–500. doi:10.1080/07481180302885

Moskowitz, J. T., Folkman, S., Collette, L., & Vittinghoff, E. (1996). Coping and mood during AIDS-related caregiving and bereavement. *Annals of Behavioral Medicine, 18*(1), 49–57.

Moskowitz, J. T., Hult, J. R., Duncan, L. G., Cohn, M. A., Maurer, S., Bussolari, C., & Acree, M. (2012). A positive affect intervention for people experiencing health-related stress: Development and non-randomized pilot test. *Journal of Health Psychology, 17*(5), 676–692. doi:10.1177/1359105311425275

Ochsner, K. N., Bunge, S. A., Gross, J. J., & Gabrieli, J. D. E. (2002). Rethinking feelings: An fMRI study of the cognitive regulation of emotion. *Journal of Cognitive Neuroscience, 14*(8), 1215–1229. doi:10.1162/089892902760807212

Ochsner, K. N., Silvers, J. A., & Buhle, J. T. (2012). Functional imaging studies of emotion regulation: A synthetic review and evolving model of the cognitive control of emotion. *Annals of the New York Academy of Sciences, 1251*(1), E1–E24. doi:10.1111/j.1749-6632.2012.06751.x

Pagano, M. E., Skodol, A. E., Stout, R. L., Shea, M. T., Yen, S., Grilo, C. M., ... Gunderson, J. G. (2004). Stressful life events as predictors of functioning: Findings from the Collaborative Longitudinal Personality Disorders Study. *Acta Psychiatrica Scandinavica, 110*(6), 421–429. doi:10.1111/j.1600-0447.2004.00398.x

Ray, R. D., McRae, K., Ochsner, K. N., & Gross, J. J. (2010). Cognitive reappraisal of negative affect: Converging evidence from EMG and self-report. *Emotion, 10*(4), 587–592. doi:10.1037/a0019015

Ryff, C. D., Singer, B., Love, G. D., & Essex, M. J. (1998). Resilience in adulthood and later life: Defining features and dynamic processes. In J. Lomranz (Ed.), *Handbook of aging and mental health: An integrative approach* (pp. 69–96). New York, NY: Plenum Press.

Schaefer, S. M., Jackson, D. C., Davidson, R. J., Aguirre, G. K., Kimberg, D. Y., & Thompson-Schill, S. L. (2002). Modulation of amygdalar activity by the conscious regulation of negative emotion. *Journal of Cognitive Neuroscience, 14*, 913–921. doi:10.1162/089892902760191135

Seligman, M. E. P., Rashid, T., & Parks, A. C. (2006). Positive psychotherapy. *American Psychologist, 61*(8), 774–788. doi:10.1037/0003-066X.61.8.774

Sheldon, K. M., & Lyubomirsky, S. (2006). How to increase and sustain positive emotion: The effects of expressing gratitude and visualizing best possible selves. *Journal of Positive Psychology, 1*(2), 73–82.

Shiota, M. N. (2006). Silver linings and candles in the dark: Differences among positive coping strategies in predicting subjective well-being. *Emotion, 6*(2), 335–339. doi:10.1037/1528-3542.6.2.335

Shiota, M. N., & Levenson, R. W. (2012). Turn down the volume or change the channel? Emotional effects of detached versus positive reappraisal. *Journal of Personality and Social Psychology, 103*(3), 416. doi:10.1037/a0029208

Sin, N. L., & Lyubomirsky, S. (2009). Enhancing well-being and alleviating depressive symptoms with positive psychology interventions: A practice-friendly meta-analysis. *Journal of Clinical Psychology, 65*(5), 467–487. doi:10.1002/jclp.20593

Smith, E. E., & Jonides, J. (1999). Storage and executive processes in the frontal lobes. *Science, 283*(5408), 1657–1661. doi:10.1126/science.283.5408.1657

Tamir, M. (2009). What do people want to feel and why? Pleasure and utility in emotion regulation. *Current Directions in Psychological Science, 18*(2), 101–105. doi:10.1111/j.1467-8721.2009.01617.x

Tennant, C. (2002). Life events, stress and depression: A review of the findings. *Australian and New Zealand Journal of Psychiatry, 36*(2), 173–182. doi:10.1046/j.1440-1614.2002.01007.x

Thompson, R. A. (1994). Emotion regulation: A theme in search of definition. *Monographs of the Society for Research in Child Development, 59*(2–3), 25–52, 250–283. doi:10.2307/1166137

Tomaka, J., Blascovich, J., Kibler, J., & Ernst, J. M. (1997). Cognitive and physiological antecedents of threat and challenge appraisal. *Journal of Personality and Social Psychology, 73*(1), 63–72. doi:10.1037//0022-3514.73.1.63

Tosevski, D. L., & Milovancevic, M. P. (2006). Stressful life events and physical health. *Current Opinion in Psychiatry, 19*(2), 184–189. doi:10.1097/01.yco.0000214346.44625.57

Troy, A. S., Wilhelm, F. H., Shallcross, A. J., & Mauss, I. B. (2010). Seeing the silver lining: Cognitive reappraisal ability moderates the relationship between stress and depression. *Emotion, 10*(6), 783–795. doi:10.1037/a0020262

Tugade, M. M., & Fredrickson, B. L. (2007). Regulation of positive emotions: Emotion regulation strategies that promote resilience. *Journal of Happiness Studies, 8*(3), 311–333.

Wager, T. D., Davidson, M. L., Hughes, B. L., Lindquist, M. A., & Ochsner, K. N. (2008). Prefrontal-subcortical pathways mediating successful emotion regulation. *Neuron, 59*(6), 1037–1050. doi:10.1016/j.neuron.2008.09.006

Watson, D., Wiese, D., Vaidya, J., & Tellegen, A. (1999). The two general activation systems of affect: Structural findings, evolutionary considerations, and psychobiological evidence. *Journal of Personality and Social Psychology, 76*(5), 820–838. doi:10.1037//0022-3514.76.5.820

Whalen, P. J. (1998). Fear, vigilance, and ambiguity: Initial neuroimaging studies of the human amygdala. *Current Directions in Psychological Science, 7*(6), 177–188. doi:10.1111/1467-8721.ep10836912

Wrosch, C., Heckhausen, J., & Lachman, M. E. (2000). Primary and secondary control strategies for managing health and financial stress across adulthood. *Psychology and Aging, 15*(3), 387–399. doi:10.1037//0882-7974.15.3.387

11

Could Meditation Modulate the Neurobiology of Learning Not to Fear?

BRITTA K. HÖLZEL, SARA W. LAZAR,
AND MOHAMMED R. MILAD ■

Mindfulness meditation, the way it is currently introduced into contemporary psychology, has been derived from ancient Asian traditions, dating back approximately 2,500 years in Indian philosophy (Satipatthana Sutta, 2008). Although mindfulness meditation has most systematically been described in the Buddhist meditation literature (e.g., Satipatthana Sutta, 2008; Thera, 1962), its essence, the nonjudgmental attention to experiences in the present moment, also lies at the heart of other ancient and contemporary spiritual traditions (cf., Kabat-Zinn, 2003; Krishnamurti, 1999; Maharshi, 1959). Mindfulness is defined as the awareness that emerges through deliberately and nonjudgmentally paying attention to present-moment experiences, such as thoughts, emotions, and body sensations (Kabat-Zinn, 2003). Bishop and colleagues (2004) suggest a two-component model of mindfulness. The first component focuses on the self-regulation of attention so that it is maintained on immediate experience. The second involves approaching one's experience with an orientation of curiosity, openness, and acceptance toward the encountered experiences, regardless of their valence and desirability.

BENEFICIAL EFFECTS OF MINDFULNESS PRACTICE
ON MENTAL AND PHYSICAL HEALTH

Mindfulness meditation has been reported to produce beneficial effects on a number of psychiatric, functional somatic, and stress-related symptoms and has therefore increasingly been incorporated into psychotherapeutic programs (Baer, 2003; Grossman, Niemann, Schmidt, & Walach, 2004). A growing body of research documents the efficacy of mindfulness-based interventions in the treatment of a number of clinical disorders, including depression (Hofmann, Sawyer, Witt, & Oh, 2010; Teasdale et al., 2000), substance abuse (Bowen et al., 2006), eating disorders (Tapper et al., 2009), and chronic pain (Grossman, Tiefenthaler-Gilmer, Raysz, & Kesper, 2007). Mindfulness techniques have also been proven successful in the treatment of anxiety disorders (Hoge et al., 2013; Roemer, Orsillo, & Salters-Pedneault, 2008) and have been demonstrated to reduce anxiety symptoms (Hofmann et al., 2010). Furthermore, mindfulness meditation positively influences aspects of physical health, including improved immune function (Carlson, Speca, Faris, & Patel, 2007; Davidson et al., 2003) and reduced blood pressure and cortisol levels (Carlson et al., 2007). Not only has mindfulness successfully been used in the treatment of disorders and improvement of health, it has also been shown to produce positive effects on psychological well-being in healthy participants (Carmody & Baer, 2008; Chiesa & Serretti, 2009) and to enhance cognitive functioning (Jha, Krompinger, & Baime, 2007; Ortner, Kilner, & Zelazo, 2007; Pagnoni & Cekic, 2007; Slagter et al., 2007). Historically, mindfulness has been practiced to achieve enduring happiness (Ekman, Davidson, Ricard, & Wallace, 2005) and to gain insight into a view of the true nature of existence (Olendzki, 2010).

UNDERSTANDING THE UNDERLYING MECHANISMS
OF MINDFULNESS

It is striking that this seemingly simplistic practice can have such a wide range of applications and effects. Along with the many positive implications of mindfulness arises the question: How does mindfulness work, and what are its mechanisms? While there is a growing body of empirical literature, covering a wide range of research, including qualitative research, feasibility trials, controlled clinical trials, behavioral studies, and neuroscientific research, there is a relative paucity of theoretical models that address the mechanisms underlying its beneficial effects (but see Baer, 2003; Brown, Ryan, & Creswell, 2007; Lutz, Slagter, Dunne, & Davidson, 2008; Shapiro, Carlson, Astin, &

Freedman, 2006). We have recently suggested that mindfulness works by positively impacting several mechanisms that enhance self-regulation, including attention regulation, body awareness, emotion regulation, and a change in the perspective on the "self" (Hölzel, Lazar, et al., 2011). In the remainder of this chapter, we will discuss the hypothesis that mindfulness works in part by enhancing the ability to extinguish conditioned emotional responses.

MINDFULNESS AS AN EXPOSURE SITUATION

During mindfulness, practitioners expose themselves to "whatever is present in the field of awareness," including external stimuli as well as body sensations and emotional experiences. They let themselves be affected by the experience, refraining from engaging in internal reactivity toward it, and instead bring acceptance to bodily and affective responses (Hart, 1987). Practitioners are instructed to meet unpleasant emotions (such as fear, sadness, anger, aversion) by turning towards them, rather than turning away (Santorelli, 2000).

Parallels between the process described here and exposure therapy are evident. Exposure therapy is a highly effective behavioral therapy technique for reducing fear and anxiety responses (Chambless & Ollendick, 2001). Its core element is to expose patients to fear-provoking stimuli and prevent their usual response in order for them to extinguish the fear response, and instead to acquire a sense of safety in the presence of the formerly feared stimuli (Öst, 1997). Clinical studies on exposure therapy show that access to safety behaviors can interfere with the beneficial effects of an exposure situation (Lovibond, Mitchell, Minard, Brady, & Menzies, 2009; Wells et al., 1995). Safety behaviors include not only overt behavior (such as avoiding eye contact in social phobia) but also cognitive avoidance (such as suppressing thoughts related to the feared situation, or distracting attention). Mindfulness meditation includes refraining from engaging in cognitive avoidance or other safety behaviors by using enhanced attention regulation skills, thereby maximizing the exposure to the experienced emotion.

Additionally, meditation is often associated with high levels of relaxation in the form of increased parasympathetic tone and decreased sympathetic activity (Benson, 1975). Peripheral physiological changes have been observed with some consistency, including decreased heart rate (Zeidan, Johnson, Gordon, & Goolkasian, 2010), decreased blood pressure (De la Fuente, Franco, & Salvator, 2010), decreased breathing rate (Lazar et al., 2005), decreased skin conductance response (Austin, 2006), and decreased muscle tension (Benson, 1975). Because extinction mechanisms are thought to be supported by the experience of a state of relaxation while encountering the feared stimuli (Wolpe, 1958), the relaxation component of meditation might serve to maximize the effects of the extinction process.

EXTINCTION OF CONDITIONED FEAR

Fear conditioning has been much investigated in numerous species. It is a learning process in which a neutral stimulus (such as a light or a tone, conditioned stimulus, CS) is paired with an aversive unconditioned stimulus (such as an aversive electric shock, US). After a few pairings, the presentation of the CS comes to illicit various conditioned fear responses, such as freezing in rodents and enhanced skin conductance response (SCR) in humans. Repeated presentations of the CS in the absence of the US result in the extinction of all conditioned responses. Extinction does not erase the initial association between conditioned and unconditioned stimuli, but it is thought to form a new memory trace (Quirk, 2002; Rescorla, 2001) or reconsolidate the old memory with new contextual associations (Inda, Muravieva, & Alberini, 2011; Nader & Einarsson, 2010; Rossato, Bevilaqua, Izquierdo, Medina, & Cammarota, 2010). After extinction training, extinction memory is thought to compete with conditioned memory for control of fear expression (Myers & Davis, 2007). Recent research has shown that successful extinction memory reliably differentiates healthy from pathological conditions (Holt et al., 2009; Milad et al., 2008; reviewed in Graham & Milad, 2011). Extinction learning and its retention may thus be a critical process in the transformation of maladaptive states. It allows individuals to learn not to have a fear response to neutral stimuli, when there is no adaptive function for the fear response. Therefore, fear extinction brings individuals in a position where they experience a sense of safety and can flexibly elicit other emotional and behavioral reactions.

BRAIN REGIONS INVOLVED IN FEAR EXTINCTION AND EXTINCTION RETENTION

Recent magnetic resonance imaging (MRI) research on fear conditioning, including that from our team, has identified a network of brain regions that are crucial for the extinction of conditioned fear responses and its retention (reviewed in Milad & Quirk, 2012). As we will outline next, this network seems to strengthen through mindfulness practice.

The ventromedial prefrontal cortex (vmPFC) has been shown to be important for a successful recall of the extinction, with the magnitude of vmPFC activation positively correlated with extinction recall (Milad et al., 2007).

Milad et al. (2005) also found that cortical thickness of the vmPFC in healthy humans is positively correlated with the magnitude of extinction recall; the thicker the vmPFC, the better the extinction recall, suggesting that its size might explain individual differences within the normal healthy range in the ability to modulate fear. Similarly, findings from rodent studies also support the importance of the vmPFC in extinction recall. It has been shown that rats with vmPFC lesions are able to extinguish fear within a session but are unable to recall extinction memory 24 hours later (Lebron, Milad, & Quirk, 2004; Quirk, Russo, Barron, & Lebron, 2000).

In addition to the vmPFC, hippocampal activation has also been found to be involved in fear extinction. We have shown that hippocampal activation was observed in healthy subjects during the recall of extinction memory, and functional connectivity analysis reveals that the vmPFC and hippocampus work in concert during extinction recall to inhibit fear (Milad et al., 2007). The magnitude of activation in both brain regions was positively correlated with the magnitude of extinction memory (usually measured by SCR). Given the documented role of the hippocampus in context-modulated extinction recall in rodents (Corcoran, Desmond, Frey, & Maren, 2005; Corcoran & Maren, 2001), hippocampal activation during extinction recall is likely related to signaling the extinguished context (contextual safety). The significant functional correlation between the vmPFC and hippocampus as well as their positive correlation with extinction memory recall suggests that they comprise a network that mediates the expression of extinction memory in the appropriate context (Milad et al., 2007).

The amygdala has been implicated in both human and animal studies as playing a crucial role during the acquisition and expression of conditioned fear (Davis & Whalen, 2001; LeDoux, 2000; Pare, Quirk, & Ledoux, 2004; Phelps & LeDoux, 2005), including the detection of stressful and threatening stimuli and the initiation of adaptive coping responses. When individuals regulate their emotions, the amygdala is thought to be down-regulated by the vmPFC and the hippocampus (Banks, Eddy, Angstadt, Nathan, & Phan, 2007; Davidson, Jackson, & Kalin, 2000), which both have extensive connections to the amygdala. This inhibition of the amygdala serves to suppress fear (Milad, Rauch, Pitman, & Quirk, 2006; Rauch, Shin, & Phelps, 2006), thereby allowing control over behavioral reactions to emotions (Price, 2005). Furthermore, there are several recent rodent studies that have also implicated the amygdala in fear extinction learning (Herry et al., 2008; Likhtik, Popa, Apergis-Schoute, Fidacaro, & Pare, 2008).

Deficits in fear extinction are thought to contribute to several psychiatric disorders. Several neuroimaging studies have shown that all of the aforementioned structures are dysfunctional across several anxiety disorders. For example, Milad and colleagues have shown that patients with posttraumatic stress disorder (relative to controls) exhibit deficient fear extinction, and such deficiency is associated with amygdala hyperactivity during extinction learning and hypoactivity in the vmPFC and hippocampus (Milad et al., 2009). Neuroimaging studies have also shown that the aforementioned structures are dysfunctional in obsessive-compulsive disorder (Milad & Rauch, 2012), depression (Anand et al., 2005), and schizophrenia (Holt et al., 2009).

EFFECTS OF MEDITATION PRACTICE ON THE NEURAL NETWORK UNDERLYING EXTINCTION

There is recent evidence from anatomical MRI studies that the aforementioned brain regions show structural changes following mindfulness meditation training. Cross-sectional studies comparing mindfulness meditators and nonmeditators found that meditators showed greater gray matter concentration in the hippocampus (Hölzel et al., 2008; Luders, Toga, Lepore, & Gaser, 2009). Furthermore, we recently observed that structural changes in the hippocampus were detectable within a period of only 8 weeks in participants that underwent Mindfulness-Based Stress Reduction (Hölzel, Carmody, et al., 2011), and that cumulative hours of meditation training were positively correlated with gray matter concentration in the vmPFC in experienced meditators (Hölzel et al., 2008). In a longitudinal study enrolling participants in an 8-week Mindfulness-Based Stress Reduction course, we found an impact of the stress-reducing effects of mindfulness meditation on the amygdala; the greater the decrease in a participant's perceived stress scores over the 8 weeks, the greater a decrease the participant showed in gray matter concentration in the right amygdala (Hölzel et al., 2010). Modified gray matter concentration in these regions dependent on meditation training might potentially be related to the improved ability to regulate emotional responses. Furthermore, functional MRI studies show that meditation involves activation of the hippocampus and medial prefrontal cortex (Hölzel et al., 2007; Lazar et al., 2000; Lou et al., 1999; Newberg et al., 2001), suggesting that regular meditation practice enhances the function of these brain regions. Additionally, amygdala activation is reduced following 8 weeks of mindfulness practice in social anxiety disorder (Goldin & Gross, 2010). We have recently published the first study to elucidate the neural correlates of anxiety symptom reductions in patients with generalized anxiety disorder following mindfulness training, and we have found that a change in amygdala-prefrontal connectivity was correlated with symptom improvements (Hölzel et al., 2013). Furthermore, in a cross-sectional study, we applied unpleasant transcutaneous stimuli to experienced mindfulness meditators and nonmeditators. During stimulus anticipation, meditators showed stronger vmPFC activation and decreased fear when compared to nonmeditators (Gard et al., 2012).

OVERLAP BETWEEN BRAIN REGIONS INVOLVED IN FEAR EXTINCTION AND MINDFULNESS MEDITATION

As reviewed earlier, there appear to be striking similarities in the brain regions being influenced by mindfulness meditation and those involved in mediating fear extinction. These findings suggest that mindfulness meditation could directly influence one's capacity to extinguish conditioned fear by enhancing the structural and functional integrity of the brain network involved in safety signaling. The neuroscientific considerations described here support the previously held view that extinction might contribute to some of the beneficial effects of mindfulness practice (Baer, 2003; Brown et al., 2007).

THE RELEVANCE OF ENHANCED EXTINCTION PROCESSES THROUGH MINDFULNESS MEDITATION

The role of extinction processes in the improvements following mindfulness-based treatments is most obvious in the treatment of anxiety disorders, which have reliably been found to benefit from mindfulness practice (Hoge et al., 2013; Kabat-Zinn et al., 1992; Roemer et al., 2008). Fear extinction forms the basis for common behavioral therapies (i.e., exposure therapy) that are employed to treat patients with anxiety disorders. As such, there has been a substantial increase in the interest of exploring mechanisms by which fear extinction can be facilitated to aid patients with anxiety disorders. Several recent studies have provided very exciting data showing the potential for pharmacological agents that could improve fear extinction. Others have shown that fear extinction may also be improved in a nonpharmacological way (Monfils, Cowansage, Klann, & LeDoux, 2009; Schiller et al., 2010). If the hypothesis put forth here that mindfulness meditation might enhance the ability to extinguish conditioned fear holds true, mindfulness could provide an additional nonpharmacological method by which fear extinction can be facilitated. Nonreactivity and the successive extinction mechanism might also be highly relevant for the benefits of mindfulness in the treatment of substance abuse (Brewer et al., 2009), where patients can learn to replace previously established stimulus-response associations with more adaptive responses to overcome craving.

Beyond that, exposure is pursued toward "whatever emotions present themselves," including sadness, anger, and aversion, as well as pleasant emotions, such as happiness. We therefore suggest that extinction is effective during all of these emotional experiences, leading to an overwriting of previously learned stimulus-response associations. Buddhist teachings claim that the noncling-ing to unpleasant and pleasant experiences leads to liberation (Olendzki, 2010). Framed in Western psychological terminology, one could say that nonreactivity leads to unlearning of previous connections (extinction and reconsolidation), and thereby to liberation from being bound to habitual emotional reactions.

THE POSITIVE NEUROSCIENCE PROJECT

The hypothesis put forth here remains to be tested empirically through experimental studies that directly investigate the impact of meditation practice on the ability to extinguish conditioned emotional responses. In our research under the Positive Neuroscience project, we are investigating the impact of participation in the Mindfulness-Based Stress Reduction (MBSR) program on fear conditioning, extinction, and extinction memory in healthy but stressed individuals. MBSR is an 8-week, manualized program (Kabat-Zinn, 1990) that consists of weekly, teacher-led group meetings plus one "day of mindfulness" in the sixth week of the course. During these sessions, mindfulness is trained via sitting and walking meditation, yoga exercises, and the "body scan," in which attention is sequentially directed through the whole body. Participants also receive stress education. In daily homework practice, participants practice mindfulness exercises at home (with the help of an audio recording). They are taught to practice mindfulness also in their daily activities, such as eating, washing the dishes, and so on, as a way to facilitate the transfer of mindfulness into daily life. In our research project, we are employing a 2-day fear conditioning, extinction, and extinction retention paradigm in the MRI scanner before and after the MBSR course, and waitlist control period. Using skin conductance response, we are investigating whether the mindfulness intervention leads to modified fear conditioning, facilitated fear extinction, and facilitated extinction retention. The functional MRI BOLD response will provide insight into underlying neural mechanisms that might facilitate emotional learning.

CONCLUSION

Whereas multiple studies have investigated impaired fear conditioning in individuals suffering from mental disorders (Holt et al., 2009; Milad et al., 2008), little is known about the positive spectrum of this dimension. Ancient Indian scriptures recommend mindfulness meditation practice for decreasing suffering and the cultivation of positive mental states that are conducive for one's own and others' well-being (Ekman et al., 2005). Potentially, mindfulness meditation might do so in part by improving emotional learning beyond the normal range. As meditation is practiced (in various forms) across most religions, testing the hypothesis put forth here could help our understanding of how a spiritual practice could lead to the positive effects often experienced by those who practice it. Thus, it could improve our knowledge on how psychological health functioning could be enhanced and cultivated by demonstrating that these psychological changes are underlined by plastic changes in the brain. Furthermore, understanding the underlying neural correlates of the positive benefits resulting from mindfulness practice will have important clinical implications, because it can inform the application of these nonpharmacological techniques for individuals suffering, for example, from anxiety disorders.

REFERENCES

Anand, A., Li, Y., Wang, Y., Wu, J., Gao, S., Bukhari, L., Mathews, V. P., . . . Lowe, M. J. (2005). Activity and connectivity of brain mood regulating circuit in depression: A functional magnetic resonance study. *Biological Psychiatry, 57*(10), 1079–1088. doi:S0006-3223(05)00186-1 [pii] 10.1016/j.biopsych.2005.02.021

Austin, J. H. (2006). *Zen-brain reflections*. Cambridge, MA: MIT Press.

Baer, R. A. (2003). Mindfulness training as a clinical intervention: A conceptual and empirical review. *Clinical Psychology: Science and Practice, 10*(2), 125–143.

Banks, S. J., Eddy, K. T., Angstadt, M., Nathan, P. J., & Phan, K. L. (2007). Amygdala-frontal connectivity during emotion regulation. *Social Cognitive and Affective Neuroscience, 2*(4), 303–12. doi:10.1093/scan/nsm029

Benson, H. (1975). *The relaxation response*. New York, NY: Morrow.

Bishop, S. R., et al. (2004). Mindfulness: A proposed operational definition. *Clinical Psychology: Science and Practice, 11*, 230–241. doi:10.1093/clipsy/bph077

Bowen, S., Witkiewitz, K., Dillworth, T. M., Chawla, N., Simpson, T. L., Ostafin, B. D., . . . Marlatt, G. A. (2006). Mindfulness meditation and substance use in an incarcerated population. *Psychology of Addiction Behavior, 20*(3), 343–347. doi:2006-10832-015 [pii] 10.1037/0893-164X.20.3.343

Brewer, J. A., Sinha, R., Chen, J. A., Michalsen, R. N., Babuscio, T. A., Nich, C., . . . Rounsaville, B. J. (2009). Mindfulness training and stress reactivity in substance abuse: results from a randomized, controlled stage I pilot study. *Substance Abuse, 30*(4), 306–317. doi:916725438 [pii] 10.1080/08897070903250241

Brown, K. W., Ryan, R. M., & Creswell, J. D. (2007). Mindfulness: Theoretical foundations and evidence for its salutary effects. *Psychological Inquiry, 18*(4), 211–237. doi:10.1080/10478400701598298

Carlson, L. E., Speca, M., Faris, P., & Patel, K. D. (2007). One year pre-post intervention follow-up of psychological, immune, endocrine and blood pressure outcomes
  of mindfulness-based stress reduction (MBSR) in breast and prostate cancer outpa-
  tients. *Brain, Behavior, and Immunity, 21*(8), 1038–1049. doi:S0889-1591(07)00085-2
  [pii] 10.1016/j.bbi.2007.04.002
Carmody, J., & Baer, R. A. (2008). Relationships between mindfulness practice and
  levels of mindfulness, medical and psychological symptoms and well-being in a
  mindfulness-based stress reduction program. *Journal of Behavioral Medicine, 31*(1),
  23–33. doi:10.1007/s10865-007-9130-7
Chambless, D. L., & Ollendick, T. H. (2001). Empirically supported psychological
  interventions: Controversies and evidence. *Annual Review of Psychology, 52*, 685–
  716. doi:10.1146/annurev.psych.52.1.685 52/1/685 [pii]
Chiesa, A., & Serretti, A. (2009). Mindfulness-based stress reduction for stress management in healthy people: a review and meta-analysis. *Journal of Alternative and
  Complementary Medicine, 15*(5), 593–600. doi:10.1089/acm.2008.0495
Corcoran, K. A., Desmond, T. J., Frey, K. A., & Maren, S. (2005). Hippocampal
  inactivation disrupts the acquisition and contextual encoding of fear extinction. *Journal of Neuroscience, 25*(39), 8978–8987. doi:25/39/8978 [pii] 10.1523/
  JNEUROSCI.2246-05.2005
Corcoran, K. A., & Maren, S. (2001). Hippocampal inactivation disrupts contextual
  retrieval of fear memory after extinction. *Journal of Neuroscience, 21*(5), 1720–1726.
  doi:21/5/1720 [pii]
Davidson, R. J., Jackson, D. C., & Kalin, N. H. (2000). Emotion, plasticity, context, and
  regulation: Perspectives from affective neuroscience. *Psychological Bulletin, 126*(6),
  890–909.
Davidson, R. J., Kabat-Zinn, J., Schumacher, J., Rosenkranz, M., Muller, D., Santorelli,
  S. F., . . . Sheridan, J. F. (2003). Alterations in brain and immune function produced
  by mindfulness meditation. *Psychosomatic Medicine, 65*(4), 564–570.
Davis, M., & Whalen, P. J. (2001). The amygdala: Vigilance and emotion. *Molecular
  Psychiatry, 6*(1), 13–34.
De la Fuente, M., Franco, C., & Salvator, M. (2010). Reduction of blood pressure in
  a group of hypertensive teachers through a program of mindfulness meditation.
  Behavioral Psychology-Psicologia Conductual, 18(3), 533–552.
Ekman, P., Davidson, R. J., Ricard, M., & Wallace, A. (2005). Buddhist and psychologi-
  cal perspectives on emotions and well-being. *Current Directions in Psychological
  Science, 14*(2), 59–63.
Gard, T., Hölzel, B. K., Sack, A. T., Hempel, H., Lazar, S. W., Vaitl, D., & Ott, U. (2012).
  Pain attenuation through mindfulness is associated with decreased cognitive con-
  trol and increased sensory processing in the brain. *Cerebral Cortex, 22*(11), 2692–
  702. doi:10.1093/cercor/bhr352
Goldin, P. R., & Gross, J. J. (2010). Effects of mindfulness-based stress reduction
  (MBSR) on emotion regulation in social anxiety disorder. *Emotion, 10*(1), 83–91.
  doi:2010-01983-016 [pii] 10.1037/a0018441
Graham, B. M., & Milad, M. R. (2011). The study of fear extinction: Implications for
  anxiety disorders. *American Journal of Psychiatry, 168*(12), 1255–1265.

Grossman, P., Niemann, L., Schmidt, S., & Walach, H. (2004). Mindfulness-based stress reduction and health benefits. A meta-analysis. *Journal of Psychosomatic Research, 57*(1), 35–43.

Grossman, P., Tiefenthaler-Gilmer, U., Raysz, A., & Kesper, U. (2007). Mindfulness training as an intervention for fibromyalgia: Evidence of postintervention and 3-year follow-up benefits in well-being. *Psychotherapy and Psychosomatics, 76*(4), 226–233. doi·000101501 [pii] 10.1159/000101501

Hart, W. (1987). *The art of living: Vipassana meditation: As taught by S. N. Goenka.* New York, NY: HarperOne.

Herry, C., Ciocchi, S., Senn, V., Demmou, L., Muller, C., & Luthi, A. (2008). Switching on and off fear by distinct neuronal circuits. *Nature, 454*(7204), 600–606. doi:nature07166 [pii] 10.1038/nature07166

Hofmann, S. G., Sawyer, A. T., Witt, A. A., & Oh, D. (2010). The effect of mindfulness-based therapy on anxiety and depression: A meta-analytic review. *Journal of Consulting and Clinical Psychology, 78*(2), 169–183. doi:2010-05835-004 [pii] 10.1037/a0018555

Hoge, E. A., Bui, E., Marques, L., Metcalf, C. A., Morris, L. K.,Robinaugh, D. J., . . . Simon, N. M. (2013). Randomized controlled trial of mindfulness meditation for generalized anxiety disorder: Effects on anxiety and stress reactivity. *Journal of Clinical Psychiatry, 74*(8), 786–792.

Holt, D. J., Lebron-Milad, K., Milad, M. R., Rauch, S. L., Pitman, R. K., Orr, S. P., . . . Goff, D. C. (2009). Extinction memory is impaired in schizophrenia. *Biological Psychiatry, 65*(6), 455–463.

Hölzel, B K, Carmody, J., Evans, K. C., Hoge, E. A., Dusek, J. A., Morgan, L., . . . Lazar, S. W. (2010). Stress reduction correlates with structural changes in the amygdala. *Social Cognitive and Affective Neuroscience, 5*, 11–17. doi:10.1093/scan/nsp034

Hölzel, B. K., Carmody, J., Vangel, M., Congleton, C., Yerramsetti, S. M., Gard, T., & Lazar, S. W. (2011). Mindfulness practice leads to increases in regional brain gray matter density. *Psychiatry Research, 191*(1), 36–43. doi:10.1016/j.pscychresns.2010.08.006

Hölzel, B. K., Hoge, E. A., Greve, D. N., Gard, T., Creswell, J. D., Brown, K. W., . . . Lazar, S. W. (2013). Neural mechanisms of symptom improvements in generalized anxiety disorder following mindfulness training. *NeuroImage: Clinical, 2*, 448–458. doi:10.1016/j.nicl.2013.03.011

Hölzel, B. K., Lazar, S. W., Gard, T., Schuman-Olivier, Z., Vago, D. R., & Ott, U. (2011). How does mindfulness meditation work? Proposing mechanisms of action from a conceptual and neural perspective. *Perspectives on Psychological Science, 6*(6), 537–559. doi:10.1177/1745691611419671

Hölzel, B. K., Ott, U., Gard, T., Hempel, H., Weygandt, M., Morgen, K., & Vaitl, D. (2008). Investigation of mindfulness meditation practitioners with voxel-based morphometry. *Social Cognitive and Affective Neuroscience, 3*(1), 55–61.

Hölzel, B. K., Ott, U., Hempel, H., Hackl, A., Wolf, K., Stark, R., & Vaitl, D. (2007). Differential engagement of anterior cingulate and adjacent medial frontal cortex in adept meditators and non-meditators. *Neuroscience Letters, 421*(1), 16–21. doi:S0304-3940(07)00451-X [pii]10.1016/j.neulet.2007.04.074

Inda, M. C., Muravieva, E. V., & Alberini, C. M. (2011). Memory retrieval and the passage of time: From reconsolidation and strengthening to extinction. *J Neurosci*, *31*(5), 1635–1643. doi:31/5/1635 [pii] 10.1523/JNEUROSCI.4736-10.2011

Jha, A. P., Krompinger, J., & Baime, M. J. (2007). Mindfulness training modifies subsystems of attention. *Cognitve, Affective, and Behavioral Neuroscience*, *7*(2), 109–119.

Kabat-Zinn, J. (1990). *Full catastrophe living*. New York, NY: Delta.

Kabat-Zinn, J. (2003). Mindfulness-based interventions in context: Past, Present, and Future. *Clinical Psychology: Science and Practice*, *10*(2), 144–156.

Kabat-Zinn, J., Massion, A. O., Kristeller, J., Peterson, L. G., Fletcher, K. E., Pbert, L., . . . Santorelli, S. F. (1992). Effectiveness of a meditation-based stress reduction program in the treatment of anxiety disorders. *American Journal of Psychiatry*, *149*(7), 936–943.

Krishnamurti, J. (1999). *The light in oneself: True meditation*. Boston, MA: Shambhala.

Lazar, S. W., Bush, G., Gollub, R. L., Fricchione, G. L., Khalsa, G., & Benson, H. (2000). Functional brain mapping of the relaxation response and meditation. *Neuroreport*, *11*(7), 1581–1585.

Lazar, S. W., Kerr, C. E., Wasserman, R. H., Gray, J. R., Greve, D. N., Treadway, M. T., . . . Fischl, B. (2005). Meditation experience is associated with increased cortical thickness. *Neuroreport*, *16*(17), 1893–1897.

Lebron, K., Milad, M. R., & Quirk, G. J. (2004). Delayed recall of fear extinction in rats with lesions of ventral medial prefrontal cortex. *Learning and Memory*, *11*(5), 544–548. doi:11/5/544 [pii] 10.1101/lm.78604

LeDoux, J. E. (2000). Emotion circuits in the brain. *Annual Review of Neuroscience*, *23*, 155–84. doi:10.1146/annurev.neuro.23.1.155

Likhtik, E., Popa, D., Apergis-Schoute, J., Fidacaro, G. A., & Pare, D. (2008). Amygdala intercalated neurons are required for expression of fear extinction. *Nature*, *454*(7204), 642–645. doi:nature07167 [pii] 10.1038/nature07167

Lou, H. C., Kjaer, T. W., Friberg, L., Wildschiodtz, G., Holm, S., & Nowak, M. (1999). A 15O-H2O PET study of meditation and the resting state of normal consciousness. *Human Brain Mapping*, *7*(2), 98–105.

Lovibond, P. F., Mitchell, C. J., Minard, E., Brady, A., & Menzies, R. G. (2009). Safety behaviours preserve threat beliefs: Protection from extinction of human fear conditioning by an avoidance response. *Behaviour Research and Therapy*, *47*(8), 716–720. doi:S0005-7967(09)00120-X [pii] 10.1016/j.brat.2009.04.013

Luders, E., Toga, A. W., Lepore, N., & Gaser, C. (2009). The underlying anatomical correlates of long-term meditation: Larger hippocampal and frontal volumes of gray matter. *NeuroImage*, *45*(3), 672–678. doi:10.1016/j.neuroimage.2008.12.061

Lutz, A., Slagter, H. A., Dunne, J. D., & Davidson, R. J. (2008). Attention regulation and monitoring in meditation. *Trends in Cognitive Sciences*, *12*(4), 163–169. doi:S1364-6613(08)00052-1 [pii] 10.1016/j.tics.2008.01.005

Maharshi, R. (1959). *The collected works of Ramana Maharshi*. New York, NY: Weiser.

Milad, M R, Orr, S. P., Lasko, N. B., Chang, Y., Rauch, S. L., & Pitman, R. K. (2008). Presence and acquired origin of reduced recall for fear extinction in PTSD: Results of a twin study. *Journal of Psychiatric Research*, *42*(7), 515–520. doi:S0022-3956(08)00026-5 [pii] 10.1016/j.jpsychires.2008.01.017

Milad, M. R., Pitman, R. K., Ellis, C. B., Gold, A. L., Shin, L. M., Lasko, N. B., . . . Rauch, S. L. (2009). Neurobiological basis of failure to recall extinction memory in posttraumatic stress disorder. *Biological Psychiatry*, *66*(12), 1075–1082. doi:S0006-3223(09)00896-8 [pii] 10.1016/j.biopsych.2009.06.026

Milad, M. R., Quinn, B. T., Pitman, R. K., Orr, S. P., Fischl, B., & Rauch, S. L. (2005). Thickness of ventromedial prefrontal cortex in humans is correlated with extinction memory. *Proceedings of the National Academy of Sciences USA*, *102*(30), 10706–10711. doi:0502441102 [pii] 10.1073/pnas.0502441102

Milad, M. R., & Quirk, G. J. (2012). Fear extinction as a model for translational neuroscience: Ten years of progress. *Annual Review of Psychology*, *63*, 129–151. doi:10.1146/annurev.psych.121208.131631

Milad, M. R, & Rauch, S. L. (2012). Obsessive-compulsive disorder: Beyond segregated cortico-striatal pathways. *Trends in Cognitive Sciences*, *16*(1), 43–51. doi:10.1016/j.tics.2011.11.003

Milad, M. R., Rauch, S. L., Pitman, R. K., & Quirk, G. J. (2006). Fear extinction in rats: Implications for human brain imaging and anxiety disorders. *Biological Psychology*, *73*(1), 61–71. doi:S0301-0511(06)00026-3 [pii] 10.1016/j.biopsycho.2006.01.008

Milad, M. R., Wright, C. I., Orr, S. P., Pitman, R. K., Quirk, G. J., & Rauch, S. L. (2007). Recall of fear extinction in humans activates the ventromedial prefrontal cortex and hippocampus in concert. *Biological Psychiatry*, *62*(5), 446–454. doi:S0006-3223(06)01298-4 [pii] 10.1016/j.biopsych.2006.10.011

Monfils, M. H., Cowansage, K. K., Klann, E., & LeDoux, J. E. (2009). Extinction-reconsolidation boundaries: Key to persistent attenuation of fear memories. *Science*, *324*(5929), 951–955. doi:1167975 [pii] 10.1126/science.1167975

Myers, K. M., & Davis, M. (2007). Mechanisms of fear extinction. *Molecular Psychiatry*, *12*(2), 120–50. doi:10.1038/sj.mp.4001939

Nader, K., & Einarsson, E. O. (2010). Memory reconsolidation: An update. *Annals of the New York Academy of Sciences*, *1191*, 27–41. doi:NYAS5443 [pii] 10.1111/j.1749-6632.2010.05443.x

Newberg, A., Alavi, A., Baime, M., Pourdehnad, M., Santanna, J., & d'Aquili, E. (2001). The measurement of regional cerebral blood flow during the complex cognitive task of meditation: A preliminary SPECT study. *Psychiatry Research*, *106*(2), 113–122. doi:S0925492701000749 [pii]

Olendzki, A. (2010). *Unlimiting mind: The radically experiential psychology of Buddhism*. Somerville, MA: Wisdom.

Ortner, C. N. M., Kilner, S. J., & Zelazo, P. D. (2007). Mindfulness meditation and reduced emotional interference on a cognitive task. *Motivation and Emotion*, *31*(4), 271–283. doi:10.1007/s11031-007-9076-7

Öst, L. G. (1997). Rapid treatment of specific phobias. In G. C. L. Davey (Ed.), *Phobias: A handbook of theory, research, and treatment* (p. 451). Chichester, UK: Wiley.

Pagnoni, G., & Cekic, M. (2007). Age effects on gray matter volume and attentional performance in Zen meditation. *Neurobiology of Aging*, *28*(10), 1623–1627. doi:10.1016/j.neurobiolaging.2007.06.008

Pare, D., Quirk, G. J., & Ledoux, J. E. (2004). New vistas on amygdala networks in conditioned fear. *Journal of Neurophysiol*, *92*(1), 1–9. doi:10.1152/jn.00153.2004 92/1/1 [pii]

Phelps, E. A., & LeDoux, J. E. (2005). Contributions of the amygdala to emotion processing: From animal models to human behavior. *Neuron*, *48*(2), 175–187. doi:S0896-6273(05)00823-8 [pii] 10.1016/j.neuron.2005.09.025

Price, J. L. (2005). Free will versus survival: Brain systems that underlie intrinsic constraints on behavior. *Journal of Comparative Neurology*, *493*(1), 132–139. doi:10.1002/cne.20750

Quirk, G. J. (2002). Memory for extinction of conditioned fear is long-lasting and persists following spontaneous recovery. *Learning and Memory*, *9*(6), 402–407. doi:10.1101/lm.49602

Quirk, G. J., Russo, G. K., Barron, J. L., & Lebron, K. (2000). The role of ventromedial prefrontal cortex in the recovery of extinguished fear. *Journal of Neuroscience*, *20*(16), 6225–6231. doi:20/16/6225 [pii]

Rauch, S. L., Shin, L. M., & Phelps, E. A. (2006). Neurocircuitry models of posttraumatic stress disorder and extinction: human neuroimaging research—past, present, and future. *Biological Psychiatry*, *60*(4), 376–382. doi:S0006-3223(06)00796-7 [pii] 10.1016/j.biopsych.2006.06.004

Rescorla, R. A. (2001). Retraining of extinguished Pavlovian stimuli. *Journal of Experimental Psychology: Animal Behavior Process*, *27*(2), 115–124.

Roemer, L., Orsillo, S. M., & Salters-Pedneault, K. (2008). Efficacy of an acceptance-based behavior therapy for generalized anxiety disorder: Evaluation in a randomized controlled trial. *Journal of Consulting and Clinical Psychology*, *76*(6), 1083–1089. doi:2008-16943-009 [pii] 10.1037/a0012720

Rossato, J. I., Bevilaqua, L. R., Izquierdo, I., Medina, J. H., & Cammarota, M. (2010). Retrieval induces reconsolidation of fear extinction memory. *Proceedings of the National Academy of Sciences USA*. doi:1016254107 [pii] 10.1073/pnas.1016254107

Santorelli, S. (2000). *Heal thy self: Lessons on mindfulness in medicine*. New York, NY: Three Rivers Press.

Satipatthana Sutta: Frames of reference. (2008). (T. Bhikku, Trans.). *Access to Insight*. Retrieved November 2015, from http://www.accesstoinsight.org/tipitaka/mn/mn.010.than.html

Schiller, D., Monfils, M. H., Raio, C. M., Johnson, D. C., Ledoux, J. E., & Phelps, E. A. (2010). Preventing the return of fear in humans using reconsolidation update mechanisms. *Nature*, *463*(7277), 49–53. doi:nature08637 [pii] 10.1038/nature08637

Shapiro, S. L., Carlson, L. E., Astin, J. A., & Freedman, B. (2006). Mechanisms of mindfulness. *Journal of Clinical Psychology*, *62*(3), 373–386. doi:10.1002/jclp.20237

Slagter, H. A., Lutz, A., Greischar, L. L., Francis, A. D., Nieuwenhuis, S., Davis, J. M., & Davidson, R. J. (2007). Mental training affects distribution of limited brain resources. *PLoS Biology*, *5*(6), e138. doi:10.1371/journal.pbio.0050138

Tapper, K., Shaw, C., Ilsley, J., Hill, A. J., Bond, F. W., & Moore, L. (2009). Exploratory randomised controlled trial of a mindfulness-based weight loss intervention for women. *Appetite*, *52*(2), 396–404. doi:S0195-6663(08)00618-1 [pii] 10.1016/j.appet.2008.11.012

Teasdale, J. D., Segal, Z. V, Williams, J. M., Ridgeway, V. A., Soulsby, J. M., & Lau, M. A. (2000). Prevention of relapse/recurrence in major depression by mindfulness-based cognitive therapy. *Journal of Consulting and Clinical Psychology, 68*(4), 615–623.

Thera, N. (1962). *The heart of Buddhist meditation.* London, UK: Rider and Company.

Wells, A., Clark, D. M., Salkovskis, P., Ludgate, J., Hackmann, A., & Gelder, M. (1995). Social phobia—The role of in-situation safety behaviors in maintaining anxiety and negative beliefs. *Behavior Therapy, 26*(1), 153–161.

Wolpe, J. (1958). *Psychotherapy by reciprocal inhibition.* Stanford, CA: Stanford University Press.

Zeidan, F., Johnson, S. K., Gordon, N. S., & Goolkasian, P. (2010). Effects of brief and sham mindfulness meditation on mood and cardiovascular variables. *Journal of Alternative and Complementary Medicine, 16*(8), 867–873. doi:10.1089/acm.2009.0321

12

The Role of Brain Connectivity in Musical Experience

PSYCHE LOUI ■

Human beings of all ages and all cultures have been creating, enjoying, and celebrating music for centuries, yet how the experiences of music are instantiated in the human brain is only beginning to be understood. To gain a full understanding of the neuroscience of positive experiences, one of the goals of positive neuroscience must entail examining how the brain subserves music appreciation. The central thesis of this chapter is that structural and functional networks in the human brain enable musical behaviors that are exceptional, resourceful, and rewarding. Here I will describe studies that characterize how the human brain implements varieties of human perceptual, cognitive, and emotional abilities that surround musically relevant behaviors. Two parallel lines of these studies investigate special populations—people with absolute pitch and synesthesia—that possess exceptional abilities in perceptual categorization and association, respectively. Another line of studies examines how the general population can learn the structure that underlies musical systems from mere exposure, and identifies neural substrates of this learning process. A third line of studies tackles neural structures that give rise to uniquely personal, intense emotional responses to music. Finally, I propose a view that music furthers our understanding of the fundamental organizational structure of the brain as an interlocking set of networked highways, and I close with speculations on what the present studies could mean for positive neuroscience and to psychology and neuroscience more generally.

ABSOLUTE PITCH—A CASE OF HYPERCONNECTIVITY

Absolute pitch (AP) is the enhanced ability to categorize musical pitches without a reference. The ability can be tested with a pitch categorization task, easily done on a piano or with computerized testing (we have implemented one such test at musicianbrain.com/aptest). In a typical trial of such a pitch categorization test, a tone is played and the subject's task is to identify the pitch class of the tone (A, B-flat, B, C, etc.). While the vast majority of the population—non-AP possessors—perform almost at chance, AP possessors are robustly able to label pitches above chance. AP is thought to be rare, ranging from 0.01% to 1% of the population (Ward, 1999), but it is relatively common among several special populations. Among the "best" Western classical composers as identified by *The New York Times* (Tommasini, 2011), more than half are AP possessors as identified by historical evidence. This high occurrence of AP among great composers has led some to suggest that AP may be a sign of genius, musical creativity, and/or exceptional ability in the musical domain (Levitin & Rogers, 2005; Ward, 1999). Despite this association with exceptional ability, however, AP is also linked to neurodevelopmental disorders. High-functioning individuals with autism perform above controls in pitch discrimination and categorization (Bonnel et al., 2003), and musicians with AP are more likely to possess autism traits than musicians without AP (Dohn, Garza-Villarreal, Heaton, & Vuust, 2012). Furthermore, individuals with Williams syndrome, a neurogenetic disorder resulting in developmental delay coupled with strong language and social skills, out-perform controls in pitch categorization tasks despite impaired general cognitive ability, suggesting that the development of AP within its critical period may be extended in children with neurogenetic disorders such as Williams syndrome (Lenhoff, Perales, & Hickok, 2001). In addition to associations with a neurogenetic disorder, evidence for genetic contributions to AP include familial aggregation of AP ability even after controlling for musical training (Baharloo, Service, Risch, Gitschier, & Freimer, 2000). People of East Asian descent are much more likely to have AP (Gregersen, Kowalsky, Kohn, & Marvin, 1999), and more recently a genome-wide linkage study has identified several loci of genetic linkage to AP, including chromosomes 8q24.21, 7q22.3, 8q21.11, and 9p21.3 (Theusch, Basu, & Gitschier, 2009).

There is also abundant evidence for developmental contributions to AP. People who speak tone languages, as well as people with early musical training, are more likely to have AP (Deutsch, Dooley, Henthorn, & Head, 2009). Furthermore, the type of musical training influences the accuracy of AP: People who train in high-pitched instruments, such as the violin, are more likely to have AP in high registers; people who train in low-pitched instruments, such as the cello, are more likely to have AP in low registers; and pianists are more likely to have AP for white keys than black keys on the piano (Miyazaki, 1989). Due to its interactions with genetic and environmental contributions, AP has been described as a new model for investigating the effects of genes and development on neural and cognitive function (Zatorre, 2003).

These genetic and developmental behavioral differences suggest that AP possessors may have structural differences in the brain even in utero, as well as functional differences that may either (a) emerge as a consequence of these structural differences or (b) develop as a compensatory mechanism or strategy around the structural differences. Using diffusion tensor imaging, a magnetic resonance imaging (MRI) technique that allows visualization and quantification of major white matter connections in the brain, we found larger white matter volumes of structural connectivity in a segment of the arcuate fasciculus—specifically the segment connecting the superior and middle temporal gyri—in AP subjects relative to well-matched controls (Loui, Li, Hohmann, & Schlaug, 2011a). Left-hemisphere connectivity was especially robustly enhanced in the AP subjects, with the volume of identified tracts being significantly and positively correlated with behavioral accuracy in pitch categorization tasks (Loui et al., 2011a).

In addition to structural differences in the AP brain, differences in brain function at rest and during the processing of musical sounds may provide further insight into the neural mechanisms of exceptional perceptual categorization. To investigate the functional underpinnings of enhanced perceptual categorization abilities, we conducted a functional MRI (fMRI) study using the sparse temporal sampling design (Hall et al., 1999) in 15 AP possessors and 15 controls matched for age, sex, ethnicity, linguistic background, and age of onset and number of years of musical training.[1] Subjects listened to short musical segments and rated the levels of emotional arousal in music, compared to a rest condition. fMRI during emotional judgments of musical stimuli showed higher activations in multiple regions in the AP group. Increased activity was observed in the left superior temporal gyrus and left postcentral gyrus, regions involved in auditory and somatosensory processing, respectively. Additionally, increased activity was observed in bilateral hippocampus, amygdala, and substantia nigra/ventral tegmental area in the AP group, regions important in emotion and reward processing. These distributed increases in auditory, sensory integration, and emotion and reward processing regions may suggest intrinsic enhancements in the functional brain network of the AP group.

What do we mean by intrinsic enhancements of a functional brain network? To motivate ideas on brain networks, consider the social networks that are familiar to human society. You might have friends from elementary school, friends from high school, friends from college, and friends from graduate school. Occasionally a friend from graduate school might also know your friend from high school, in a situation many refer to as "small-world" phenomenon (Watts & Strogatz, 1998). The ways in which we describe the small-world network of our social circles can also be applied to descriptions of the human brain (Reijneveld, Ponten, Berendse, & Stam, 2007; Sporns, Tononi, & Kötter, 2005).

The newly emerging field of connection science has produced tools for describing network properties of the human brain using graph theory and small-world networks (e.g., Rubinov & Sporns, 2010), tools that can describe network properties of the human brain as a network with nodes of brain regions (or groups of functionally defined brain regions) and edges of connections that represent significant structural or functional connections between the nodes. When applied to fMRI data, such a network analysis entails obtaining time-series data from each region in the brain (as defined, in this case, using an anatomical atlas; Tzourio-Mazoyer et al., 2002), and then performing correlations between every pair of these time-series to obtain a pairwise connection matrix to describe the connection properties of each brain region. This pairwise connection matrix can yield statistics to describe the whole brain network—the sum total of all nodes and edges in the brain. These network properties include degree (number of significant connections in the network), strengths (of significant connections), clustering (proportion of nodes connected to each node that are also connected to each other), global and local efficiency (how efficiently information exchange happens in all or part of the network—related to clustering and inversely related to the path length between two nodes; Latora & Marchiori, 2001). Applying graph theory to fMRI data in AP subjects and controls, we saw that the AP group showed increased network connectivity, especially in the left superior temporal gyrus (Figure 12.1). Specifically, fMRI data from the AP group showed increased degrees and increased clustering throughout the brain, with effects centering around the left superior temporal gyrus. These differences in network degree and clustering remained the same even when the analysis was repeated only in the silent rest condition data, suggesting that network differences in AP brain were intrinsic, rather than tied to the task of music listening per se (Loui, Zamm, & Schlaug, 2012b). The intrinsic differences of network connectivity in the AP brain may explain the phenomenon of AP possessors hearing pitch categories even in nonmusical situations, such as environmental sounds (some AP possessors report, for example, hearing that the washing machine is a G-sharp, or that the wind is an F).

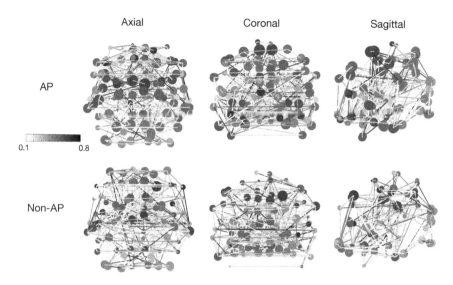

Figure 12.1 Small-world network of absolute pitch (AP) and non-AP functional magnetic resonance imaging data: Each node (circle) denotes one brain region (as defined by an atlas), and each edge (line) represents a connection, defined as a significant correlation at the $r > .5$ threshold. The size of each node denotes the degree (number of connections), whereas the shading of each node denotes the clustering coefficient (proportion of a node's connected nodes that are also connected with each other). Shading of the edges corresponds to strength of connections, with black lines denoting highest correlations. The larger nodes and darker hubs in the AP group from these visualizations show that the AP brain is an enhanced network; that is, it has more degrees and higher clustering.

SYNESTHESIA—ANOTHER CASE OF ENHANCED CONNECTIVITY

Having seen that AP is characterized by heightened structural and functional connectivity, especially in regions of the brain that subserve auditory perception, a possible follow-up question concerns which other groups or special populations might also possess similar modes of enhanced connectivity. One candidate population of increased connectivity is people with synesthesia. While AP is a neurological phenomenon where sound stimuli are perceived as belonging to categories of pitch classes, synesthesia is another neurological phenomenon where perceptual stimuli trigger concurrent perceptual sensations in other modalities. In grapheme-color synesthesia, letters and numbers trigger percepts of color, whereas in colored-music synesthesia, musical sounds (pitches, chords, timbres) trigger percepts of color. Like AP, the possession of synesthesia is sensitive to both genetic and environmental contributions: It runs in the family and is eight times more common in people in the creative industries, such as artists, composers, and poets (Ramachandran & Hubbard, 2001). Existing models posit two classes of neural mechanisms that may give rise to synesthesia: hyperconnectivity and disinhibition. Models of hyperconnectivity describe increased connectivity (both structural and functional), increased binding, or cross-wiring/cross-activation between regions involved in processing the relevant trigger and concurrent sensations (Ramachandran & Hubbard, 2001). In contrast, models pertaining to disinhibition posit that regions that normally inhibit the cross-wiring or cross-activation between trigger and concurrent processing are not in place among synesthetes (Grossenbacher & Lovelace, 2001). While most of the cognitive neuroscience literature on synesthesia has focused on grapheme-color synesthesia, studying colored-music synesthesia may be an optimal model to disentangle these competing hypotheses. This is because the regions mainly involved in color processing (visual association cortices in the occipital lobe) and in musical sound processing (auditory association cortices in the temporal lobe) are relatively distal in the brain; thus, any enhanced connections between these processing regions would be expected to bridge the clearly definable processing regions in the auditory and visual systems.

To identify potential differences in patterns of structural connectivity between synesthetes and controls, we compared diffusion tensor images of 10 colored-music synesthetes and 10 controls who were matched for age, sex, ethnicity, IQ (as determined by Shipley scores), and number of years and age of onset of musical training. We found that people with colored-music synesthesia have different hemispheric asymmetry and increased structural connectivity in the white matter tracts connecting visual and auditory association areas to the frontal lobe (Zamm, Schlaug, Eagleman, & Loui, 2013). Results are driven by enhanced white matter connectivity among synesthetes in the right hemisphere inferior frontal occipital fasciculus (IFOF—shown in three views in Figure 12.2), a white matter pathway that connects visual association regions in the occipital lobe, through auditory association regions in the temporal lobe, to attention binding or top-down modulation regions in the frontal lobe. Furthermore, fractional anisotropy (a measure of white matter integrity) of the right IFOF of the synesthete group correlated with the consistency of audiovisual synesthetic associations as defined by the Synesthesia Battery (Eagleman, Kagan, Nelson, Sagaram, & Sarma, 2007). A search within the IFOF for most significant brain–behavior correlations revealed that white matter underlying the right fusiform gyrus correlated most strongly with behavioral performance on the Synesthesia Battery, further pinpointing the role of IFOF in audiovisual associations toward white matter within the right fusiform gyrus (shown by the arrow in Figure 12.2).

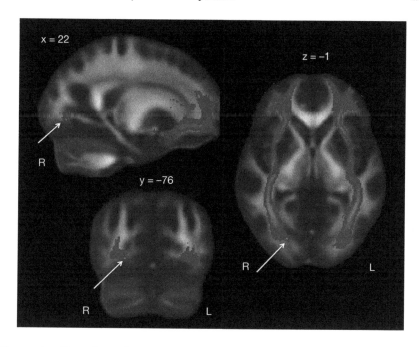

Figure 12.2 The inferior-frontal occipital fasciculus (IFOF): A pathway connecting occipital lobe to frontal lobe through the temporal lobe is shown as activated cluster. We found that colored-music synesthetes have higher white matter integrity in this pathway in the right hemisphere, with the association between white matter integrity and synesthetic behavior being highest in the fusiform gyrus, identified by the arrow.

The finding of increased IFOF connectivity in colored-music synesthetes required manual selection of regions of interest (ROIs), by coders blinded to the group assignment of each subject, that were the neuroanatomical landmarks or endpoints of the IFOF. This manual selection process, although time consuming, ensured the highest reliability in adhering to individual differences in sulcal and gyral anatomy of each individual brain, while eschewing bias by ensuring similar sizes and locations of ROIs between the synesthete and control groups. However, scaling up the manual selection of ROIs to more regions in the brain can be costly. Thus, in a follow-up diffusion tensor imaging study, we explored the use of pairwise probabilistic tractography applied on ROIs that were defined by applying the Harvard-Oxford atlas across each brain and constraining the resultant ROIs to voxels within white matter. Pairwise tractography across all 111 seed regions, as defined by the Harvard-Oxford atlas, resulted in a 111 x 111 matrix expressing the strength of all connections between any pair of regions in the brain. This bottom-up pairwise tractography result enables another application of the small-world network analysis pipeline toward structural connectivity data, as opposed to functional connectivity data, as discussed earlier in this chapter. A whole-brain comparison between synesthetes' and control subjects' structural brain networks revealed that the synesthetes' brain network had more degrees and higher strengths of connections relative to controls. Region-specific comparisons between the connectivity values from each ROI showed significantly more connections (Bonferroni-corrected for 111 ROIs) in the synesthetes' brain network in the bilateral superior and middle temporal gyri, inferior lateral occipital cortex, supracalcarine cortex, and frontal medial cortex—regions involved in auditory association, visual association, and top-down modulation that are also traversed by the IFOF (Loui, Zamm, & Schlaug, 2013).

To investigate functional differences in synesthetes hand in hand with the structural differences, we applied the previously discussed sparse-temporal sampling fMRI paradigm of emotional judgment of musical stimuli to colored-music synesthetes. Preliminary fMRI results showed shared enhancements between AP and synesthetes relative to controls, in auditory processing regions in the superior temporal lobe as well as regions responsible for top-down control in the frontal lobe. In addition, synesthetes showed higher activations in the right superior temporal gyrus, a way station of auditory perception, coupled with increased activations in bilateral color-sensitive visual association regions in the lingual gyrus of the occipital lobe, during the perception of musical stimuli that were rated by the synesthetes as highly arousing (Loui, Zamm, & Schlaug, 2012a). These functional results converge with structural differences observed in the synesthete brain in showing domain-specific enhancements in auditory and visual association, coupled with a general network of auditory and cognitive processing during music perception that is shared with the nonsynesthete control population.

In sum, exceptional audiovisual associations may be subserved by the integrity of white matter that connects visual and auditory association regions to top-down modulatory regions in the frontal lobe. The synesthete's enhanced perceptual experience of seeing colors when hearing sounds may involve both domain-general (top-down) and domain-specific (bottom-up) enhancements in structural connectivity in white matter, as well as functional connectivity in gray matter. These results offer a link between synesthesia and other populations characterized by enhanced local white matter connectivity, such as AP possessors (Loui et al., 2011a) and individuals with high cognitive intelligence, high emotional intelligence, and exceptional creativity (Chiang et al., 2009; Jung et al., 2010; Takeuchi et al., 2011), as well as in patients with auditory verbal hallucinations and autistic spectrum disorders (Fletcher et al., 2010; Hoffman & Hampson, 2011).

Results presented so far suggest that AP and synesthesia are plausible models of exceptional behavior that lie on the high end of a spectrum of individual differences in connectivity. It remains to be seen what other types of exceptional behavior fall under this category of hyperconnectivity syndromes. Mottron et al. (2013) describe savant syndrome, hyperlexia, and hypergraphia as more examples of enhanced perceptual functioning in addition to AP and synesthesia. While these special populations may possess heightened connectivity in brain structure and function, what remains to be seen is the degree to which any enhanced connectivity patterns in these special populations, if observed, may be shared with or distinct from each other.

THE HUMAN BRAIN IS RESOURCEFUL—STATISTICAL LEARNING OF MUSICAL STRUCTURE

Results presented thus far have pertained to rare populations of humans who have unusual giftedness or impairments in musical functions. What about the rest of us? What are the bases of brain connectivity that enable the learning and liking of music within our society? Here we describe the use of a novel musical system to investigate the brain connectivity substrates for learning new music in humans.

The new musical system is a finite state grammar based on the Bohlen-Pierce scale, an artificial musical scale that uses a 3:1 frequency ratio instead of the 2:1 ratio (octave) found around the world. Detailed descriptions of this new musical system exist elsewhere (Loui, 2012a, 2012b; Loui, Wessel, & Hudson Kam, 2010) and therefore will not be repeated here, but important for present purposes we note that using an artificial musical system, we can generate thousands of new melodies that can be presented to subjects, giving us high precision and experimental control in the investigation of how learning occurs in humans. After hearing a large set of (400) melodies in one of two possible artificial finite-state grammar systems only once each, participants could not only recognize the melodies they had heard but also could generalize their knowledge of the underlying grammar toward new melodies that had not been heard before, suggesting that humans exploit the statistical properties of their sound environment to acquire sensitivity toward grammatical structure when confronted with a new musical system (Loui, 2012a, 2012b; Loui et al., 2010). Event-related potential data showed two negative waveforms, the first reflecting sensory processing in the superior temporal lobe and the second reflecting further cognitive analysis in the frontal lobe, that increased after learning to differentiate statistically frequent instances of the new musical system, suggesting that the human brain rapidly and flexibly acquires musical structure by capitalizing on frequency and probability of sound events—statistical resources that are available within the auditory environment (Loui, Wu, Wessel, & Knight, 2009).

In further studies we asked which anatomical connections in the brain might be allowing this rapid statistical learning system. As the arcuate fasciculus is a major white matter pathway that connects the temporal lobe and frontal lobe structures and is diminished in people who lack musical ability (Loui, Alsop, & Schlaug, 2009), it was a prime candidate for a neuroanatomical correlate of individual differences in new music learning. We tested the possibility that the structure and morphology of the arcuate fasciculus might reflect individual differences in learning the Bohlen-Pierce scale: We correlated the volume of the arcuate fasciculus, as defined by probabilistic tractography from diffusion tensor imaging data, with individual scores in the generalization test for learning the Bohlen-Pierce scale. Results showed that the ventral branch of the right arcuate fasciculus, connecting the right middle temporal gyrus (MTG—the ventral portion of Wernicke's area) with the right inferior frontal gyrus (IFG—the Broca's area), was significantly correlated with generalization scores (Loui, Li, & Schlaug, 2011b). Control tasks showed that this correlation was specific to music learning, and not to individual differences in memory or intellectual functioning. Furthermore, white matter integrity in the turning point of the arcuate fasciculus, in white matter underlying the supramarginal gyrus, was most highly correlated with learning accuracy. This suggests that individual differences in arcuate fasciculus morphology, specifically the extent to which the arcuate fasciculus descends into the temporal lobe, may be predictive of individual differences in learning ability. This is consistent with work by Flöel and colleagues (Flöel, de Vries, Scholz, Breitenstein, & Johansen-Berg, 2009), which showed an association between white matter integrity in tracts from the Broca's area and success in learning an artificial grammar. Taken together, by combining a new learning paradigm with neuroimaging techniques that enable the visualization and comparison of individual differences in white matter pathways, we were able to identify anatomical connections in the brain that may be required for music learning.

EMPATHIZING VIA INTENSELY PLEASURABLE MUSIC—REWARDS OF THE MUSICAL EXPERIENCE

While statistical learning mechanisms in the brain are crucial for the learning of musical structures, most people do not report music learning as a primary reason for their avid consumption—even to the point of addiction—of music in their culture. Music is a multi-billion-dollar industry: People who have no formal musical training regularly enjoy intense emotional experiences at concerts where the music that is played often has only minimal structural complexity. Yet the emotional rewards of music are intensely personal and profound. What causes strong emotional responses to music?

In a recent study (Sachs, Ellis, Schlaug, & Loui, 2016), we asked if there were any structural connectivity characteristics in people who consistently experience strong emotional responses to music, compared to people who rarely experience such emotions to music. In a large sample (N – 237) of adult college-aged subjects, we administered the Aesthetic Responses to Music Questionnaire, which asked for subjects' personalities (using the Ten-Item Personality Inventory), history of music training, and demographic information, as well as their preferences for various genres of music, the frequency with which music gave them various strong emotional experiences such as chills, goosebumps, feelings of awe, tears, feelings in the pit of the stomach, and heart palpitations. Subjects also listed their favorite pieces of music and the ones that elicited these strong sensations. From these survey data we identified the 10 most emotional responders—those who consistently and reliably experienced chills and other strong emotional sensations according to their self-report—and the 10 least emotional responders—those who reportedly never experienced chills or any other strong emotional experience, despite similar age, sex, intellectual functioning, and amount and intensity of musical training (Sachs et al., 2016). These 20 individuals were brought into the lab for behavioral ratings of emotional arousal and psychophysical recordings of heart rate and skin conductance to confirm subjective reports of arousal, as well as structural neuroimaging to identify possible differences in the brain that are associated with strong emotional responses to music. We compared people who get chills from music and people who do not get chills, controlling for differences in personality, musical training, and musical exposure. Results showed greater volume of white matter connectivity between auditory regions in the superior temporal gyrus and emotion-processing regions in the insula and medial prefrontal cortex (MPFC). This three-node network of superior temporal gyrus, insula, and MPFC traverses white matter fasciculi that include the aforementioned arcuate fasciculus, which connects the superior temporal lobe to the lateral prefrontal cortex, and the uncinate fasciculus, which connects the anterior temporal lobe to the MPFC. The effects of increased white matter volume in the chill perceivers were bilateral, but stronger in the right hemisphere, consistent with existing literature showing bilateral but rightward-leaning activations during strongly emotional aesthetic responses to music (Salimpoor, Benovoy, Larcher, Dagher, & Zatorre, 2011; Trost, Ethofer, Zentner, & Vuilleumier, 2011).

The MPFC is activated by intensely pleasurable responses (Blood & Zatorre, 2001) and mental imagery of autobiographically relevant music (Janata, 2009; Janata et al., 2002; Kleber, Birbaumer, Veit, Trevorrow, & Lotze, 2007).

It is more generally engaged in emotional processing (Phan, Wager, Taylor, & Liberzon, 2002), specifically activated in self-referential mental activity (Gusnard, Akbudak, Shulman, & Raichle, 2001) and empathic accuracy—the tracking of attributions about other individuals' internal emotional state (Zaki, Weber, Bolger, & Ochsner, 2009). Recent fMRI studies also showed increased MPFC function accompanied by decreased lateral PFC function during creative improvisation, such as jazz improvisation (Limb & Braun, 2008) and freestyle rapping (Liu et al., 2012). The ventral MPFC is impoverished in connectivity among psychopathic criminals (Motzkin, Newman, Kiehl, & Koenigs, 2011). Because the MPFC plays a crucial role in creativity as well as with emotionally empathizing with others, our finding of increased auditory-to-MPFC activity in people who get chills from music may relate creativity in music to empathy, thus informing theories about the evolutionary function of music. Perhaps the reason that humans have evolved to create music is to identify emotionally with each other via an auditory mode of communication.

Debates on the evolutionary function of music have lasted for centuries, and while the current debate surrounds whether music can be an evolutionary adaptation or exaptation (Trainor, 2006), I believe these results from the study on chills can inform this debate by bringing the evolutionary function of music into a social context. If emotional experiences to music involve areas of the brain that are important for empathizing with other people, then perhaps the purpose of music is to arouse emotional responses that resonate with other minds. Music, then, is a social artifact for empathy.

The view of music as a social artifact for empathy is also supported by a recent controlled study in which children who learned to play music together significantly improved in emotional empathy, relative to an untrained control group (Rabinowitch, Cross, & Burnard, 2012). While further studies are needed to test for control interventions, this training study converges with our neuroimaging results in implicating networks of emotional response to music that are shared with social-emotional processing.

CONCLUSION

The studies presented in this chapter touch on the multiple dimensions of musical experience: pitch perception, sound production, sound categorization, audiovisual association, grammar learning, and emotional and aesthetic reception. In each of these dimensions we show that structural and/or functional connectivity plays an important role. One of the conclusions that emerge from these data is that music is a powerful tool for examining myriad brain functions, ranging from primary cortical functions (auditory perception) to the more mystical and elusive subjective experiences (aesthetic response). Music recruits a fronto-temporal network that allows sound perception, production, and categorization. This network engenders musical knowledge, which is acquired via statistical exposure. Aspects of the frontotemporal network are also implicated in creativity and emotional communication.

If studying the brain can inform our understanding of music, one might ask the inverse question: What can music teach us about the organization of the brain? Recently there has been a debate on what, if anything, might be the fundamentally unifying structure of the brain. In 2012, Wedeen et al. published in *Science* findings from diffusion spectral imaging, concluding that the brain is organized in grid-like structures, like a woven fabric or like the streets of Manhattan. This claim was criticized by Catani et al. (2012), who contended that the findings were due to the imaging technique used rather than to the intrinsic structure of the brain per se, and that if anything, the unifying structure of the brain is as a series of small paths that might enlarge due to use and reuse, thus resembling the streets of Victorian London.

How can the findings here contribute to such a debate? Is there anything that music and neuroimaging research is telling us about the unifying structure of the brain that is separate from all the neuroimaging methods we use? My view is that if musical function must rapidly, flexibly, and resourcefully recruit entire continua of mental operations, from the most basic pitch discrimination functions to the most intensely personal subjective experiences such as aesthetics, then perhaps the structure of the brain that enables music is as an interlocking set of networked highways and byways that connect regions that subserve various functions. Certainly the arcuate fasciculus plays a prominent role as a superhighway linking perception and action operations, but the entrances and exits from such a superhighway may interface with other highways such as the inferior frontal occipital fasciculus and the uncinate fasciculus, which correlate with top-down modulation of audiovisual associations and social-emotional processing, respectively. A comprehensive model of musical experience, then, must incorporate most if not all of the principal structures and functions of the human brain. Future work will continue to characterize components of musical experience that may be engendered by networks and clusters within the connectome, defined as a sum total of all connections in the brain. By relating the varieties of exceptional, resourceful, and rewarding human experiences, as instantiated in musical behavior, to systems and networks of the human brain, the neuroscience of music perception and cognition addresses the core goal of positive neuroscience in advancing our understanding of human flourishing.

NOTE

1. Sparse temporal sampling refers to the temporally sparse (e.g., once every 15 seconds, as opposed to once every 2 seconds in a regular design) acquisition of functional magnetic resonance images in an environment where auditory presentations are important to the experiment. Auditory stimuli are presented in silence, and as the brain's hemodynamic response associated with the auditory event is recruited, which typically requires 4 to 8 seconds, the functional magnetic resonance images are acquired, thus allowing the presentation of auditory stimuli in silence.

REFERENCES

Baharloo, S., Service, S. K., Risch, N., Gitschier, J., & Freimer, N. B. (2000). Familial aggregation of absolute pitch. *American Journal of Human Genetics, 67*(3), 755–758.

Blood, A. J., & Zatorre, R. J. (2001). Intensely pleasurable responses to music correlate with activity in brain regions implicated in reward and emotion. *Proceedings National Academy of Sciences USA, 98*(20), 11818–11823.

Bonnel, A., Mottron, L., Peretz, I., Trudel, M., Gallun, E., & Bonnel, A. M. (2003). Enhanced pitch sensitivity in individuals with autism: A signal detection analysis. *Journal of Cognitive Neuroscience, 15*(2), 226–235.

Catani, M., Bodi, I., & Dell'Acqua, F. (2012). Comment on "The geometric structure of the brain fiber pathways." *Science, 337*(6102), 1605; author reply 1605.

Chiang, M-C., Barysheva, M., Shattuck, D. W., Lee, A. D., Madsen, S. K., Avedissian, C., . . . Thompson, P. M. (2009). Genetics of brain fiber architecture and intellectual performance. *Journal of Neuroscience, 29*(7), 2212–2224.

Deutsch, D., Dooley, K., Henthorn, T., & Head, B. (2009). Absolute pitch among students in an American music conservatory: Association with tone language fluency. *Journal of the Acoustical Society of America, 125*(4), 2398–2403.

Dohn, A., Garza-Villarreal, E. A., Heaton, P., & Vuust, P. (2012). Do musicians with perfect pitch have more autism traits than musicians without perfect pitch? An empirical study. *PLoS One, 7*(5), e37961.

Eagleman, D. M., Kagan, A. D., Nelson, S. S., Sagaram, D., & Sarma, A. K. (2007). A standardized test battery for the study of synesthesia. *Journal of Neuroscience Methods, 159*(1), 139–145.

Fletcher, P. T., Whitaker, R. T., Tao, R., DuBray, M. B., Froehlich, A., Ravichandran, C., . . . Lainhart, J. E. (2010). Microstructural connectivity of the arcuate fasciculus in adolescents with high-functioning autism. *Neuroimage, 51*(3), 1117–1125.

Flöel, A., de Vries, M. H., Scholz, J., Breitenstein, C., & Johansen-Berg, H. (2009). White matter integrity in the vicinity of Broca's area predicts grammar learning success. *Neuroimage, 47*(4), 1974–1981.

Gregersen, P. K., Kowalsky, E., Kohn, N., & Marvin, E. W. (1999). Absolute pitch: Prevalence, ethnic variation, and estimation of the genetic component. *American Journal of Human Genetics, 65*(3), 911–913.

Grossenbacher, P. G., & Lovelace, C. T. (2001). Mechanisms of synesthesia: cognitive and physiological constraints. *Trends in Cognitive Science*, 5(1), 36–41.

Gusnard, D. A., Akbudak, E., Shulman, G. L., & Raichle, M. E. (2001). Medial prefrontal cortex and self-referential mental activity: Relation to a default mode of brain function. *Proceedings of the National Academy of Sciences USA*, 98(7), 4259–4264.

Hall, D. A., Haggard, M. P., Akeroyd, M. A., Palmer, A. R., Summerfield, A. Q., Elliott, M R , Bowtell, R. W. (1999). "Sparse" temporal sampling in auditory fMRI. *Human Brain Mapping*, 7(3), 213–223.

Hoffman, R. E., & Hampson, M. (2011). Functional connectivity studies of patients with auditory verbal hallucinations. *Frontiers in Human Neuroscience*, 6, 6.

Janata, P. (2009). The neural architecture of music-evoked autobiographical memories. *Cerebral Cortex*, bhp008.

Janata, P., Birk, J. L., Van Horn, J. D., Leman, M., Tillmann, B., & Bharucha, J. J. (2002). The cortical topography of tonal structures underlying Western music. *Science*, 298(5601), 2167–2170.

Jung, R. E., Segall, J. M., Bockholt, H. J., Flores, R. A., Smith, S. M., Chavez, R. S., & Haier, R. J. (2010). Neuroanatomy of creativity. *Human Brain Mapping*, 31, 398–409.

Kleber, B., Birbaumer, N., Veit, R., Trevorrow, T., & Lotze, M. (2007). Overt and imagined singing of an Italian aria. *Neuroimage*, 36(3), 889–900.

Latora, V., & Marchiori, M. (2001). Efficient behavior of small-world networks. *Physical Review Letters*, 87(19), 198701.

Lenhoff, H. M., Perales, O., & Hickok, G. (2001). Absolute pitch in Williams syndrome. *Music Perception*, 18(4), 491–503.

Levitin, D. J., & Rogers, S. E. (2005). Absolute pitch: Perception, coding, and controversies. *Trends in Cognitive Science*, 9(1), 26–33.

Limb, C. J., & Braun, A. R. (2008). Neural substrates of spontaneous musical performance: An fMRI study of jazz improvisation. *PLoS One*, 3(2), e1679.

Liu, S., Chow, H. M., Xu, Y., Erkkinen, M. G., Swett, K. E., Eagle, M. W., . . . Braun, A. R. (2012). Neural correlates of lyrical improvisation: An fMRI study of freestyle rap. *Science Reports*, 2, 834.

Loui, P. (2012a). Learning and liking of melody and harmony: Further studies in artificial grammar learning. *Topics in Cognitive Science*, 4, 1–14.

Loui, P. (2012b). Statistical learning—What can music tell us? In P. Rebuschat & J. Williams (Eds.), *Statistical learning and language acquisition* (pp. 433–462). Berlin, Germany: Mouton de Gruyter.

Loui, P., Alsop, D., & Schlaug, G. (2009). Tone deafness: A new disconnection syndrome? *Journal of Neuroscience*, 29(33), 10215–10220.

Loui, P., Li, H. C., Hohmann, A., & Schlaug, G. (2011a). Enhanced connectivity in absolute pitch musicians: A model of hyperconnectivity. *Journal of Cognitive Neuroscience*, 23(4), 1015–1026.

Loui, P., Li, H. C., & Schlaug, G. (2011b). White matter integrity in right hemisphere predicts pitch-related grammar learning. *NeuroImage*, 55(2), 500–507.

Loui, P., Wessel, D. L., & Hudson Kam, C. L. (2010). Humans rapidly learn grammatical structure in a new musical scale. *Music Perception*, 27(5), 377–388.

Loui, P., Wu, E. H., Wessel, D. L., & Knight, R. T. (2009). A generalized mechanism for perception of pitch patterns. *Journal of Neuroscience*, 29(2), 454–459.

Loui, P., Zamm, A., & Schlaug, G. (2012a). Absolute pitch and synesthesia: Two sides of the same coin? Shared and distinct neural substrates of music listening. In *Proceedings of the 12th International Conference for Music Perception and Cognition* (pp. 618–623).

Loui, P., Zamm, A., & Schlaug, G. (2012b). Enhanced functional networks in absolute pitch. *NeuroImage, 63*(2), 632–640.

Loui, P., Zamm, A., & Schlaug, G. (2013). *Oboes are red, violins are blue: Network connectivity of white matter in colored-Music synesthesia.* Paper presented at the Organization for Human Bran Mapping, Seattle, WA.

Miyazaki, K. I. (1989). Absolute pitch identification: Effects of timbre and pitch region. *Music Perception, 7*(1), 1.

Mottron, L., Bouvet, L., Bonnel, A., Samson, F., Burack, J. A., Dawson, M., & Heaton, P. (2013). Veridical mapping in the development of exceptional autistic abilities. *Neuroscience and Biobehavioral Reviews, 37*(2), 209–228.

Motzkin, J. C., Newman, J. P., Kiehl, K. A., & Koenigs, M. (2011). Reduced prefrontal connectivity in psychopathy. *Journal of Neuroscience, 31*(48), 17348–17357.

Phan, K. L., Wager, T., Taylor, S. F., & Liberzon, I. (2002). Functional neuroanatomy of emotion: A meta-analysis of emotion activation studies in PET and fMRI. *Neuroimage, 16*(2), 331–348.

Rabinowitch, T-C., Cross, I., & Burnard, P. (2012). Long-term musical group interaction has a positive influence on empathy in children. *Psychology of Music.* doi:10.1177/0305735612440609.

Ramachandran, V. S., & Hubbard, E. M. (2001). Synaesthesia—A window into perception, thought and language. *Journal of Consciousness Studies, 8*(12), 3–34.

Reijneveld, J. C., Ponten, S. C., Berendse, H. W., & Stam, C. J. (2007). The application of graph theoretical analysis to complex networks in the brain. *Clinical Neurophysiology, 118*(11), 2317–2331.

Rubinov, M., & Sporns, O. (2010). Complex network measures of brain connectivity: Uses and interpretations. *Neuroimage, 52*(3), 1059–1069.

Sachs, M. E., Ellis, R. J., Schlaug, G., & Loui, P. (2016). Brain connectivity reflects human aesthetic responses to music. *Social, Cognitive, and Affective Neuroscience.* In press.

Salimpoor, V. N., Benovoy, M., Larcher, K., Dagher, A., & Zatorre, R. J. (2011). Anatomically distinct dopamine release during anticipation and experience of peak emotion to music. *Nature Neuroscience, 14*(2), 257–262.

Sporns, O., Tononi, G., & Kötter, R. (2005). The human connectome: A structural description of the human brain. *PLoS Computational Biology, 1*(4), e42.

Takeuchi, H., Taki, Y., Sassa, Y., Hashizume, H., Sekiguchi, A., Nagase, T., . . . Kawashima, R. (2011). White matter structures associated with emotional intelligence: Evidence from diffusion tensor imaging. *Human Brain Mapping, 34*(5), 1025–1034.

Theusch, E., Basu, A., & Gitschier, J. (2009). Genome-wide study of families with absolute pitch reveals linkage to 8q24.21 and locus heterogeneity. *American Journal of Human Genetics, 85*(1), 112–119.

Tommasini, A. (2011, January 7). The Greatest. *The New York Times*, Retreved from http://www.nytimes.com.

Trainor, L. J. (2006). Innateness, learning, and the difficulty of determining whether music is an evolutionary adaptation. *Music Perception*, *24*(1), 105–110.

Trost, W., Ethofer, T., Zentner, M., & Vuilleumier, P. (2011). Mapping aesthetic musical emotions in the brain. *Cerebral Cortex*, *22*(12), 2769–2783.

Tzourio-Mazoyer, N., Landeau, B., Papathanassiou, D., Crivello, F., Etard, O., Delcroix, N., . . . Joliot, M. (2002). Automated anatomical labeling of activations in SPM using a macroscopic anatomical parcellation of the MNI MRI single subject brain. *Neuroimage*, *15*(1), 273–289.

Ward, W. D. (1999). Absolute pitch. In D. Deutsch (Ed.), *The psychology of music* (pp. 265–298). New York, NY: Academic Press.

Watts, D. J., & Strogatz, S. H. (1998). Collective dynamics of /'small-world/' networks. *Nature*, *393*(6684), 440–442.

Wedeen, V. J., Rosene, D. L., Wang, R., Dai, G., Mortazavi, F., Hagmann, P., . . . Tseng, W-Y. I. (2012). The geometric structure of the brain fiber pathways. *Science*, *335*(6076), 1628–1634.

Zaki, J., Weber, J., Bolger, N., & Ochsner, K. (2009). The neural bases of empathic accuracy. *Proceedings National Academy of Sciences USA*, *106*(27), 11382–11387.

Zamm, A., Schlaug, G., Eagleman, D. M., & Loui, P. (2013). Pathways to seeing music: Enhanced structural connectivity in colored-music synesthesia. *NeuroImage*, *74*, 359–366.

Zatorre, R. J. (2003). Absolute pitch: A model for understanding the influence of genes and development on neural and cognitive function. *Nature Neuroscience*, *6*(7), 692–695.

13

The Function of Positive
Emotions in Exploration

HANS L. MELO AND ADAM K. ANDERSON ■

A large empirical literature shows that people who are happier achieve better life outcomes, including financial success, supportive relationships, mental health, effective coping, and even physical health and longevity. Unlike negative emotions (e.g., anger, fear), which focus attention, cognition, and physiology toward coping with an immediate threat or problem (Derryberry & Tucker, 1994; Easterbrook, 1959), positive emotions are not critical to one's immediate safety, well-being, or survival but may function to discover and build survival-promoting personal resources. These resources can be *cognitive*, such as the ability to attend mindfully to the present moment; *psychological*, such as the ability to regulate flexibly one's own behavior to fit current circumstances; *social*, such as the ability to give and receive affection and social support; or *physical*, such as the ability to rebound from stress-induced peaks in blood pressure. Having greater resources, in turn, helps people effectively meet life's challenges and take advantage of its opportunities.

At present, it is unknown how the brain represents the capacity for positivity. Prior psychological theories have posited dopaminergic mediation of the cognitive sequelae of positive emotion (Ashby, Isen, & Turken, 1999). However, the dopaminergic system is not monolithic but is composed of multiple pathways (e.g., mesolimbic, mesocortical, nigrostriatal) and numerous receptor types (D1–D5) and their variants that support equally diverse functions (Burgdorf & Panksepp, 2006; Panksepp, 1998). Furthermore, dopamine transmission is not directly related to pleasure or well-being, which have often been confused with approach or appetitive motivation (Berridge & Robinson, 1998). Our thesis is that positivity is associated with activation of dopaminergic "play" systems (Panksepp, 1998) that correspond to flexible exploration (Cohen, McClure, & Yu, 2007; Daw, O'Doherty, Dayan, Seymour, & Dolan, 2006), rather than engaging dopaminergic "seeking" systems that motivate approach toward events predicting reward (Panksepp, 1998). Seeking systems are associated with variations in dopaminergic release, which support exploitation of fixed routines that maximize reward via reinforcement learning substrates (Bilder, Volavka, Lachman, & Grace, 2004). These include reward prediction error in the ventral and dorsal striatum (O'Doherty et al., 2004), value-related activity in the medial orbitofrontal cortices (O'Doherty, Kringelbach, Rolls, Hornak, & Andrews, 2001), and predictions of future rewards in the adjacent medial prefrontal cortex (Gottfried, O'Doherty, & Dolan, 2003).

The capacity for stability and exploitation of learned regularities, versus that for flexibility and exploration of new possibilities, reflects fundamental opposing demands on cognitive control, both of which are essential for successful goal-directed actions. While one must guard goals and actions against distraction, one has to respond flexibly and eventually switch between goals in response to significant changes in the environment (Dreisbach et al., 2005). Whereas exploitation involves relying on strategies that reliably maximize currently available rewards, exploration entails gathering information about alternative courses of action, which may be more risky but potentially more profitable (Cohen, McClure, & Yu, 2007). Results suggest that the frontopolar (BA10) cortices play a key role in exploratory action selection and improvisation (e.g., Daw et al., 2006). We predict that positivity is associated with such frontally mediated exploratory capacities to alter the flexibility and scope of cognition, from focusing on what is to what could be. Thus, with state- and trait-positive emotions, people may become increasingly flexible, discerning, and creative in their approach to present experience, while building their resources for coping with setbacks and obstacles for the future.

COGNITION AND POSITIVE EMOTION

Positive Emotions and Selective Attention

A burgeoning amount of evidence indicates that affective states have a measurable impact on attention, such that diverse affective states are associated with changes in attention that may impact perception and cognition (Rowe, Hirsh, & Anderson, 2006). Attention refers to those cognitive processes that allow an individual to focus selectively on one aspect of the environment while ignoring, or devoting fewer resources to, others. It is therefore thought that this cognitive faculty underpins the control of perception, thought, and behavior, and it is generally acknowledged to depend on inhibitory control, such as suppression of irrelevant information and response inhibition (Hasher, Lustig, & Zacks, 2006; Rowe et al., 2006). For instance, a vastly confirmed finding is the narrowing of attention during negative affective states, sometimes referred to as "weapon focus," where the breadth of attention is constricted to a smaller focal region and thus peripheral details are not encoded (Christianson, 1990; Derryberry, 1988; Easterbrook, 1959). In case of a life-threatening situation, this narrowing of attention may facilitate quick and decisive action trajectories that would improve chances of survival (Fredrickson, 2001). This interaction between negative affect and attention may have important consequences for clinical research where such attentional biases are used to study disorders such as anxiety and depression (Oaksford, Morris, Grainger, & Williams, 1996). By contrast, recent work examining the role of positive affect on attention reveals an opposing effect of negative and positive affect, whereby induction of positive mood is associated with increase in attentional breadth (Rowe et al., 2006). We have identified robust behavioral effects and begun to elucidate the associated neural mechanisms (Schmitz, De Rosa, & Anderson, 2009). In this section we describe some of this work and aim to situate our findings within the greater context of positive psychology and specifically the broaden-and-build theory (Fredrickson, 2001).

From the perspective of information processing, the notion of broadened awareness translates into differential modes of attentional processing critical for controlling thought, behavior, and perception. It follows that if affective states are able to influence attention differentially, then such influence may reflect fundamental changes in the mode of information processing. Thus, altering the capacity for attention (e.g., via mood induction) has broad implications for shaping the contents of awareness, and it influences internal conceptual as well as external perceptual processing. Specifically, this suggests that the increased cognitive flexibility and creative thinking associated with positive mood may reflect a fundamental change in information processing, namely to broaden the scope of selective attention. This is, of course, in direct contrast to the narrowing of attention associated with negative affect (Derryberry, 1998). Indeed, support for this assertion comes from studies examining global versus local cognitive strategies, whereby positive mood is associated with greater global or holistic processing (i.e., seeing the forest before the trees) versus local processing (i.e., the trees before the forest) (Basso, Schefft, Ris, & Dember, 1996; Gasper & Clore, 2002). For example, individuals under positive mood indicate a square made of triangles is more similar to a square than a triangle. However, such affective biases have been interpreted within the affect-as-information framework (Schwarz & Clore, 1983), whereby positive moods increase access to what is in mind during the task at hand, rather than an underlying change in the manner or breadth of how attention may be allocated (Rowe et al., 2006).

More recently, however, work in our lab has examined the impact of affective states on attention, with the aim of testing whether positive emotions underpin a fundamental change in mode of information processing whereby attentional breadth is enhanced across cognitive domains. In a recent study (Rowe et al., 2006), we investigated whether positive affect may result in a relaxation of attentional filters across the semantic and visuospatial cognitive domains. In the visuospatial domain, positive affect resulted in greater interference from adjacent flanking distractors in an Ericksen Flanker task, thus suggesting impairment in selective attention associated with positive affect. These findings are consistent with previous observations that selective attention is associated with the inhibitory filtering of task-irrelevant distraction (Friedman & Miyake, 2004), such that decreased attentional selection would allow encoding of peripheral information and thus decrease capacity to inhibit processing of spatially adjacent irrelevant information. Thus, positive affect resulted in a "leaky" attentional filter—impairing spatial selective attention performance and allowing peripheral irrelevant information to be more fully encoded. In the conceptual domain, positive affect was associated with increased capacity to generate remote associates for familiar words (e.g., mower, atomic, foreign = POWER) in a Remotes Associates Task (RAT), such that participants under positive mood solved significantly more problems than when under negative mood. This indicated that access to internal semantic information was facilitated by positive affect, in a way that more distant semantic relationships seemed closer and more easily accessible. Furthermore, for positive affect, individual differences in enhanced semantic access were correlated with the degree of impaired visual selective attention, such that under positive mood, individuals with the greatest breadth in semantic access (indexed by performance on the RAT) demonstrated the most pronounced visuospatial attentional breadth (indexed by slower performance on the Flanker task).

In a more recent study (Schmitz, De Rosa, & Anderson, 2009), we used functional magnetic resonance imaging to examine whether the opposing influences of positive and negative affective states extend to perceptual encoding in the visual cortices. Participants viewed brief presentations of face/place concentric stimuli and were asked to attend to the faces while leaving the places unattended. As face and place information was presented at different visual eccentricities, our physiological metric of visual field of view (FOV) was a valence-dependent modulation of place processing in the parahippocampal place area (PPA). Consistent with our predictions, positive affective states increased PPA response to novel places as well as adaptation to repeated places, as compared to negative states. Individual differences in self-reported positive and negative affect correlated inversely with PPA encoding of peripheral places, as well as with activation in the mesocortical prefrontal cortex and amygdala. Psychophysiological interaction analyses further demonstrated that valence-dependent responses in the PPA arose from opponent coupling with extrafoveal regions of the primary visual cortex during positive and negative states. These findings indicate that affective valence differentially biases gating of early visual inputs, fundamentally altering the scope of perceptual encoding. Thus, we have found that positive affect can literally alter the spotlight of visual attention, making it more diffuse and encompassing.

Taken together, these findings suggest that this broadening in informational access associated with positive affect is not restricted to a particular cognitive domain, but rather that it may underlie a more global shift in mode of information processing present at even early stages of perceptual encoding. As such, we propose that positive affect results in a fundamental change in information processing whereby span of attentional allocation to both external visual and internal conceptual space is enhanced.

Linking these findings to the greater context of research in positive psychology, we propose that this shift in information processing may facilitate more open, flexible, and exploratory cognition expanding both exteroceptive and interoceptive domains. This assertion resonates strongly with the broaden-and-build theory, which proposes that positive emotions serve to adaptively broaden awareness and thought-action repertoires, which in turn build enduring personal resources, ranging from physical and intellectual resources to social and psychological resources (Fredrickson, 2001; Fredrickson et al., 2003). As converging evidence for this theory accrues, a picture has begun to emerge in which positive affect engenders a creative and more generative mindset that results in greater cognitive flexibility across diverse situations, including medical diagnosis (Estrada, Isen, & Young, 1994), industrial negotiations (Carnevale & Isen, 1986), intuitive judgments (Bolte, Goschke, & Kuhl, 2003), decision making (Isen, 2001), and creative problem-solving tasks (Isen, Daubman, & Nowicki, 1987). For example, participants experiencing positive mood are more readily able to solve the Duncker candle task (Duncker, 1945; Isen et al., 1987), a classic problem-solving task, which asks participants to fix a lit candle on the wall using only a candle, a book or matches, and a box of thumbtacks. This task is devised in such a way that participants must overcome functional fixedness and use the materials in unconventional ways in order to solve the problem. Similarly, people are more likely to solve unusual word associations when they are in a positive mood, compared with a negative or neutral mood (Ashby et al., 1999; Bolte et al., 2003; Isen et al., 1987), a test of creative problem solving. This evidence strongly links positive affect with an increased capacity for creativity and novel thinking.

Exploration and Positive Affect

Exploration is a ubiquitous phenomenon in nature. Exploratory behavior has been documented in a wide range of species, including insects, snakes, lizards, birds, rats, mice, great apes, and humans (Power, 2000). While researchers in different fields have used different definitions of exploration, common among these definitions is a behavior leading to information gathering, especially of novel information or changes in the environment, such that uncertainty about the external environment is reduced. For example, animal researchers have noted that exploration typically occurs upon an animal's initial exposure to an environment, or when some change in the environment has occurred (Power, 2000). It is important to note, however, that exploration is not the only response to novelty; other responses, including fear and avoidance (neophobia), are also frequently observed.

Scholars have long proposed an adaptive evolutionary role for exploration such that an animal's ability to explore might be tightly connected with its chances of survival. For example, exploration of an environment would lead to greater familiarization with the resources available, and become instrumental in procuring food, building shelters, and identifying and protecting oneself from danger, all of which have important implications for an organism's survival. Of course, such potential benefits must be weighed against current resources, energy expenditure, and risks in the environment. As we will discuss in more detail, this trade-off has been examined and further developed in terms of exploration versus exploitation within the field of reinforcement learning. While all of these considerations are well reasoned and have been carefully studied, we argue that exploration is more than just a response to fulfilling life-supporting needs such as food and shelter, but that at least in humans it may also facilitate the development of higher cognitive resources (such as flexibility and creativity) associated with positive affect and which support enhanced levels of well-being.

From the perspective of cognitive psychology, one possible way of defining exploration is as an interaction between motivation and attention, such that exploration results when attention allocated to a certain region or object in the environment is combined with a positive motivational state. Thus, exploration may take place when an animal in a high motivational state encounters an appetitive object or environment. Critically, whether an object is investigated depends on its perceived valence and the degree of motivation, such that an appetitive object will result in an approach response, whereas an aversive object will result in a withdrawal or flee response. It has long been proposed that affect may have evolved from such opposing approach and withdrawal responses. However, it is important to note that exploration has also been observed to occur in the absence of appetitive objects (rewards) (Tolman, 1948), or motivation, as when animals are satiated. In fact, rats may even choose to delay eating when hungry in order to explore, suggesting that exploration may be rewarding in itself (Berlyne, 1955, 1966). For the purpose of this discussion, whether motivation is elicited by an appetitive object (extrinsic) or already present in the individual (intrinsic) will be treated equally. However, we make a distinction between reward-based exploration, which may be driven by extrinsic motivation associated with an external reward, and exploration in the absence of reward—*play exploration*—which may be driven by intrinsic motivation such as in free exploration. What is important from this perspective is that exploration may arise as a result of the interaction between attention and motivation mediated by affective state.

As we discussed in the previous section, positive states are associated with broader, more diffuse attention and negative states with narrower, more focused attention. With regard to motivation, high positive motivational states may lead to approach behavior and negative motivational states to withdrawal or avoidance. Thus, positive affect will result in more diffuse, broadened attention and approach motivation, which together may enhance exploratory behavior, predisposing the mind and body to wonder. By contrast, negative affect will narrow attention and promote avoidance motivational states, leading to decreased exploratory behavior, predisposing the mind and body to focus and stay put. Thus, we propose that exploration relies on an interaction between attention and motivational states mediated by affect, such that positive affect will be associated with enhanced exploratory tendencies.

Evidence from diverse sources supports this assertion. For example, it has long been observed that rodents are more likely to explore an environment after being satiated, and less likely to explore after experiencing aversive stimuli (such as a shock) (Berlyne, 1966). Rat analogues of depression also exhibit decreased exploratory tendency (Dong et al., 2012), and indeed depressed humans show decreased motivational drive and impaired exploratory behavior (Krishnan & Nestler, 2011). Children in a mildly stressful situation (such as withdrawal from their caregivers) are less likely to engage in exploration of new toys than when in presence of their caregivers (Rheingold & Eckerman, 1969).

From the perspective of reinforcement learning, exploration of new actions is essential for learning, but it must be weighed against the cost of bypassing more reliable alternatives with known value and facing potential risks in the environment (Sutton & Barto, 1998). As an organism (agent) interacts with its environment, it must learn which actions lead to good outcomes, with the overall goal of maximizing reward. For this purpose, an agent must try different actions—*explore*—and determine which lead to greater rewards. Over time, learning will take place and the agent will choose the most rewarding actions—*exploit*. However, in a changing environment, as it is the rule in nature, there is greater uncertainty and an agent must continue to explore different options, even if previously sampled, in order to update itself about the current state of the environment. Thus, a challenge arises as the agent must choose whether to exploit a reliable option or explore a new one which may be more risky but potentially more profitable (Sutton & Barto, 1998). This dilemma is known as the trade-off between exploration and exploitation. Decades of research in reinforcement learning have demonstrated that while an optimal solution for this kind of problem is often hard or in fact impossible to find, under certain assumptions it is possible to create computational models that test different strategies and may even determine optimal strategies for certain problems. In fact, such models have been used to show that animals are capable of utilizing optimal foraging strategies (Charnov, 1976).

Recent work with humans has combined modern neuroimaging techniques with such well-defined computational models to examine the neural mechanisms associated with this trade-off between exploration and exploitation. In a recent study, Daw and colleagues (2006) collected functional magnetic resonance imaging data of participants while completing a gambling task inside a magnetic resonance imaging scanner. The gambling task, a four-armed bandit, was set up in such a way that participants had to choose between four slots, each yielding a different reward, which varied from trial to trial. Participants learned a reward only by actively sampling a specific slot. This feature of the experiment forced the participants to actively exploit or explore in different trials in order to maximize reward. Using decision rules derived from reinforcement learning models, researchers were able to classify decisions as exploitative or exploratory. Functional magnetic resonance imaging revealed some of the underlying neural mechanisms. Activation in the frontopolar cortex and intraparietal sulcus was associated with exploratory decisions, whereas activation of the striatum and ventromedial prefrontal cortex was associated with exploitative decisions. This study provided a characterization of exploration and exploitation in a value-based setting, and it provided evidence for distinct networks associated with exploratory and exploitative behavior. These results add to a wealth of evidence for a primary role of dopaminergic networks in appetitive choice, with striatal (Delgado, Nystrom, Fissell, Noll, & Fiez, 2000; Knutson, Westdorp, Kaiser, & Hommer, 2000; McClure, Berns, & Montague, 2003; O'Doherty et al., 2004) and medial prefrontal networks mediating learning to exploit, underpinned by computational reinforcement learning theory.

While such work provides a strong computational framework for the study of exploration, and elucidates some of the associated neural mechanisms, it has been limited to reward-based exploratory behavior and thus does not incorporate exploration in the absence of reward.

It has long been acknowledged that learning and exploration can take place in the absence of reinforcement. A clear example of this is latent learning (Blodgett, 1929; Tolman, 1948). In a classical experiment, three groups of rats were placed in a maze: Group 1 was reinforced every time they got to the end of the maze, group 2 was allowed to explore the maze and only presented with rewards at a later stage, and group 3 was allowed to explore the maze but never reinforced. As expected, group 1 improved its performance (indexed by number of wrong turns) through the maze with trials, and group 3 showed no evidence of improvement. The surprising results were that as soon as rewards were introduced for group 2, performance improved much more rapidly than expected, and in some cases surpassed that of the extrinsically rewarded group. The researchers interpreted these results as evidence that the rats had been learning all along, generating a "cognitive map" of the environment, but expression of learning was not manifest until it was called upon.

We propose that this type of learning and exploration is related to "play exploration" described by psychologists as behavior that appears not to have a specific purpose or not to serve an immediately relevant function, lacks obvious motivation or consummatory activities, exhibits a degree of flexibility or randomness in behavioral sequences, and carries an element of pleasure (Archer & Birke, 1983). Examples of this type of exploration include play fighting, locomotive exercise, and object play. For example, when a satiated rat is placed in a maze, even if in the presence of food, it will first investigate the environment. However, the purpose of such behavior is not obvious to the observer. It is not clear whether the animal is trying to escape, checking for predators, searching for shelter or water, and so on. In fact, the animal might even bypass the opportunity of eating in order to keep exploring. Indeed, the animal is acting without an obvious motivation, other than perhaps the intrinsic motivation of learning more about its environment.

In humans it has been reported that play exploration may be associated with creativity, enhanced problem solving, social adjustment, and general intellectual and language development (Archer & Birke, 1983). For example, children who are allowed to play with materials later to be used in a problem-solving task perform better than children for whom the properties of the materials have been explained (Archer & Birke, 1983; Smith & Dutton, 1979; Sylva et al., 1976). Similarly, children who spent a period of free play with a set of everyday objects were able to suggest more possible uses for objects than children who spent the same length of time watching or imitating the actions of an experimenter with the objects (Dansky, 1980; Dansky & Silverman, 1973, 1975). This finding suggests that play exploration facilitates creative thinking necessary for problem solving.

We propose that positive affect facilitates both reward-based exploration and play exploration. In both cases, we see exploration as the result of an interaction between attention and motivation, which is mediated by affective state such that positive affect will result in diffuse attentional scope, positive motivational state, and enhanced exploratory tendency. With regard to reward-based exploration, reinforcement learning theory indicates that in order to maximize profit an individual must learn how to balance the trade-off between exploration and exploitation. Indeed, recent work using such computational formalizations have tested these types of models in humans and successfully identified associated neural mechanisms. With regard to play exploration, we propose this kind of behavior promotes flexibility and creative problem solving. Future work in the field should examine in more detail the interaction between exploration, motivation, and attention, and further how they relate to other cognitive functions such as flexibility, creativity, problem solving, and more generally to well-being. This work should also aim to identify the associated neural mechanisms using neuroimaging techniques, and more directly test whether positivity is associated with positive emotions. We suggest that play exploration is central to well-being and the function of positive emotions.

RESILIENCE

A life well lived is not one without adversity, but rather adaptive responses to life's slings and arrows. Resilience is the ultimate expression of cognitive and emotional flexibility. From minor stressful events such as failing an exam to major tragedies such as the loss of a loved one, life presents us with many emotional challenges. A natural and intuitive strategy to deal with them might be to try to minimize and avoid such challenges, but while some challenges might be foreseeable and preventable, many are not. Thus, it might not only be the number of negative events that we face, but how we deal with them that is critical for our well-being. Researchers have pointed out that people differ vastly in their ability to "bounce back" from a negative experience; while some individuals are deeply affected by life stressors and develop poor mental health, others seem to overcome even major traumatic events quickly (Bonanno, Papa, Lalande, Westphal, & Coifman, 2004). In fact, some individuals even seem to thrive in response to strong emotional challenges (Tedeschi & Calhoun, 2004). This ability to "bounce back" or to effectively cope and adapt in the face of loss, hardship, or adversity is referred to as resilience (Block & Kremen, 1996; Waugh, Wager, Fredrickson, Noll, & Taylor, 2008).

Much work on this topic has revolved around identifying risks and implications for mental health and psychopathy. For example, resilient individuals are less likely to exhibit enduring grief symptoms after losing a loved one. Researchers have further shown that while resilient individuals do experience grief, just as their nonresilient counterparts, they are better able to remain functioning in their lives (Bonanno et al., 2002). Other studies have shown that resilient people exhibit reduced depressive symptoms in response to a financial crisis (Fredrickson, Tugade, Waugh, & Larkin, 2003) and reduced mental distress after returning from combat (Florian, Mikulincer, & Taubman, 1995). Researchers have also identified many factors that play a role in an individual's ability to cope with odds, including socioeconomic status and physical health (Schooler & Caplan, 2009), social support (Florian, Mikulincer, & Taubman, 1995), self-esteem, problem-solving ability (Dumont & Provost, 1999), intelligence (Masten, 2001), and positive emotions (Tugade & Fredrickson, 2004).

Surprisingly little work, however, has been devoted to understanding the underlying psychological and neurological mechanisms associated with this faculty. In recent years, psychologists have proposed emotional flexibility as a possible psychological mechanism. Resilient individuals might recover from distress by adapting flexibly to the changing demands of stressful events. For example, a study showed that when faced with the prospect of a stressful event, such as having to give a public speech, high-resilience individuals exhibited faster cardiovascular recovery (Tugade & Fredrickson, 2004). Similarly, individuals who were better able to enhance or suppress their emotions experienced less distress in the aftermath of the September 11 events (Bonanno et al., 2004). Converging evidence suggests that resilient individuals enjoy superior ability to regulate their emotions and may further be able to make strategic use of this capacity to adapt flexibly to their current emotional need. At the same time, a growing body of evidence suggests a close relationship between resilience and positive affect. For example, resilient people are optimistic, curious and open to new experiences, and characterized by high positivity (Block & Kremen, 1996; Fredrickson, Mancuso, Branigan, & Tugade, 2000). Indeed, studies indicate that positive emotions help individuals to cope with distress (Folkman & Moskowitz, 2000) and predict enhanced health and psychological well-being (Affleck & Tennen, 1996).

From the perspective of cognitive psychology, resilience might be related to different modes of information processing, with low resilience associated with more stable, "sticky," cognitive states, and high resilience associated with more flexible and adaptive cognitive states. Stable cognitive states refer to those cognitive functions that promote maintenance of current actions through focused and sustained attention, such as holding a thought in working memory or continuing to apply a specific problem-solving strategy. By contrast, flexible cognitive states promote adaptability and change with regard to current actions, such as adopting a new strategy for problem solving. Previous studies have shown that positive affect may be associated with flexible cognitive states, while negative affect might be associated with stable cognitive states (Fredrickson et al., 2003; Tugade & Fredrickson, 2004). We propose that such interaction also impacts an individual's ability to regulate his or her emotions. In line with the broadening of attention and access to information, positive emotions may allow access to a greater conceptual-action space in response to emotional challenge. Individuals with enhanced positive affect may thus have access to a larger pool of thoughts and strategies, which might then be used to adapt and regulate their emotions in the event of a negative experience. Thus, we would expect high-resilience individuals to also exhibit high positive affectivity, and low-resilience individuals to exhibit low positive affectivity. Indeed, studies supporting this hypothesis show that positive emotions may help individuals achieve efficient emotion regulation by flexibly adapting their physiological response and by reappraising a negative experience in terms of positive meaning (Tugade & Fredrickson, 2004). Further studies have begun to identify associated neural correlates with the finding that prolonged activation of the anterior insula in response to negative stimuli might characterize low resilience (Waugh et al., 2008). Such studies have been seen in the light of the broaden-and-build theory, which consistent with our line of thought, proposes that positive emotions help individuals overcome stressful experiences by expanding their thought-action repertoires and promoting emotional flexibility (Tugade & Fredrickson, 2004).

Future studies should examine more directly the interaction between affect and trait resilience. For example, it might be fruitful to test directly whether induction of positive affect might help individuals recover more effectively from a negative experience, while induction of negative mood might impair their ability to recover from emotional challenge. Given the established finding that depressed individuals, who also score low in trait resilience, tend to ruminate, it might also be interesting to examine the relation between affect, trait resilience, and rumination. One way of formulating this relation is that as a result of a negative experience an individual's attentional scope is narrowed, which in turn reduces his or her thought-action repertoire. Being stuck in such a negative, narrow, but stable cognitive state would result in rumination and, over time, in depression. As such, low-resilience individuals would be more likely to experience such narrow but stable cognitive states in response to a negative event and thus exhibit a higher risk of developing depression.

GENETICS

Research literature on well-being consistently reveals that the characteristics and resources valued by society correlate with subjective well-being. For example, marriage (Mastekaasa, 1994), a comfortable income (Diener & Biswas-Diener, 2002), superior mental health (Koivumaa-Honkanen et al., 2004), and physical health and longevity (Danner, Snowdon, & Friesen, 2001) all correlate with reports of high happiness levels. Such associations between desirable life outcomes and happiness have led most investigators to assume that success makes people happy. This assumption is ubiquitous in the general population and can be found throughout the literature. However, what is often overlooked is that these associations are correlational and do not necessarily imply a success-happiness causal link. In other words, it is not clear whether success engenders happiness or perhaps happiness engenders success. This is not to reject the notion that resources and success may lead to well-being but to also consider the alternative path—that people with natural predispositions for higher levels of well-being are more likely to achieve favorable life circumstances. This alternative path suggests the possibility that some people may have a genetic predisposition for experiencing positive affect and higher levels of subjective well-being.

A recent meta-analytical study (Sin & Lyubomirsky, 2009) looking at over 200 studies on the subject found substantial evidence for positive emotions promoting success. The authors concluded that positive affect—the hallmark of well-being—may be the cause of many of the desirable characteristics, resources, and successes correlated with happiness. From a different perspective, recent research shows that, while variables such as socioeconomic status, income, marriage, level of education, and religiosity are significantly associated with individual happiness, none typically accounts for more than 3% of the variance (Frey, 2008; Layard, 2005). Moreover, changes in these variables appear to yield only short-term changes to happiness. For example, researchers have noted that increases in income either have little or no lasting effect on happiness (Clark, 2008; Easterlin, 1974; Stevenson & Wolfers, 2008) and, furthermore, that happiness levels tend to revert toward a "set point" or "baseline" of happiness (Kahneman, Diener, & Schwarz, 1999). The bases for this phenomenon are not well understood, but theorists believe genetic predispositions may play an important role (Diener, Suh, Lucas, & Smith, 1999; Kahneman et al., 1999).

Indeed, previous studies have shown that baseline happiness is significantly heritable. For example, a seminal study by Lykken and Tellegen (1996), using a sample of several thousand middle-aged twins, estimated heritability of subjective well-being at about 50%. Subsequent estimates have ranged from 33%

(De Neve, 2011) and 38% (Stubbe, Posthuma, Boomsma, & De Geus, 2005) to 36%–50% (Bartels & Boomsma, 2009) and 42%–56% (Nes, Roysamb, Tambs, Harris, & Reichborn-Kjennerud, 2006).

While twin studies are an important step in establishing the influence of genes in subjective well-being, they tell us nothing about the specific genes involved, let alone the biological or neurological mechanisms through which they have an influence on well-being. Surprisingly, very little effort has been made to identify specific genes associated with subjective well-being. Only a single study has presented evidence of a specific gene that is associated with life satisfaction (De Neve, 2011). In this study investigators found that individuals with a transcriptionally more efficient version of the serotonin transporter gene (SLC6A4, also known as 5-HTT) were significantly more likely to report higher levels of life satisfaction. In this case the researchers looked only at a single candidate gene.

It is important to highlight that it is extremely unlikely that a single gene will be responsible for well-being. Such a high-level construct is likely to depend on myriad neural processes, complex brain networks that include affective and cognitive components. Thus, it is likely that hundreds, if not thousands, of genes and their interactions influence the many processes that give rise to subjective well-being. Nevertheless, it is possible that certain genes may carry more weight than others.

Given the myriad of potential genes that could influence well-being, it may be tempting to propose a genome-wide association study (GWAS) to scan the entire human genome in an effort to identify these genes. However, such methods often provide weak conclusions because of a number of statistical limitations, including multiple comparisons, type I errors, and the correlational nature of genetic findings (Frank & Fossella, 2010). Indeed, recent GWASs looking at common psychiatric disorders have reported small effects (risk explained by specific genes) (Purcell et al., 2009; Shi et al., 2009; Stefansson et al., 2009), and researchers have pointed out limitations for this kind of study (Frank & Fossella, 2010).

A promising alternative method is to select a candidate genetic polymorphism based on what is known about its dynamics in local neural circuits and large networks, and test its effect on potential cognitive systems and behavior. This approach is particularly well suited for constraining genetic analysis to specific genes that are known to act in brain regions critical for certain cognitive processes (Frank & Fossella, 2010).

A genetic polymorphism of particular interest, which has been studied extensively, is the COMT Val158Met. This polymorphism codes for the COMT enzyme, which breaks down extracellular dopamine in the prefrontal cortex—affecting dopamine levels in that region, and impacting prefrontal cortex–dependent cognitive processes such as executive function. Critically, the Valine-to-Methionine substitution results in differences in activity of the enzyme degrading dopamine (Lachman et al., 1996), with the Met allele showing slower degradation of dopamine as compared to the Val allele. Thus, Met carriers exhibit higher dopamine in the prefrontal cortex than Val/Val homozygous individuals (Chen et al., 2004). Converging evidence suggests that this polymorphism may differentially influence tasks involving cognitive flexibility and cognitive stability. Specifically, relatively high levels of tonic dopamine in the prefrontal cortex allow Met carriers to maintain information on working memory relevant to their present task, and thus may benefit cognitive stability. On the other hand, low levels of tonic dopamine exhibited by Val/Val homozygotes may be beneficial for tasks requiring rapid adjustments in behavior to keep up with a rapidly changing environment, and thus it may enhance cognitive flexibility. Consistent with this picture, research indicates that Met/Met carries do indeed show more stable prefrontal activation states, and enhanced performance in tasks relying on working memory, at the cost of impoverished cognitive flexibility (Durstewitz, Seamans, & Sejnowski, 2000). Val/Val participants show the opposite tendency of enhanced cognitive flexibility, and impoverished cognitive stability (Colzato, Waszak, Nieuwenhuis, Posthuma, & Hommel, 2010; Diaz-Asper et al., 2008; Egan et al., 2001; Goldberg et al., 2003).

Most of this work, however, has been done in the light of reward processing, executive control, or working memory, and little is known with regard to how COMT may affect emotional processing. An experience sampling study found that Met carriers reported more positive experiences, and reported higher positive experience to similar situations, as compared to Val carriers. Another study by Bishop and colleagues (Bishop, Cohen, Fossella, Casey, & Farah, 2006) reported increased activation of ventrolateral prefrontal cortex and orbitofrontal cortex for Val carriers in response to negative distractors in a house-matching paradigm. However, this result appears to conflict with findings by Smolka and colleagues (2005) that showed enhanced activation of ventrolateral prefrontal cortex during passive viewing of negative images.

Perhaps, rather than testing differential effects of processing negative versus neutral stimuli, future studies should investigate differences in emotional flexibility. For example, ongoing studies in our lab are testing whether Val carriers exhibit faster adaptation to emotional challenge as compared to their Met counterparts. This would relate more directly to the findings regarding cognitive flexibility explained by the differential dopamine metabolism associated with COMT. Current efforts in our lab investigate whether the enhanced cognitive flexibility exhibited by Val homozygotes is also related to emotional flexibility.

Finally, it is also important to point out that finding genes associated with emotional information processing, cognitive and emotional flexibility, and subjective well-being does not imply a deterministic view of well-being, since it is the interaction between genes and the environment that ultimately shapes our experience and behavior. Instead, such genes may simply inform us of our predispositions and allow us to make better decisions with regard to our environment.

CONCLUSION

Though still in its infancy, research looking at the interaction between positive affect and cognition has already begun to present a picture of the psychological and neurological underpinnings of positive affect and their effect on well-being. First, with regard to attention, converging evidence shows that positive emotions alter attentional focus across cognitive domains. Positive emotions have been shown to increase the breadth of perceptual visuospatial field of focus, allowing individuals to encode task-irrelevant peripheral information, and to increase access to internal semantic information, allowing individuals to generate connections among semantically distant concepts. We propose that these findings may underlie a more global shift in mode of information processing, whereby positive affect results in greater allocation of attentional resources to both external and internal information.

Based on these findings, we have proposed that this increase in attentional breadth may further impact other behavioral tendencies and, in particular, exploration. We discussed how positive affect may facilitate both reward-based exploration and exploration in the absence of reward ("play exploration"). We frame exploration as the result of an interaction between attention and motivation that is moderated by affective state. Specifically, positive affect results in more diffuse attentional scope and a positive motivational state, which we propose may lead to enhanced exploratory tendency. With regard to reward-based exploration, reinforcement learning theory indicates that in order to maximize profit an individual must learn how to balance the trade-off between exploration and exploitation. Play exploration, on the other hand, may be more closely related to latent learning, and we propose this kind of behavior promotes flexibility and creative problem solving. Future work in the field should examine in more detail the interaction between exploration, motivation, and attention, and further how they relate to other cognitive functions such as flexibility, creativity, problem solving, and more generally to well-being.

We have discussed how our ability to recover from emotional challenges might be directly related to emotional flexibility. Impoverished resilience may be associated with "sticky" cognitive states, and high resilience associated with more flexible and adaptive cognitive states. By flexibly adapting their emotions to the moment-to-moment changes in the affective landscape of their environment, resilient individuals may be able to recover quickly from negative experiences. Critically, we propose that positive emotions may be a key factor facilitating such emotional adaptability. Future work should examine more directly the interaction between affect, attention, and trait resilience.

We also discussed the possibility that some people may have a genetic predisposition for experiencing positive emotions and experience higher levels of subjective well-being. Several studies looking at data from monozygotic twins have found strong hereditary links to subjective well-being of up to 50%. However, very little work has examined the specific genes and biological mechanisms involved. Nevertheless, one gene of particular interest, COMT Val158Met, stands out as a potential candidate. Converging evidence suggests that this polymorphism may differentially influence tasks involving cognitive flexibility and cognitive stability, supporting the thesis that the function of positive emotions is related to a particular state of information processing, potentially exploration, as we propose. However, the link between this gene and its impact on affect has not been explored and remains a promising avenue for future research.

A challenge for the future is to develop a framework that successfully characterizes well-being as a product of our genetic endowment and its interaction with the environment. To this end, it may be helpful to look at recent efforts in the field of psychiatry that aim to characterize mental disease as a function of observable traits (phenotype) underpinned by genetic markers (genotype) interacting with the environment. Researchers in this field use the term "endophenotype" to refer to measurable components unseen by the unaided eye along the pathway between disease and distal genotype (Gottesman & Gould, 2003). The idea is to find common biological denominators of behavioral symptoms across individuals suffering from a specific mental illness in an effort to deconstruct and simplify psychiatric disorders. The advantage of this method is that it opens the possibility of redefining complex conditions in terms of a few stable phenotypes, which have a clear genetic component and may be more specific to the disorder and thus allow a more direct study of biological underpinnings associated with that condition. Despite the inherent complexity of psychiatric disorders, promising findings for conditions such as schizophrenia indicate clear genetic bases for known symptoms, including deficits in sensory gating (Watanabe et al., 2007) and working memory (Wedenoja et al., 2008). However, for the most part, the field has had limited success in its search for definite genetic markers associated with other mental disorder, and researchers point to the complexity of the brain itself, complex interactions not just among genes, proteins, cells, and circuits of cells but also between individuals and their changing experiences (Gottesman & Gould, 2003). We expect similar challenges in identifying the gene–environment interactions that give yield to the resources that support good mental health. The examination of genes and gene–environment interactions that give rise to the presence of positive emotions and associated cognitive states is greatly limited compared to studies of poor mental health, and thus are in great demand. Well-being genes are not merely the absence of genes predisposing one toward psychopathology.

As such, we propose that this approach may be suitable for the study of well-being. Just like many of the disorders psychiatrists are interested in, well-being is a complex construct defined primarily by observable behavioral characteristics that correlate with subjective evaluation, which has been shown to be strongly heritable, but ultimately is likely to arise from a complex interaction between an individual's genetic make-up and his or her environment. To explore this possibility further, we might consider the criteria suggested by researchers in psychiatry for identifying reliable biological markers or endophenotypes (Gottesman & Gould, 2003).

1. The endophenotype is associated with illness in the population.
2. The endophenotype is heritable.
3. The endophenotype is primarily state independent (manifests in an individual whether or not illness is active).
4. Within families, endophenotype and illness cosegregate.
5. The endophenotype found in affected family members is found in nonaffected family members at a higher rate than in the general population.

While these criteria were developed with the aim of examining mental illness, we believe that they can be easily reformulated to study mental health, well-being, and human flourishing. For example, the following could be used by researchers as a guideline for finding endophenotypes associated with well-being:

1. The endophenotype is associated with well-being (WB) in the population.
2. The WB endophenotype is heritable.
3. The WB endophenotype is primarily state independent (manifests in an individual whether or not high levels of well-being are currently observed).
4. Within families, the WB endophenotype and well-being cosegregate.

This approach thus calls for identifying biological markers of behavioral characteristics associated with well-being and associated cognitive capacities across healthy populations. For example, cognitive processes associated with positivity and well-being such as diffuse attention and cognitive flexibility may also have a genetic basis and are thus strong candidates for well-being endophenotypes. In the same way, given the established connection between positive affectivity and well-being, it might be fruitful to examine more closely its genetic underpinnings. This approach opens the possibility of characterizing well-being in terms of biologically well-defined stable phenotypes, with a clear genetic component and whose neurological underpinnings may be better understood. Such characterization must bear in mind the complex interactions between such biological markers and the ever-changing nature of our environments. Finally, this implies that while we may not have control over our genetic make-up, we may be able to use this information to understand our natural predispositions and to make better use of our resources to promote well-being.

REFERENCES

Affleck, G., & Tennen, H. (1996). Construing benefits from adversity: Adaptational significance and dispositional underpinnings. *Journal of Personality, 64*, 899–922.

Archer, J., & Birke, L. I. (1983). *Exploration in animals and humans.* Berkshire, UK: Van Nostrand Reinhold.

Ashby, F. G., Isen, A. M., & Turken, A. U. (1999). A neuropsychological theory of affect and its influence on cognition. *Psychological Review, 106*, 529–550.

Bartels, M., & Boomsma, D. I. (2009). Born to be happy? The etiology of subjective well-being. *Behavior Genetics, 39*(6), 605–615.

Basso, M., Schefft, B., Ris, M., & Dember, W. (1996). Mood and global-local visual processing. *Journal of the International Neuropsychological Society, 2*(3), 249–55.

Berlyne, D. (1966). Curiosity and exploration. *Science, 153* (3731), 25–33.

Berlyne, D. (1955). The arousal and satiation of perceptual curiosity in the rat. *Journal of Comparative and Physiological Psychology, 48*, 238–246.

Berridge, K., & Robinson, T. (1998). What is the role of dopamine in reward: Hedonic impact, reward learning, or incentive salience? *Brain Research and Brain Research Review, 28* (3), 309–369.

Bilder, R., Volavka, J., Lachman, H., & Grace, A. (2004). The catechol-O-methyltransferase polymorphism: Relations to the tonic-phasic dopamine hypothesis and neuropsychiatric phenotypes. *Neuropsychopharmacology, 29*, 1943–1961.

Bishop, S. J., Cohen, J. D., Fossella, J., Casey, B. J., & Farah, M. J. (2006). COMT genotype influences prefrontal response to emotional distraction. *Cognitive Affective and Behavioral Neuroscience, 6*(1), 62–70, 6 (1), 62–70.

Block, J., & Kremen, A. M. (1996). IQ and ego-resiliency: Conceptual and empirical connections and separateness. *Journal of Personality and Social Psychology, 70*, 349–361.

Blodgett, H. (1929). The effect of the introduction of reward upon the maze performance of rats. *University of California Publications in Psychology, 4*, 113–134.

Bolte, A., Goschke, T., & Kuhl, J. (2003). Emotion and intuition. *Psychological Science, 14*(5), 416–421.

Bonanno, G., Papa, A., Lalande, K., Westphal, M., & Coifman, K. (2004). The importance of being flexible: The ability to both enhance and suppress emotional expression predicts long-term adjustment. *Psychological Science, 15*(7), 482–487.

Bonanno, G., Wortman, C., Lehman, D., Tweed, R. G., Haring, M., Sonnega, J., . . . Nesse, R. M. (2002). Resilience to loss and chronic grief: A prospective study from preloss to 18-months postloss. *Journal of Personality and Social Psychology, 83*(5), 1150–1164.

Burgdorf, J., & Panksepp, J. (2006). The neurobiology of positive emotions. *Neuroscience and Biobehavioral Reviews, 30*(2), 173–187.

Carnevale, P., & Isen, A. (1986). The influence of positive affect and visual access on the discovery of integrative solutions in bilateral negotiation. *Organizational Behavior and Human Decision Processes, 37*, 1–13.

Charnov, E. L. (1976). Optimal foraging: The marginal value theorem. *Theoretical Population Biology, 9*, 129–136.

Chen, J., Lipska, B. K., Halim, N., Ma, Q. D., Matsumoto, M., Melhem, S., . . . Weinberger, D. R. (2004). Functional analysis of genetic variation in catechol-O-methyltransferase (COMT): Effects on mRNA, protein, and enzyme activity in postmortem human brain. *American Journal of Human Genetics, 75*, 807–821.

Christianson, S., Loftus, E. (1990). Some characteristics of people's traumatic memories. *Bulletin of the Psychonomic Society, 28*, 195–198.

Clark, P. F. (2008). Relative income, happiness, and utility: An explanation for the easterlin paradox and other puzzles. *Journal of Economic Literature, 46*(1), 95–144.

Cohen, J. D., McClure, S. M., & Yu, A. (2007). Should I stay or should I go? How the human brain manages the trade-off between exploitation and exploration. *Philosophical Transactions of the Royal Society B, Biological Sciences, 362*(1481), 933–942.

Colzato, L. S., Waszak, F., Nieuwenhuis, S., Posthuma, D., & Hommel, B. (2010). The flexible mind is associated with the catechol-O-methyltransferase (COMT) Val-158- Met polymorphism: Evidence for a role of dopamine in the control of task-switching. *Neuropsychologia, 48*(9), 2764–2768.

Danner, D. D., Snowdon, D. A., & Friesen, W. V. (2001). Positive emotions in early life and longevity: Findings from the nun study. *Journal of Personality and Social Psychology, 80*(5), 804–813.

Dansky, J. L. (1980a). Cognitive consequences of sociodramatic play and exploration training for economically disadvantaged preschoolers. *Journal of Child Psychology and Psychiatry, 21*, 47–58.

Dansky, J. L., & Silverman, I. W. (1973). Effects of play on associative fluency in preschool-aged children. *Developmental Psychology, 9*, 38–43.

Dansky, J. L., & Silverman, I. W. (1975). Play: A general facilitator of associative fluency. *Developmental Psychology, 11*, 104.

Daw, N. D., O'Doherty, J. P., Dayan, P., Seymour, B., & Dolan, R. J. (2006). Cortical substrates for exploratory decisions in humans. *Nature, 441*(7095), 876–879.

De Neve, J. (2011). Functional polymorphism (5-HTTLPR) in the serotonin trans-porter gene is associated with subjective well-being: Evidence from a U.S. nationally representative sample. *Journal of Human Genetics, 56*, 456–459.

Delgado, M. R., Nystrom, L. E., Fissell, C., Noll, D. C., & Fiez, J. A. (2000). Tracking the hemodynamic responses to reward and punishment in the striatum. *Journal of Neurophysiology, 84*(6), 3072–3077.

Derryberry, D., & Reed, M. A. (1998) Anxiety and attentional focusing: Trait, state, and hemispheric influences. *Personality and Individual Differences, 25*, 745–761.

Derryberry, D., & Tucker, D. M. (1994). Motivating the focus of attention. In P. Neidenthal, & S. E. Kitayama (Eds.), *The heart's eye: Emotional influences in percep-tion and attention* (pp. 167–196). San Diego, CA: Academic Press.

Diaz-Asper, C., Goldberg, T., Kolachana, B., Straub, R., Egan, M., & Weinberger, D. (2008). Genetic variation in catechol-o-methyltransferase: Effects on working memory in schizophrenic patients, their siblings, and healthy controls. *Biological Psychiatry, 63*, 72–79.

Diener, E., & Biswas-Diener, R. (2002). Will money increase subjective well-being? *Social indicators research, 57* (2), 119–169.

Diener, E., Suh, E. M., Lucas, R. E., & Smith, H. L. (1999). Subjective well-being: Three decades of progress. *Psychological Bulletin, 125*(2), 276.

Dong, Z., Gong, B., Li, H., Bai, Y., Wu, X., Huang, Y., . . . Wang, Y. T. (2012). Mechanisms of hippocampal long-term depression are required for memory enhancement by novelty exploration. *Journal of Neuroscience, 29*(35), 11980–11990.

Dreisbach, G., Müller, J., Goschke, T., Strobel, A., Schulze, K., Lesch, K. P., & Brocke, B. (2005). Dopamine and cognitive control: The influence of spontaneous eyeb-link rate and dopamine gene polymorphisms on perseveration and distractibility. *Behavioral Neuroscience, 119*, 483–490.

Dumont, M., & Provost, M. A. (1999). Resilience in adolescents: Protective role of social support, coping strategies, self-esteem, and social activities on experience of stress and depression. *Journal of Youth and Adolescence, 28*(3), 343–363.

Duncker, K. (1945). On problem solving. *Psychological Monographs, 58*, 5.

Durstewitz, D., Seamans, J., & Sejnowski, T. (2000). Dopamine-mediated stabiliza-tion of delay-period activity in a network model of prefrontal cortex. *Journal of Neurophysiology, 83*, 1733–1750.

Easterbrook, J. A. (1959). The effect of emotion on cue utilization and the organization of behavior. *Psychological Review, 66* (3), 183–201.

Easterlin, R. (1974). Does economic growth improve the human lot? Some empiri-cal evidence. In P. David & M. Reder (Eds.), *Nations and households in eco-nomic growth: Essays in honor of Moses Abramovitz* (pp. 89–124). New York, NY: Academic Press.

Egan, M., Goldberg, T., Kolachana, B., Callicott, J., Mazzanti, C., Straub, R., . . . Weinberger, D. R. (2001). Effect of COMT val108/158 met genotype on frontal lobe function and risk for schizophrenia. *Proceedings of the National Academy of Sciences, 98*, 6917–6922.

Estrada, C., Isen, A. M., & Young, M. J. (1994). Positive affect influences creative prob-lem solving and reported source of practice satisfaction in physicians. *Motivation and Emotion, 18*, 285–299.

Florian, V., Mikulincer, M., & Taubman, O. (1995). Does hardiness con- tribute to mental health during a stressful real-life situation? The roles of appraisal and coping. *Journal of Personality and Social Psychology, 68*(4), 687–695.

Folkman, S., & Moskowitz, J. (2000). Positive affect and the other side of coping. *American Psychologist, 55*(6), 647–654.

Frank, M. J., & Fossella, J. A. (2010). Neurogenetics and pharmacology of learning, motivation, and cognition. *Neuropsychopharmacology, 36*(1), 133–152.

Fredrickson, B. L. (2001). The role of positive emotions in positive psychology: The broaden-and-build theory of positive emotions. *American Psychologist, 56*(3), 218–226.

Fredrickson, B. L. (2003). The value of positive emotions. *American Scientist, 91*, 330–335.

Fredrickson, B. L., Mancuso, R. A., Branigan, C., & Tugade, M. M. (2000). The undoing effect of positive emotions. *Motivation and Emotion, 24*(4), 237–258.

Fredrickson, B. L., Tugade, M. M., Waugh, C. E., & Larkin, G. R. (2003). What good are positive emotions in crisis? A prospective study of resilience and emotions following the terrorist attacks on the United States on September 11th, 2001. *Journal of Personality and Social Psychology, 84*(2), 365–376.

Frey, B. S. (2008). *Happiness: A revolution in economics.* Cambridge, MA: MIT Press.

Friedman, N., & Miyake, A. (2004). The relations among inhibition and interference cognitive functions: A latent variable analysis. *Journal of Experimental Psychology: General, 133*, 101–135.

Gasper, K., & Clore, G. L. (2002). Attending to the big picture: Mood and global versus local processing of visual information. *Psychological Science, 13*, 33–39.

Goldberg, T., Egan, M., Gscheidle, T., Coppola, R., Weickert, T., Kolachana, B., . . . Weinberger, D. R. (2003). Executive subprocesses in working memory: Relationship to catechol-O- methyltransferase val158met genotype and schizophrenia. *Archives of General Psychiatry, 60*(9), 889–896.

Gottesman, I. I., & Gould, T. D. (2003). The endophenotype concept in psychiatry: Etymology and strategic intentions. *American Journal of Psychiatry, 160*(4), 636–645.

Gottfried, J., O'Doherty, J., & Dolan, R. (2003). Encoding predictive reward value in human amygdala and orbitofrontal cortex. *Science, 301*, 1104–1107.

Green, A., Munafo, M., Deyoung, C., Fossella, J., Fan, J., & Gray, J. (2008). Using genetic data in cognitive neuroscience: From growing pains to genuine insights. *Nature Reviews Neuroscience, 9*, 710–720.

Hasher, L., Lustig, C., & Zacks, R. (2006). Inhibitory mechanisms and the control of attention. In A. R. A. Conway, C. Jarrold, M. J. Kane, A. Miyake, & J. N. Towse (Eds.), *Variation in working memory* (pp. 227–249). New York, NY: Oxford University Press.

Isen, A. M. (2001). An influence of positive affect on decision making in complex situations: Theoretical issues with practical implications. *Journal of Consumer Psychology, 11*(2), 75–85.

Isen, A. M., Daubman, K. A., & Nowicki, G. (1987). Positive affect facilitates creative problem solving. *Journal of Personality and Social Psychology, 52*, 1122–1131.

Kahneman, D., Diener, E., & Schwarz, N. (1999). *Well-being: The foundations of hedonic psychology.* New York, NY: Russel Sage.

Knutson, B., Westdorp, A., Kaiser, E., & Hommer, D. (2000). FMRI visualization of brain activity during a monetary incentive delay task. *Neuroimage, 12*(1), 20–27.

Koivumaa-Honkanen, H., Koskenvuo, M., Honkanen, R. J., Viinamäki, H., Heikkilä, K., & Kaprio, J. (2004). Life dissatisfaction and subsequent work disability in an 11-year follow-up. *Psychological Medicine, 34*(2), 221–228.

Krishnan, V., & Nestler, E. (2011). Animal models of depression: Molecular perspectives. *Current Topics in Behavioral Neuroscience, 7,* 121–147.

Lachman, H. M., Papolos, D. F., Saito, T., Yu, Y. M., Szumlanski, C. L., & Weinshilboum, R. M. (1996). Human catechol-O-methyltransferase pharmacogenetics: Description of a functional polymorphism and its potential application to neuropsychiatric disorders. *Pharmacogenetics, 6,* 243–250.

Layard, R. (. (2005). *Happiness: Lessons from a new science.* New York, NY: Penguin.

Lykken, D., & Tellegen, A. (1996). Happiness is a stochastic phenomenon. *Psychological Science, 7*(3), 186–189.

Mastekaasa, A. (1994). The subjective well-being of the previously married: The importance of unmarried cohabitation and time since widowhood or divorce. *Social Forces, 73*(2), 665–692.

Masten, A. S. (2001). Ordinary magic: Resilience processes in development. *American Psychologist, 56,* 227–238.

McClure, S. M., Berns, G. S., & Montague, P. R. (2003). Temporal prediction errors in a passive learning task activate human striatum. *Neuron, 38*(2), 339–346.

Nes, R. B., Roysamb, E., Tambs, K., Harris, J. R., & Reichborn-Kjennerud, T. (2006). Subjective well-being: Genetic and environmental contributions to stability and change. *Psychological Medicine, 36*(7), 1033–1042.

Oaksford, M., Morris, F., Grainger, B., & Williams, J. M. (1996). Mood, reasoning, and central executive processes. *Journal of Experimental Psychology: Learning, Memory, and Cognition, 22,* 476–492.

O'Doherty, J., Dayan, P., Schultz, J., Deichmann, R., Friston, K., & Dolan, R. (2004). Dissociable roles of ventral and dorsal striatum in instrumental conditioning. *Science, 304*(5669), 452–454.

O'Doherty, J., Kringelbach, M., Rolls, E., Hornak, J., & Andrews, C. (2001). Abstract reward and punishment representations in the human orbitofrontal cortex. *Nature Neuroscience, 4,* 95–102.

Panksepp, J. (1998). Attention deficit hyperactivity disorders, psychostimulants, and intolerance of childhood playfulness: A tragedy in the making? *Current Directions in Psychological Science, 7,* 91–98.

Power, T. G. (2000). *Play and exploration in children and animals.* Mahwah, NJ: Erlbaum.

Purcell, S., Wray, N., Stone, J., Visscher, P., O'Donovan, M., Sullivan, P., . . . Sklar, P. (2009). Common polygenic variation contributes to risk of schizophrenia and bipolar disorder. *Nature, 460,* 748–752.

Rheingold, H. L., & Eckerman, C. O. (1969). The infant's free entry into a new environment. *Journal of Experimental Child Psychology, 8,* 271–283.

Rowe, G., Hirsh, J., & Anderson, A. (2006). Positive affect increases the breadth of attentional selection. *Proceedings of the National Academy of Sciences USA, 104*(1), 383–388.

Schmitz, T., De Rosa, E., & Anderson, A. (2009). Opposing influences of affective state valence on visual cortical encoding. *Journal of Neuroscience, 29*(22), 7199–7207.

Schooler, C., & Caplan, L. J. (2009). How those who have, thrive: Mechanisms underlying the well-being of the advantaged in later life. In H. B. Bosworth & C. Hertzog, *Aging and cognition: Research methodologies and empirical advances. Decade of behavior (2000-2010)* (pp. 121-141). Washington, DC: American Psychological Association.

Schwarz, N., & Clore, G. L. (1983). Mood, misattribution and judgement of well-being. Informative and directive functions of affective states. *Journal of Personality and Social Psychology, 45*, 513–523.

Shi, J., Levinson, D., Duan, J., Sanders, A., Zheng, Y., Pe'er, I., . . . Gejman, P. V. (2009). Common variants on chromosome 6p22.1 are associated with schizophrenia. *Nature, 460*, 753–757.

Sin, N. L., & Lyubomirsky, S. (2009). Enhancing well-being and alleviating depressive symptoms with positive psychology interventions: A practice-friendly meta-analysis. *Journal of Clinical Psychology, 65*, 467–487.

Smith, P. K., & Dutton, S. (1979). Play and training in direct and innova- tive problem solving. *Child Development, 50*, 830–836.

Smolka, M. N., Schumann, G., Wrase, J., Grüsser, S. M., Flor, H., Mann, K., . . . Heinz, A. (2005). Catechol-O-methyltransferase val158met genotype affects processing of emotional stimuli in the amygdala and prefrontal cortex. *Journal of Neuroscience, 25*(4), 836–842.

Stefansson, H., Ophoff, R., Steinberg, S., Andreassen, O., Cichon, S., Rujescu, D., . . . Collier, D. A. (2009). Common variants conferring risk of schizophrenia. *Nature, 460*, 744–747.

Stevenson, B., & Wolfers, J. (2008). Economic growth and subjective well-being: Reassessing the Easterlin paradox. *Brookings Papers on Economic Activity, 2*, 1–87.

Stubbe, J., Posthuma, D., Boomsma, & De Geus, E. (2005). Heritability of life satisfaction in adults: A twin-family study. *Psychological Medicine, 35*(11), 1581–1588.

Sutton, R. S., & Barto, A. G. (1998). *Reinforcement learning: An introduction* (Vol. 1). Cambridge, MA: MIT Press.

Sylva, K., Bruner, J., & Genova, P. (1976). The role of play in the problem-solving of children 3–5 years old. In A. J. J. Bruner & K. Sylva (Eds.), *Play: Its role in development and evolution* (pp. 244–257). New York, NY: Basic Books.

Tedeschi, R. G., & Calhoun, L. G. (2004). Posttraumatic growth: Conceptual foundations and empirical evidence. *Psychological Inquiry, 15*(1), 1–18.

Tolman, E. (1948). Cognitive maps in rats and men. *Psychological Review, 55*(4), 189–208.

Tugade, M., & Fredrickson, B. (2004). Resilient individuals use positive emotions to bounce back from negative emotional experiences. *Journal of Personality and Social Psychology, 86*(2), 320–33.

Watanabe, A., Toyota, T., Owada, Y., Hayashi, T., Iwayama, Y., Matsumata, M., . . . Yoshikawa, T. (2007). Fabp7 maps to a quantitative trait locus for a schizophrenia endophenotype. *PLoS Biology, 5*(11), 297.

Waugh, C. E., Wager, T. D., Fredrickson, B. L., Noll, D. C., & Taylor, S. F. (2008). The neural correlates of trait resilience when anticipating and recovering from threat. *Social Cognitive and Affective Neuroscience, 3*(4), 322–332.

Wedenoja, J., Loukola, A., Tuulio-Henriksson, A., Paunio, T., Ekelund, J., Silander, K., . . . Peltonen, L. (2008). Replication of linkage on chromosome 7q22 and association of the regional Reelin gene with working memory in schizophrenia families. *Molecular Psychiatry, 13*(7), 673–684.

Note: Page numbers followed by the italicized letters *f* indicate material found in figures.

Printed in the USA/Agawam, MA
June 1, 2021

775616.002